Undergraduate Obstetrics and Gynaecology

Michael Hull MD FRCOG

Professor of Reproductive Medicine and
Surgery, Department of Obstetrics and
Gynaecology, University of Bristol, UK

David Joyce MA DM FRCOG

Consultant Gynaecologist, Southmead Hospital,
Bristol, UK

Gillian Turner MB BS FRCOG

Professor of Obstetrics and Gynaecology,
University of Auckland, New Zealand

Peter Wardle MD FRCS FRCOG

Consultant Senior Lecturer in Obstetrics and
Gynaecology, University of Bristol, UK

Third Edition

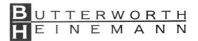

Butterworth-Heinemann
Linacre House, Jordan Hill, Oxford OX2 8DP
A division of Reed Educational and Professional Publishing Ltd

ℛ   A member of the Reed Elsevier plc group

OXFORD   BOSTON   JOHANNESBURG
MELBOURNE   NEW DELHI   SINGAPORE

First edition 1980
Reprinted 1982
Second edition 1986
Reprinted 1991, 1992
Third edition 1997
Reprinted 1997

British Library Cataloguing in Publication Data
Undergraduate obstetrics and gynaecology – 3rd ed.
   1. Gynaecology   2. Obstetrics
   I. Hull, M. G. R.
   618

ISBN 0 7506 1351 3

Library of Congress Cataloguing in Publication Data
Undergraduate obstetrics and gynaecology/Michael Hull ... [et al.].
   p.   cm.
Includes index.
Rev. ed. of: Undergraduate obstetrics and gynaecology/M. G. R.
Hull, D. N. Joyce, Gillian Turner. 2nd ed. 1986.
ISBN 0 7506 1351 3
   1. Obstetrics.   2. Gynecology.   I. Hull, Michael G. R.
Undergraduate obstetrics and gynaecology.
[DNLM: 1. Genital Diseases, Female.   2. Pregnancy.   3. Pregnancy
Complications.   WP 140 U55]
RG101.U53   96–24741
618–dc20   CIP

Origination by David Gregson Associates, Beccles, Suffolk
Printed and bound in Great Britain by MPG Books Ltd, Bodmin, Cornwall

Contents

Preface   vii
1   Modern obstetrics and gynaecology – an introduction   1
2   Obstetric and gynaecological history-taking
    and case presentation   6
3   Reproductive embryology   14
4   Reproductive anatomy   29
5   Reproductive physiology   50
6   Physiology of pregnancy, labour and lactation   74
7   Antenatal care   94
8   Intrapartum care   150
9   Postnatal care   196
10 Maternal and perinatal mortality   211
11 Contraception, sterilization and therapeutic abortion   219
12 Fertility and infertility   236
13 Miscarriage, ectopic pregnancy and hydatidiform mole   257
14 Gynaecological problems of childhood and puberty   264
15 Amenorrhoea, oligomenorrhoea and other endocrine
    problems   276
16 Abnormal genital bleeding   296
17 Endometriosis and adenomyosis   305
18 Genital infections, pruritus and discharge   315
19 Chronic pelvic pain   336
20 Premenstrual syndrome   346
21 Sexual problems   353
22 Prolapse, urinary problems and retroversion   361
23 The climacteric, menopause and postmenopause   375
24 Genital neoplasia and tumours   389
25 Obstetric and gynaecological procedures   428
Abbreviations   443
Index   447

Preface

There have been such major advances in the specialty of obstetrics and gynaecology during the last decade that it has been difficult to choose the right time to update this very successful volume. It has now been thoroughly revised and reorganized and new illustrations added, and has been strengthened by an additional expert author. We have also taken account of General Medical Council recommendations on undergraduate medical education to promote the relevant links between basic and clinical knowledge in the syllabus.

The book remains true to our original aims to write a concise but rationalized, readable and unified text, to meet the needs of practical knowledge and understanding of general medical practitioners and other specialists in caring for their women patients. Much of the use of health services by women concerns or is affected by pregnancy, conception and contraception in the young, and reproductive hormonal state after the menopause, apart from specific diseases and defects of the genital tract. Practical details needed only by specialist obstetricians and gynaecologists have not been included, but sufficient surgical information is given to assist the general practitioner in caring for their patients. We have also not included any coverage of breast disease despite connections with reproductive endocrinology, nor of neonatal paediatric care of ill babies despite overlapping interests of perinatology, because those subjects are well-covered in practice and textbooks by the respective specialists.

Major recent advances in our specialty have included new understanding of reproductive physiology, and technical refinements like single sperm injection into an oocyte, fetal diagnostic sampling and therapeutic surgical procedures, endoscopic surgery within the abdomen and uterus, high-resolution ultrasound imaging and blood flow measurement, and increasing pharmaceutical specificity. These specialist advances have been accompanied by better evaluation of diagnostic and therapeutic efficacy and safety, and this critical knowledge has led to simplification of practice and increased collaborative care between specialists and general practitioners.

Accompanying these technical and organizational advances has been increasing sensitivity to the emotional impact of caring for women in obstetrical and gynaecological practice. There have also come fundamental ethical challenges which are the concern of everyone in society, and in some instances – such as generation of embryos, egg donation to ageing women, and use of fetal tissues for research and treatment – have required the introduction of formal regulation. We have tried to recognize and draw attention to these important issues, although lacking room for adequate discussion. They are issues which should be woven into everyday clinical teaching.

M.G.R.H
D.N.J.
G.M.T.
P.G.W.

1
Modern obstetrics and gynaecology – an introduction

Anyone who has experienced the thrill and wonder of being present at the birth of a baby, or even of lambs or calves on a farm, cannot help but be excited by obstetrics. It is full of hope and joy. Labour proceeds apace and often demands an urgency and life-or-death decisions, which make obstetrics also a compelling clinical specialty. However, there can be pain and despair, and doctors must be able to deal with those too. The clinical attractions of gynaecology usually come to be appreciated later.

Together, obstetrics and gynaecology offer every type of clinical interest and challenge. In obstetrics there is the intellectual challenge of understanding the profound physiological changes during pregnancy, affecting every system of the body and in turn affecting the clinical management of any concurrent medical disorder ranging from diabetes to cardiopulmonary disorders or epilepsy. The management of fetal disorders like inherited biochemical disturbances, haemolytic anaemia or urinary tract obstruction presents special challenges because the fetus is difficult to reach and profoundly affected by its stage of maturity. Instrumental delivery of a baby, requiring diagnosis and manipulation within the blind confines of the vagina, remains a surgical art.

By contrast, antenatal care is essentially an exercise in preventive medicine, which requires a very different type of clinical discipline. It is more akin to public health medicine, whose specialists are the unsung heroes of any national health service. One of the great medical heroes in history was an obstetrician (or accoucheur) of the early 19th century, Dr Ignaz Semmelweis, who practised in Budapest and Vienna during the great days of the Austro-Hungarian empire. Destitute women were packed into the first 'lying-in' hospitals in order to deliver their babies off the street, and one-quarter of them died from 'child-bed fever'. Before Pasteur's discovery of bacteria, Semmelweis showed that the fever was linked to overcrowding of the beds and the procession of obstetricians and their students straight from the purulent postmortem room to their ward rounds. Semmelweis was the first to apply the principle of controlled prospective study to show the link and how deaths from puerperal sepsis could be largely prevented by simple hygienic measures. Read his fascinating story in *The Cry and the Covenant* by Morton Thompson (Heinemann, first published 1951) if you can still find a library copy.

There is much to be learned from history. The newcomer to an obstetric delivery suite (or 'labour ward') may wonder why obstetricians and midwives bring such close attention and sense of urgency to the care of women in labour, when so little seems to go seriously wrong and maternal death is a rarity. History shows that the greatest danger is from prolonged labour – sometimes lasting many days in times past – leading to dehydration, debilitation, infection and adrenal failure. Potentially infecting vaginal examination was avoided, thus the progress of labour – or lack of it – could often not be assessed, and caesarean section was held as a fearful last resort because so many – already desperately ill – died of it! With the advent of antibiotics, blood transfusion and oxytocic preparations to stimulate a failing uterus, modern obstetric and midwifery care aims to detect failure as soon as possible by regular examination, early correction of inefficient uterine activity if necessary, and caesarean section without delay if required. The philosophy underlying modern care is essentially the avoidance of prolonged labour. That involves close attention but is sometimes perceived as intrusive and a potential cause of iatrogenic problems, leading some women to seek the emotional sanctuary of their home to give birth, and to trust in nature. The challenge today is to combine safety with emotional satisfaction.

Gynaecology involves some of the commonest cancers, requiring radical pelvic surgery and both cytotoxic and hormonal chemotherapy, as well as population screening for preinvasive cancer of the cervix. It also involves the surgical arts of vaginal prolapse repair to retain good sexual function, and of bladder neck support to alleviate the misery of urinary incontinence, and the technical skills of conservative pelvic microsurgery and laparoscopic surgery for infertility or pelvic pain, as well as endoscopic surgery within the uterine cavity – and in pregnancy, even fetal surgery. In addition, the scope of surgery extends to ultrasound-guided procedures such as to collect eggs for *in vitro* fertilization or to drain cysts; also in pregnancy to biopsy trophoblast, sample amniotic fluid or fetal blood, or transfuse the fetus.

Gynaecology also involves the intellectual challenges of endocrinology in the management of menstrual disorders, ovulatory failures and associated conditions like hirsutism, as well as infertility and the everyday requirements of contraception. Those are the most common conditions in young adults requiring medical help, from general practitioners and hospital specialists. Some reproductive endocrine disorders also carry implications for health far beyond the reproductive system. They can involve risks of osteoporosis on the one hand and, on the other, of coronary artery disease or diabetes. Even the everyday choice of hormonal contraception or postmenopausal hormone replacement therapy requires specific consideration of the potential risks of thrombosis, stroke and cancer.

Sexuality is a major aspect of obstetrics and gynaecology. Of course, sexuality affects all our lives, young and old, and all of medicine. Old people remain keenly, if differently, interested in sex and for example after myocardial infarction or stroke their fears of sexual exertion are often forgotten by doctors. Obstetrics and gynaecology involves sexuality in every aspect. There are not only women's fears of their sex lives being harmed by operations like the common episiotomy (perineal incision to assist childbirth), hysterectomy or vaginal prolapse repair. Some routine questioning and the routine vaginal examination involve at the very least an invasion of the patient's sexual privacy. It may be necessary but must be done with politeness and sensitivity. The enormous emotional impact often goes unrecognized by doctors. Many women feel sexually despoiled, abused or virtually raped by the routine vaginal examination. By contrast, some may entertain fantasies which put the doctor at risk. The vaginal examination is never routine. On the other hand, some women present with complaints such as vaginal discharge which are really surrogates for sexual worries, and doctors need to be sensitive to those possibilities too. In their training doctors need to come to terms with their own sexuality, or at least learn to put aside their own, often narrow, perception of sexuality before they can deal confidently and sensitively with their women patients.

Womanhood, as distinct from sexuality, is another key personal, emotional and psychological feature to be appreciated in obstetric and gynaecological practice. The ability to conceive, bear children naturally and raise a family are for most women vital aspects of their lives by which they can feel fulfilled and regard themselves in high esteem. Obstetric interventions to assist them in labour and delivery, for example epidural analgesia, caesarean section, forceps delivery or even a simple episiotomy, can make them feel a failure. Sometimes that happens because their expectations of natural childbirth were raised too high and blinkered. There may thus be a psychological dilemma between home or hospital delivery. Some clamour for home delivery but many prefer what they perceive as the convenience, safety and certainty of adequate pain relief in hospital. All women are different and their individual needs for childbirth to be a satisfying and happy event should be recognized.

Infertility causes deep and unending distress, which is often kept hidden away because of desperate loss of self-esteem and sense of personal worth as a woman. It undermines a woman's sense of value to her husband and her enjoyment of sex. But when infertility is due to a sperm defect the man's self-esteem can also be severely damaged, and in turn the woman may become doubly anxious, both for him and because she may feel she cannot be fulfilled except perhaps by pressing him to accept donor insemination.

That brings us to complex and fascinating ethical, social and legal issues which affect almost every aspect of obstetric and gynaecological practice, adding to the richness and variety of the specialty. There are the issues of under-age contraception and confidentiality, and of termination of pregnancy, and even sterilization can be contentious. There are issues of screening for fetal abnormality, of occasional conflicts between fetal and maternal interests, and sometimes whether to strive excessively to keep alive a damaged baby. In infertility practice, does everyone have a right to a child, and therefore treatment? There are fundamental issues of creating and storing embryos, and of gamete donation, all of which are governed by law in the UK. There are also political issues of resource allocation and what priority society in general gives to funding services for population control on the one hand and for infertility on the other.

There are great opportunities in obstetrics and gynaecology for positive health promotion. Antenatal care has already been mentioned, and there are often opportunities for prepregnancy advice to promote fetal health. Cervical screening has also been mentioned to enable treatment to prevent cervical cancer. Possible screening for early ovarian cancer is a major challenge for the future. Contraception provides an opportunity in nearly every woman to educate about venereal disease and responsible sexual behaviour, and of an open door to discuss sexual worries. Even termination of pregnancy offers a positive opportunity for a young and often immature woman to explore her own behaviour and learn from it for the better. After the menopause, as women live longer and their expectations rise of enjoying their retirement years, they can greatly benefit from long-term prophylactic hormone replacement therapy to maintain their health and well-being. Indeed, the social costs of cardiovascular disease and osteoporotic hip fractures are enormous and an important economic consideration. Developing hormone preparations and finding the ones that suit individuals for acceptable long-term use are an important challenge for positive health promotion in the future.

What more can any doctor want than is offered by the practice of obstetrics and gynaecology? In fact, in its fullest development the specialty is beyond the scope of any individual and there are now fully fledged subspecialties of fetal and maternal medicine, reproductive medicine, gynaecological oncology and urogynaecology. Perhaps we should add that in some countries diseases and surgery of the breast are included, but not in the UK. In specialist practice the continuum of fetal and neonatal care, often involving close collaboration and decision-making by obstetricians and neonatologists, is embraced in the idea of perinatology as though it were a unified specialty. Whilst that is so in principle, in practice there are no complete perinatologists. Therefore in this book care of the newborn will be limited to coverage of the basic examination and initial care of normal babies. The student is therefore directed to texts specifically on neonatology for information about the care of ill babies.

We hope you will enjoy obstetrics and gynaecology, and that it will bring you as much professional fulfilment as it has us. We hope this book will illuminate the subject for you and stimulate you to seek deeper knowledge and understanding, and indeed perhaps a specialist career in the subject in the future. We hope too that it will help you to become a more thoughtful doctor, particularly when caring for the reproductive problems of women.

2

Obstetric and gynaecological history-taking and case presentation

History-taking and case presentation are important skills for the student and young doctor. They form a major part of the assessment of your work on a firm and in clinical examinations at MB, or higher levels. For the very best histories and presentations a sound clinical knowledge is needed in order to direct questions and shape the presentation appropriately, but the basic framework is readily acquired and will carry the student far in spite of a modest degree of ignorance! Ideally you would have read the rest of this book before tackling history-taking and case presentation, but in the real world you are very likely to be asked to perform these tasks on the first or second days on the firm and are unlikely to have had the foresight to have read the book - hence the position of this section.

It is a basic politeness and also a help to you in establishing a rapport with the patient to introduce yourself and your role (as student or examination candidate). The skills of history-taking are very similar across the specialties but the important components differ widely. Below are listed the main components of the history followed by a sample case presentation for obstetric and gynaecological patients.

OBSTETRIC HISTORY-TAKING

Introduction	Name. Age. Marital status. Parity. Gestational age.
Presenting complaint or problem	Complaint, if any, or abnormality found.
Present pregnancy	Date of last menstrual period. Normal period? Cycle. Whether recently on oral contraception. Estimated date of delivery (EDD).

	Ultrasound estimation of EDD? Symptoms at any stage, particularly bleeding, pain.
Past obstetric history	Babies. Modes of delivery. Dates. Gestations. Baby weights. Complications of all pregnancies, labours and deliveries, particularly damage or infection. Outcome: children alive and well? Miscarriages or terminations.
Past gynaecological history	Operations (e.g. cervical dilatation or conization, uterine myomectomy, vaginal repair). Infertility.
Family history	Diabetes. Recent tuberculosis. Congenital abnormalities.
General	Past and present illnesses, particularly cardiovascular, renal, endocrine. Blood transfusions. Drugs. Allergies. Social. Smoking. Alcohol. Intended baby-feeding method. Future contraceptive needs. Last cervical smear.

Obstetric case presentation

After the introduction and description of the presenting problem the most important information required is, first, the full history of the present pregnancy, one of the most important practical aspects of which is reliability of the estimated gestational age. Second is the past obstetric history because of the recurring nature of many complications. Poor fetal growth – therefore the weights of previous babies – is particularly important. Amongst the general points you need to demonstrate your understanding of the importance of social factors in determining risks not only for the fetus but subsequently to the baby through possible lack of care, and of the need for contraceptive advice for the future.

The order need not be rigidly fixed, and priority might be given to the medical history, for instance in patients with diabetes or mitral stenosis.

Table 2.1 shows how a case of polyhydramnios associated with suspected diabetes might be presented.

Table 2.1   Presentation of a case of polyhydramnios with suspected diabetes

History	Key components
This is Mrs Smith who is a 29-year-old housewife in her third pregnancy who has been admitted at 38 weeks with an unstable lie and polyhydramnios	*Introduction*: Personal description. Presenting complaint or problem
Her first pregnancy in 1992 was straightforward with a normal term delivery of a boy weighing 3.5 kg after an 8-hour labour. She had an 8-week spontaneous miscarriage in March 1994, followed by surgical evacuation of the uterus	*Past obstetric history*: Factors (or lack of them) likely to recur or add risk to present pregnancy
Mrs Smith's last period started on 15.11.95. She was certain of that date and she had a regular 28-day cycle off the contraceptive pill which she had stopped several months earlier, therefore her calculated EDD is 22.8.96. However, her last period was scanty and she was felt to be rather large for her menstrual dates, and scans at 16 and 34 weeks have put her about 4 weeks ahead with an EDD of 25.7.96. These scans showed a single fetus with a fundal placenta. An α-fetoprotein (AFP) at 16 weeks showed a normal result, with a Down's risk estimate of 1:1500	*Present pregnancy*: Reliability of EDD. Scan results, including screen for abnormality
The pregnancy was normal until 34 weeks when she was noted to have glycosuria, a transverse lie and excess amniotic fluid. The fetal lie has varied since then on each occasion seen, and the amount of fluid has continued to be excessive	Problems developing in the pregnancy
A glucose tolerance test gave a normal result, however, and detailed scanning of the fetus has shown a normal fetus, although the stomach could not be demonstrated	Investigations relevant to problems

Mrs Smith was concerned why she
was being investigated and has been
told that the baby may have a
blockage of the oesophagus, but
that this should be treatable

*What the patient knows if
relevant to discussion*

The baby is active and Mrs Smith has
been keeping a kick chart. She has
put on 13 kg during the pregnancy
and is still gaining. She is 5 ft 5 in
(1.63 m), takes size 5 shoes and
weighs 71 kg

*Fetal activity. Maternal weight
gain. Build, and predictors
of possible cephalopelvic
disproportion*

She has had no serious illnesses in the
past, no operations and no blood
transfusions

*General and past medical history:
Features relevant to pregnancy*

Her grandmother had maturity-onset
diabetes, but there is no other
history of diabetes in the family,
and no history of congenital
abnormality, recent tuberculosis,
or other serious illness

Family history: Include important
negatives, concentrating on
conditions requiring specific
action

Mrs Smith lives with her husband
and little boy in their own
three-bedroom house. Her husband
works as a computer programmer.
She does not smoke and has only
the occasional social drink

Social history: Housing and
financial situation suitable for
a baby? Social habits of risk to
fetus, baby?

Her mother is staying with them
until after she has had the baby,
so that there are no problems with
looking after the other child. She
wants to breast-feed, and will
probably return to the contraceptive
pill afterwards

Arrangements for other children.
Plans to feed this baby and for
contraception

Mrs Smith appears healthy. General
examination reveals no abnormality.
Her blood pressure is 110/70 mmHg,
there is no protein or sugar in her
urine, and there is no significant
oedema

General: Pre-eclampsia? Possible
diabetes?

Abdominal examination shows a
pregnant uterus and fetal movements. The uterus feels unusually
large for 38 weeks and she has a
fundal height of 44 cm. There seems
to be excessive amniotic fluid, with a

Obstetric: Fetal size. Lie and
presentation important from 32
weeks' gestation. Is the head
engaged or will it engage, from
36 weeks? Is the fetus still alive?
The position (of the back and

transmitted thrill, but it is not very tense and the fetus can be felt in a longitudinal lie with cephalic presentation four-fifths above the pelvic brim. Movements can be felt and the heart heard

head) is of no critical importance

In summary, this is Mrs Smith who is a 29-year-old housewife, para 1+1 at 38 weeks, and has been admitted with unstable lie and polyhydramnios

Summary: After your detailed case presentation it is helpful to finish with a brief summary giving the essential positive points

In addition, you should be ready to show that you know that antenatal care includes certain routine laboratory investigations as follows.

Investigations

Critical to the pregnancy
Haemoglobin
Rhesus, ABO groups and antibodies
Wassermann Reaction (WR), Venereal Disease Research Laboratory (VDRL) test
Sickle test/haemoglobin typing (in relevant races)
Urine culture
AFP
Ultrasonography
Opportunistic screening
Rubella antibody assay
Cervical cytology (if due)

GYNAECOLOGICAL HISTORY-TAKING

Introduction	Name. Age. Marital status. Parity.
Presenting complaint	As given by the patient, and developed appropriately.
Menstrual history	Age at menarche or menopause. Cycle. Loss (clots? number of pads or tampons, flooding?). Pain, severity and timing.
Non-menstrual bleeding	Postcoital. Intermenstrual. Postmenopausal.

Contraception	Requirement. Past and present methods.
Pregnancies	Babies. Complications, especially damage or infection. Miscarriages. Terminations.
Coitus	Ever? Difficulty. Pain, superficial or deep. Frequency, if infertile.
Vaginal discharge	Colour. Irritation. Offensive odour?
Micturition	Frequency. Dysuria. Incontinence. Delay.
Bowel action	Constipation. Pain. Blood. Mucus.
General	Present, past and family illnesses. Drugs. Allergies. Social. Smoking. Alcohol. Last cervical smear.
Special	The reader is referred to particular sections of the book dealing with histories for special cases such as infertility, endocrine disorders, psychosexual problems, etc.

Gynaecological case presentation

The presentation can be similar in structure to any other medical or surgical case. However, after the introduction and developing the particular presenting complaint you will be expected to demonstrate understanding of the possible relevance of all the other common gynaecological features listed above. You should therefore mention them all, even if negative. You should also show awareness of the possible contribution of contraceptive, social or psychosexual problems to the primary complaints.

Table 2.2 shows how a case of prolapse might be presented.

Table 2.2   Presentation of a case of prolapse

History	Key components
This is Mrs Jones, who is a 45-year-old teacher with three children who complains of a lump coming down in the vagina	*Introduction*: Personal description. Presenting complaint

She first noticed a feeling of pressure in the vagina about a year ago and this has become more noticeable in recent months, and for the last 6 weeks she has noticed a lump protruding through the introitus. She also has low backache and this symptom is worse when she is up and about and relieved when she is in bed. She has had no urinary stress incontinence or hesitancy and no problems with defecation

History of presenting complaint: Include closely related symptoms (e.g. stress incontinence for prolapse) even if negative

Mrs Jones has had three children, the oldest now 18 and the youngest 15. She had forceps for the first delivery, but the others were spontaneous deliveries. The babies weighed between 7 and 8 lb (about 3.5 kg) and the longest labour was about 8 hours. She has had no other pregnancies

Obstetric history: Possible damage from difficult deliveries?

Mrs Jones's periods began at 14 and her cycle is fairly regular, every 28–30 days, with each period lasting 6 days. The loss is not excessive and she has no intermenstrual or postcoital bleeding or abnormal discharge. She has no significant dysmenorrhoea or dyspareunia. Her last period was 2 weeks ago and she had a normal cervical smear in June last year

Menstrual history: Any reason to need hysterectomy along with vaginal repair (if necessary)?

She took the contraceptive pill until the age of 34 when she had a laparoscopic sterilization performed. She and her husband have regular intercourse without any problems except that she thinks the vagina feels rather slack

Contraceptive and coital history: Still young and sexually active: would need adequate vagina after repair

Her general health is good and she has no other symptoms on review of systems. She is not on any drugs and is not allergic to anything. Her weight is normal and she does not smoke, nor does she have a chronic cough or constipation

General health: Factors affecting operative or anaesthetic risks. Factors risking operative failure due to strain on vagina

She has had no serious illnesses in the past and no operations except the laparoscopic sterilization

Past medical history: Points relevant as above

Mrs Jones lives with her husband and three children in their own four-bedroom house. Her 18-year-old daughter is quite capable of running the house should Mrs Jones need to come into hospital

Social history: Possible need for special arrangements to allow patient to be admitted to hospital or for convalescence

Examination
Mrs Jones appears healthy. General examination reveals no abnormality and her blood pressure is 120/80 mmHg. She is not obese and there is no swelling or mass in her abdomen

General examination: Fit for operation? Any specific factor contributing to prolapse?

Vaginal examination (if you are required to do it) reveals a healthy looking vulva and vagina, but a marked cystocele, moderate rectocele, and deficient perineum. The cervix looks healthy and there is no demonstrable uterine descent. The uterus feels normal in size and is upright and mobile, and there is no adnexal swelling or tenderness

Vaginal examination: Describe your findings but also be prepared to discuss whether the prolapse requires treatment. Would physiotherapy suffice? Does she require anterior and/or posterior vaginal repair? Does she need operative support for the uterus, or hysterectomy?

In summary, Mrs Jones is a 45-year-old parous teacher with a year's history of vaginal prolapse. Her general health is good. Examination reveals a marked cystocele with some rectocele and a deficient perineum but no demonstrable uterine descent and no other abnormality

Summary: After your detailed case presentation it is helpful to finish with a brief summary giving the essential positive points

3

Reproductive embryology

INTRODUCTION

The distinction between gestational age and embryonal or fetal age needs to be carefully made when considering events in early pregnancy relating to embryonic development. In clinical practice gestational age is used, being simply dated from the last menstrual period.

The fetus is called an embryo until it shows obvious external human form (after about 8 weeks). Fetal and embryonal age are thus the same and are calculated from the moment of fertilization or, being so close, of ovulation. Average human fetal life lasts 266 days (38 weeks) until birth.

In clinical practice, however, the duration of pregnancy is expressed as the gestational age, which, by convention, is calculated from the last menstrual period (LMP), the so-called duration of amenorrhoea. Since in the usual 28-day menstrual cycle ovulation occurs on about day 14 of the cycle (day 1 being the first day of menstruation), gestational age is thus 14 days greater than fetal age and the average length of gestation until birth is 280 days (40 weeks, or about 9 calendar months and 7 days).

Fetal age is, of course, what really matters, but it is rarely feasible to define when ovulation occurred; the LMP is the only readily available reference point, hence the use of gestational age. Unfortunately, due to variation in the menstrual cycle, gestational age is often not simply equal to the duration of amenorrhoea, while other misleading factors are also common in practice. The calculation of gestational age often has to be corrected in the light of new evidence during pregnancy or afterwards. The correction is always aimed, however, at bringing gestational age into line with fetal age (i.e. the latter plus 14 days).

THE GONADS

Development of the gonad into a testis or ovary is normally determined by the presence or absence, respectively, of a Y chromosome. However, whilst a Y chromosome determines germ cell differentiation into spermatogonia, differentiation of the testis depends on a specific histocompatibility antigen, the H-Y antigen, absence of which can lead to gonadal dysgenesis and female development in an XY individual. In the female, ovarian follicles would be rapidly lost by atresia unless maintained by the presence of a second X chromosome. Thus Turner syndrome due to 45,X0 is characterized by ovarian dysgenesis.

Both gonads develop from **three elements**: germ cells and two distinct types of somatic cells. In addition the efferent ductules of the testis develop from branches of the mesonephric duct.

1 The large primordial **germ cells** differentiate very early in fetal life, no later than 3 weeks (5 weeks' gestation). They develop at the root of the yolk sac situated ventrally and migrate by amoebic movement, probably directed by chemotaxis, via the gut mesentery to the urogenital ridges situated dorsally (Fig. 3.1).

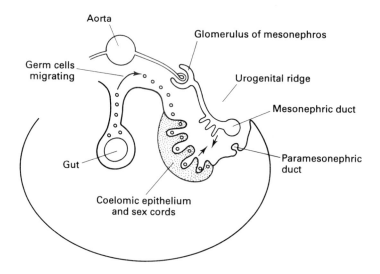

Fig. 3.1 Abdominal cross-section showing development of the primordial urogenital structures between 4 and 6 weeks' embryonic age.

2 **Coelomic** epithelium of the genital ridges proliferates deeply to form **sex cords** which envelop the germ cells (Fig. 3.1). The sex cords arrive in two waves. The primary wave reaches the medulla of the gonad and is of critical importance in the testis, giving rise to the seminiferous tubules. The secondary wave remains at the cortex and is of critical importance in the development of the ovary later, giving rise to the ovarian follicles.

(a) The sex cord cells form the **Sertoli cells** of seminiferous tubules or **granulosa cells** of ovarian follicles, in each case acting in support of the germ cells, being intimately connected with them, and separating them from the surrounding mesenchyme.

(b) The deeper reaches of the sex cords contain no germ cells but in the testis will form the **straight tubules of the rete testis**, which will link with outgrowing mesonephric tubules (Fig. 3.2).

(c) The sex cords become separated from the surface coelomic epithelium, which in the case of the testis becomes condensed to form the covering **tunica albuginea**.

3 **Mesenchymal** cells situated close around the sex cords, but separated from them by their basal lamina, differentiate into the **steroid-producing interstitial cells** – in the ovary **theca cells**, and in the testis **Leydig cells**. These have receptors to human chorionic gonadotrophin which is at peak levels when the testis is

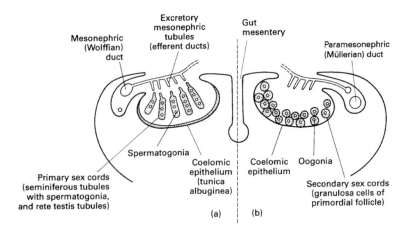

Fig. 3.2 Differentiation of (a) the testis at about 7 weeks' embryonic age, and (b) the ovary at about 8 weeks. In the ovary the secondary sex cords have divided into discrete follicles around each oogonium.

differentiating – ahead of the ovary – and is able to respond by secreting testosterone. That is of critical importance and timing in the differentiation of the genital tract and external genitalia in the male (see below).

Gonadal oncogenesis

When it comes to the clinical pathology of ovarian neoplasms (see Chapter 24), it is worth relating them to their distinct cellular ontogeny: germ cells (e.g. teratomas), sex cord cells (e.g. granulosa cell tumour, which can secrete oestrogen) and mesenchymal cells (e.g. thecoma-fibromas, which can also secrete steroids, and anomalous Leydig cell tumours which secrete testosterone); though by far the commonest benign and malignant tumours originate from the coelomic epithelium (the so-called epithelial cysts, filled with secretions which are specifically serous or mucinous in type).

THE GENITAL DUCTS

Originally two ducts are present on each side by 6 weeks of fetal age:

1 The **mesonephric duct** or Wolffian system extends from the excretory tubules of the mesonephros (Fig. 3.1) to open into the urogenital sinus. It is destined to develop into the male genital tract in the presence of the testes. The Leydig cells produce testosterone which stimulates the development of the mesonephric duct into the **efferent ductules** of the testis (now becoming linked with the tubules of the rete testis arising from the sex cords: see Fig. 3.2), and **epididymis**, **vas deferens** and **seminal vesicles**.

Close to its opening into the urogenital sinus the mesonephric duct sprouts the **ureteric bud** which grows laterally and upwards to form the collecting system of the definitive kidney by linking with the metanephros (Fig. 3.3). Differential growth of the urogenital sinus leads to separate opening of the ureters into it above and lateral to the mesonephric ducts (Fig. 3.4). The ureters now open into the definitive bladder and, in the male, the seminal vesicles open into the urethra. When the testes descend into the scrotum via the inguinal canals the vasa deferentia must loop over the ureters, as shown later in Figure 3.7.

In the male the Sertoli cells also produce anti-Müllerian hormone (or Müllerian inhibiting substance) which inhibits development of the paramesonephric ducts.

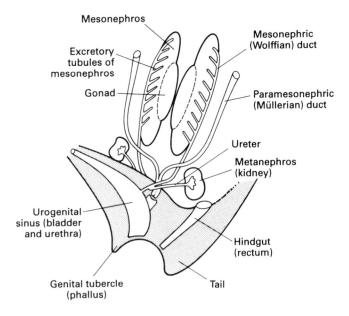

Fig. 3.3 Sagittal–oblique view showing development of the complete urogenital systems at about 8 weeks' embryonic age, just before sexual differentiation.

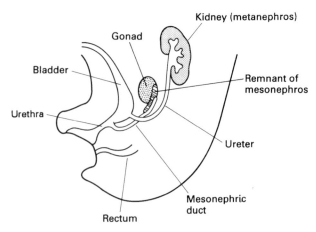

Fig. 3.4 Differentiation of the bladder and urethra from the urogenital sinus at about 9 weeks' embryonic age. Differential growth of the sinus has led to separate openings into the bladder of the ureter and mesonephric duct (seminal vesicle in the male) and crossing of the ducts. Differential growth of the trunk has carried the kidney up into the abdomen, leaving the gonad in the pelvis.

2 The **paramesonephric duct** or Müllerian system develops parallel to the mesonephric duct by invagination of the coelomic epithelium, as shown in Figure 3.1. At its upper extremity it remains open into the coelomic cavity (Fig. 3.3), where in the female it will form the fimbrial opening of the **Fallopian tube**. It passes downwards and medially to fuse with its opposite number to form the **uterus** (Fig. 3.3). The fused paramesonephric ducts do not open into the urogenital sinus, but fuse with the sinovaginal bulbs (see below).

Development of the genital tract in the female is a neutral process resulting from the absence of testicular hormone signals. The paramesonephric ducts develop due to lack of anti-Müllerian hormone, and the mesonephric ducts fail to develop due to lack of testosterone. The hormonal influence is strictly paracrine (i.e. local) rather than endocrine because it acts only on the same side as the testis, as shown by unilateral transplantation experiments in animals. The ovary has no specific influence and differentiates later. The relative timing of gonadal development and control of genital tract development is summarized in Table 3.1.

Table 3.1 Summary of stages, timing and hormonal control of embryonic development of the urogenital systems. Note that the key determinants are the earlier development of the testis than the ovary, and its consequent early secretion of testosterone and anti-Müllerian hormone. The timing of events is given by embryonic age rather than gestational age, and by crown–rump length (CRL, in brackets)

Male and female

3 weeks
(CRL 2 mm)
Primordial germ cells develop at root of yolk sac

4–6 weeks
(5–22 mm)
Urogenital ridges develop, germ cells migrate, and primitive sex cords and genital ducts (mesonephric and paramesonephric) are formed
Urogenital sinus and genital tubercle appear

6–9 weeks
(22–50 mm)
Urinary system differentiated (kidney from metanephros, ureter from mesonephric duct)

Male
6–7 weeks
(22–27 mm)
Testis differentiated
Secretion of testosterone (by Leydig cells) and anti-Müllerian hormone (Sertoli cells), leading to:

7–8 weeks
(27–40 mm)
Mesonephric ducts (Wolffian system) differentiated
Paramesonephric ducts and sinovaginal bulbs (Müllerian system) inhibited

Table 3.1 *cont.*

8–12 weeks (40–90 mm)	External genitalia differentiated (dependent on dihydrotestosterone converted at receptor sites from testosterone)
8 weeks	Testis 'descended' into pelvis (due to differential growth of body; held by gubernaculum testis)
28 weeks	Testis at deep inguinal ring
32 weeks	Testis descended into scrotum
Female 7–8 weeks (27–40 mm)	Ovary differentiated, depends on secondary wave of sex cord development
8–12 weeks (40–90 mm)	Paramesonephric ducts and sinovaginal bulbs (Müllerian system) differentiated Mesonephric ducts regress
9–12 weeks (50–90 mm)	External genitalia differentiated

THE VAGINA

The **sinovaginal bulbs** are a pair of solid outgrowths of the urogenital sinus (Fig. 3.5), which fuse together in the midline and meet the fused paramesonephric ducts above. The sinovaginal bulbs give rise to the **vagina** by hollowing out and then merging into one (Fig. 3.5). It is uncertain whether the paramesonephric ducts contribute to the vagina – possibly to the epithelial lining. (They were once thought to contribute the upper third of the vagina.)

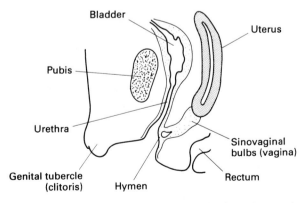

Fig. 3.5   Differentiation of the vagina from the two sinovaginal bulbs, which are fused and starting to become hollowed at about 10 weeks' embryonic age.

The mesonephric ducts probably do not contribute to the vagina, but remnants are clearly present in the vaginal wall anterolaterally, where congenital cysts arising from the mesonephric ducts sometimes occur. However, in the female the mesonephric ducts though undeveloped may have an inductor action on the Müllerian system. Thus absence of the mesonephric duct on one side may lead to one-sided uterine anomaly and one-sided blind vagina, along with ipsilateral absent kidney due to lack of a ureteric bud (which normally arises from the lower end of the mesonephric duct) (see below on clinically important anomalies).

THE EXTERNAL GENITALIA

The external genitalia in both male and female develop from the same primordial structures as shown in Figure 3.6: the genital tubercle (penis or clitoris); the urogenital groove (urethra) from the urogenital sinus; the urethral folds, one on each side (cavernous bodies of the penis or labia minora); and the genital swellings, one on each side (scrotum or labia majora).

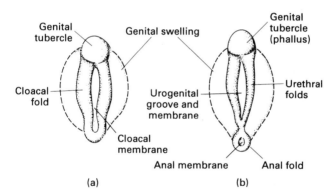

Fig. 3.6   Initial differentiation of the primordial (still neutral) structures of the external genitalia from the cloaca between (a) 4 weeks' embryonic age and (b) 6 weeks.

In the male, differentiation of the external genitalia depends on dihydrotestosterone converted locally in the receptor target tissues from circulating testosterone. For that to occur the target tissues must be able to bind testosterone and contain the enzyme 5α-reductase to achieve the conversion. Failure of either mechanism can lead to varying degrees of impaired male genital development despite plentiful testosterone. The classical example is the so-called testicular feminization syndrome (see later).

Normally the genital tubercle grows into a phallus which carries on its ventral aspect the extended urogenital groove, which becomes enclosed to form the penile urethra by fusion of the urethral folds from each side, which also form the cavernous bodies of the penis. The external genital swellings also fuse, to form the scrotum, and the line of fusion is marked by the scrotal raphe. Differentiation is completed with closure of the urethra to the tip of the penis after 12 weeks but the testes do not descend into the scrotum until 32 weeks.

In the female, differentiation of the external genitalia is determined by the absence of testosterone (or strictly dihydrotestosterone). As with the internal genitalia, it is a neutral process in hormonal terms. Thus in males unable to utilize testosterone as in the classical testicular feminization syndrome mentioned above, the external genitalia develop as in the normal female. The phallus remains small (clitoris), the urethral folds and genital swellings do not fuse and remain separate paired structures (the labia minora and majora, respectively), and the urogenital sinus remains open (the vestibule) and receives the openings of the urethra (external meatus) and vagina (introitus). The remnant of the urogenital membrane forms the hymen. The complete sequence of events in the development of the urogenital tracts is summarized in Table 3.2.

Table 3.2.   Summary of ontogeny of urogenital systems

Structure	Primordium
URINARY SYSTEM	
Kidney	Metanephros
Ureter and renal pelvis	Ureteric bud from lower end of mesonephric duct
GENITAL SYSTEM	
Male	
Testis	
Spermatids (secondary, haploid spermatocytes)	Germ cells (from root of sac)
	Urogenital ridge
Tunica albuginea	Coelomic epithelium
Seminiferous tubules, including Sertoli cells	Sex cords (primary, medullary cords)
Rete testis tubules	
Interstitial (Leydig) cells	Mesenchyme
Efferent ductules	Mesonephros, excretory ducts
Epididymis	
Vas deferens	Mesonephric duct
Seminal vesicles	(Wolffian system)

Table 3.2 *cont.*

External genitalia

Penis	
Dorsum	Genital tubercle
Ventral part	
enclosing urethra	Urethral folds (fused)
Cavernous bodies	
Penile urethra	Urogenital groove
Scrotum	Genital swellings (fused)

Female

Ovary	
Oocytes (primary, diploid)	Germ cells
	Urogenital ridge
Epithelial covering	Coelomic epithelium
Follicles	
Granulosa cells	Sex cords (secondary, cortical)
Theca cells	
Stroma	Mesenchyme
Fallopian tube	
Uterus	Paramesonephric (Müllerian)
? Upper vagina	ducts*
? Vaginal epithelium	
Vagina	Sinovaginal bulbs (from urogenital sinus)*
External genitalia	
Clitoris	Genital tubercle
Vestibule	Urogenital groove
Labia minora	Urethral folds
(including cavernous bodies)	
Labia majora	Genital swellings
Hymen	Urogenital membrane

* The paramesonephric ducts and sinovaginal bulbs together constitute the Müllerian system.

GONADAL DESCENT

Both ovary and testis descend from the abdomen into the pelvis by 8 weeks of age, not by active migration but due to differential growth of the body. The gonads are held down by a mesenchymal condensation called the caudal genital ligament, which is continuous with ligamentous condensations leading via the inguinal region (and future inguinal canal) to the external genital swelling (the future scrotum or labium major).

The complete ligament in the male is called the gubernaculum testis. In the female it forms the suspensory ligament of the ovary (to the uterus) and the round ligament (from the uterus to the inguinal canal; see Chapter 4, Fig. 4.4).

Passage of the testis into the scrotum depends on evagination of the peritoneum through the inguinal canal alongside the gubernaculum. The so-called vaginal process of peritoneum persists as the tunica vaginalis enveloping the testis in the scrotum (Fig. 3.7). It normally becomes obliterated in the inguinal canal, but may persist as a congenital hernia or cyst.

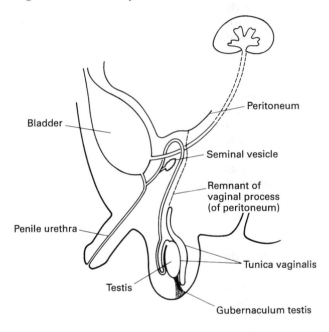

Fig. 3.7 Depiction of the path of descent of the testis and vas deferens from the pelvis through the inguinal canal, originally accompanied by evagination of the peritoneum, looping over the ureter.

The final descent of the testis into the scrotum during late fetal life is accompanied by shortening of the gubernaculum but may not be due to that. It is, however, an active process controlled by hormones, probably both gonadotrophins and androgens. Failure of the testis to descend, called cryptorchidism, is discussed below.

DEVELOPMENTAL ABNORMALITIES

These can occur due to structural failures of indeterminate cause or abnormal hormonal actions on the primordial systems.

1 **Agenesis or hypoplasia of a urogenital ridge** will result in absence of the gonad, genital tract, kidney and renal tract on the affected side. In the female there will be an apparently normal vagina but obviously abnormal uterus (unicornute, i.e. single-horned), being rather narrow and diverted to the side.

   Ovarian dysgenesis is characterized by tiny 'streak' ovaries without any follicles, typically (but often not) occurring with Turner syndrome due to a missing X chromosome. The abnormality is not due to original absence of germ cells but to excessive germ cell atresia (see Chapter 5 on oogenesis).

2 **Mesonephric duct anomalies** can lead in the male to occlusion or extensive deficiency of the vas deferens and epididymis. If bilateral, it will result in obstructive azoospermia despite normal-functioning testes.

   Anomalies affecting the opening of the mesonephric duct into the urogenital sinus may also be associated with an absent kidney due to lack of the ureteric bud.

   In the female normal remnants of the mesonephric system can give rise to cysts. Mesonephric excretory tubules (analogous with the efferent ductules of the testis: see Fig. 3.2) persist in the ovarian mesentery as the epoophoron and can give rise to paraovarian cysts. Caudal remnants of the mesonephric duct can give rise to cysts of Gartner's duct alongside the vagina.

3 **Paramesonephric duct anomalies** include unilateral agenesis or hypoplasia but the commonest are due to failure of fusion in the formation of the uterus. There are numerous variations and degrees of uterine anomaly, some of which are illustrated in Figure 3.8.

   In addition, anomalous development of the sinovaginal bulbs can lead to fusion failures in vaginal development (Fig. 3.8) or to partial or complete vaginal aplasia. The commonest type of vaginal aplasia is limited to membrane-like occlusion of the lower vagina, sometimes incorrectly called imperforate hymen. It becomes membrane-like partly due to the build-up of menses behind it (cryptomenorrhoea).

   Because of the inductor role of the mesonephric duct on the paramesonephric duct and sinovaginal bulb, the underlying cause of some uterovaginal abnormalities is mesonephric anomaly, and is therefore often associated with urinary tract

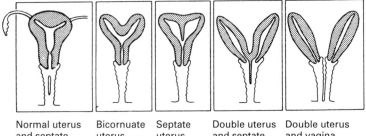

| Normal uterus and septate vagina | Bicornuate uterus | Septate uterus | Double uterus and septate vagina | Double uterus and vagina ('uterus didelphis') |

Fig. 3.8   Common anomalies of the uterus and vagina due to varied degrees of non-fusion of the paired embryonic structures from which they originate.

anomalies (due to lack of a ureteric bud from the mesonephric duct), which should also be sought in practice.

4 **Gonadal maldescent**. In the male, failure of the testis to descend into the scrotum, called cryptorchidism, often occurs as an isolated anomaly despite otherwise normal testicular development, testosterone secretion and consequent sexual development. It is often associated however with defective spermatogenesis and infertility. That may not be simply due to overheating of the testes by remaining within the body, but could be a direct result of defective hormonal control causing failure of testicular descent in the first place. That may also explain why surgical correction of cryptorchidism often fails to restore spermatogenesis.

The ovary may also fail to descend fully. In the adult it is normally suspended loosely deep in the pelvis behind the uterus. Failure of development of the Müllerian system, such as an absent uterine horn on one side, is often associated with the ovary on that side remaining at the level of the pelvic brim (just in front of the ureter).

5 **Hormonal disorders**. In genetic males with normal testes various androgen insensitivity syndromes can occur due to enzyme defects in the receptor tissues preventing conversion of testosterone to dihydrotestosterone, though in varying degrees. The testes produce normal amounts of testosterone, oestradiol and anti-Müllerian hormone, but the peripheral tissues cannot respond to testosterone and effectively 'see' only the other hormones. In the classic complete testicular feminization syndrome there are thus normal female external genitalia (due to ineffective testosterone), but absent internal female genitalia and

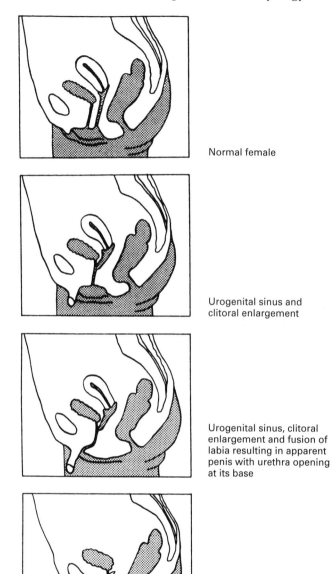

Normal female

Urogenital sinus and clitoral enlargement

Urogenital sinus, clitoral enlargement and fusion of labia resulting in apparent penis with urethra opening at its base

Normal male

Fig. 3.9 Complete and incomplete differentiation of the female and male genitalia seen in sagittal section.

a short blind vagina (due to anti-Müllerian hormone); and after pubertal maturation of the testes there is normal breast development (due to oestrogen) but lack of pubic, axillary and facial hair (due to ineffective testosterone). In addition, the testes remain within the abdomen.

Intermediate maldevelopments of the external genitalia can occur due to partial defects of androgen metabolism in males, or due to androgen excess in females (see below). Simple examples are illustrated in Figure 3.9.

Androgen excess in females can be due to various enzymic defects of the adrenal gland. Some can be associated with serious mineralocorticoid deficiency which threatens the life of the newborn. Others primarily affect androgen production, which may become apparent only after puberty but the classic syndrome of congenital adrenal hyperplasia presents at birth by ambiguous external genitalia and later by steadily increasing hirsutism and clitoral enlargement. Treatment is required by pituitary–adrenal suppression using glucocorticoids, though it cannot alter the genital changes that have already developed.

FURTHER READING

Ancien, P. (1992) Embryological observations on the female genital tract. *Human Reproduction* 7: 437–445.

Duncan, S.L.B. (1997) Embryology of the female genital tract: its genetic defects and congenital abnormalities. In: *Gynaecology*, 2nd edn, edited by Shaw, R.W., Soutter, W.P. and Stanton, S.L. Churchill Livingstone, Edinburgh, pp. 3–21.

England, M.A. (1990) *A Colour Atlas of Life Before Birth*. Wolfe Medical Publications, London.

Hillier, S.G., Kitchener, H.C., Neilson, J.P. (eds) (1996) *Scientific Essentials of Reproductive Medicine*. W.B. Saunders, London.

Langman, J. (1990) *Medical Embryology*, 6th edn. Williams & Wilkins, Baltimore.

4

Reproductive anatomy

THE VULVA

The vulva is the name for the female external genitalia and is depicted in Figure 4.1. It is bordered by the mons veneris anteriorly and the labiocrural folds posterolaterally. The vaginal introitus is usually closed due to apposition of the labia majora but may gape to some degree in parous women. The labia minora are hairless and virtually simple folds of skin, but they contain highly vascular tissue which may become turgid when sexually excited. The labia minora fuse anteriorly to form the prepuce of the clitoris, which is thus usually hidden. The clitoris consists of erectile tissue analogous with the penis and also becomes turgid (to a varying degree) when sexually excited (see Chapter 21). The vestibular bulbs, analogous with the corpus spongiosum in the male, extend backwards from the clitoris deep to the bulbocavernosus muscle (Fig. 4.2).

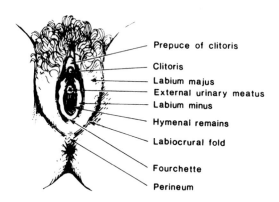

Prepuce of clitoris

Clitoris

Labium majus

External urinary meatus

Labium minus

Hymenal remains

Labiocrural fold

Fourchette

Perineum

Fig. 4.1 The vulva.

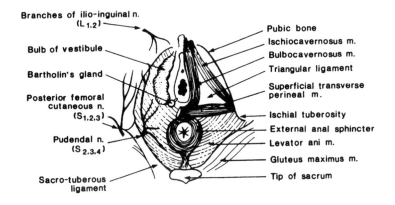

Fig. 4.2   Structures lying deep to the vulva.

The depression between the labia minora, into which open the urethra and vagina, is called the vestibule. The ducts of Bartholin's glands also open on to it posterolaterally (Fig. 4.2). The anterior limit of the vestibule is the clitoral prepuce and the posterior limit is the fourchette (Fig. 4.1). The latter is a skinfold at the posterior aspect of the vaginal introitus. To allow delivery of a baby the fourchette has to stretch greatly, and the perineum has to stretch both laterally and anteroposteriorly, the anus being pushed backwards.

The vulva is supplied by nerves and vessels as follows:

1 Innervation of the vulva is illustrated in Figure 4.2
2 Arterial supply is mainly by the internal pudendal artery (from the internal iliac artery) which accompanies the pudendal nerve from the ischial spine, and anteriorly by the superficial external pudendal artery (from the femoral artery).
3 Venous drainage accompanies the arteries.
4 Lymphatic drainage accompanies the blood vessels and is mainly to the superficial inguinal nodes, thence to the deep inguinal and external iliac nodes; from deeper structures lymphatics accompany the pudendal vessels to the internal iliac nodes. There is free cross-drainage between the two sides, but due to the distinct embryological origin of the vulva the lymphatic field is sharply demarcated peripherally by the labiocrural folds (Fig. 4.1).

THE PELVIC FLOOR

The pelvic floor consists of all tissues from (and including) the pelvic peritoneum to the vulva and perineum, but in terms of support the most important structures are the levator ani muscles and the pelvic fascia.

The muscles

The perineal group of muscles (Fig. 4.2) are minor structures of little importance in the woman. They share common insertion with some fibres of the anal sphincter, and in particular with the levator ani muscles, into a midline raphe called the perineal body (Fig. 4.3a). This is a fibromuscular structure which has to stretch greatly with the perineum to allow delivery of a baby (Fig. 4.3b), and is then frequently torn or deliberately incised (episiotomy; see Chapter 25).

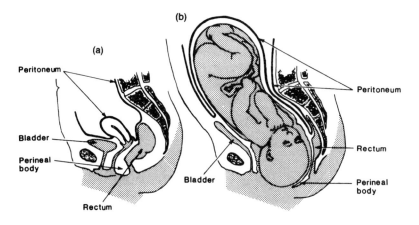

Fig. 4.3 Sagittal view of the genital tract in (a) the non-pregnant state, and (b) pregnancy, as the fetal head is distending the vagina and perineum just before delivery.

The levator ani muscles (Fig. 4.2) form a sling from the lateral pelvic walls, the fibres passing downwards and posteriorly to their insertion in the perineal body, coccyx and sacrum. They form a floor for the pelvis which slopes downwards, medially and forwards, this shape having an important influence on the way the fetal head is channelled in the process of delivery. The levator ani muscles pull the perineal body upwards and forwards, thus acting as a sphincter and support for the vagina, which is consequently normally held in a slight S-shape (Fig. 4.3a); by supporting the vagina they also support and raise the bladder neck and can be used to prevent micturition. The levator ani muscles are voluntary but are reflexly relaxed during micturition and defecation and are reflexly contracted when otherwise straining, such as when coughing. Their innervation is from S2–4 via the pudendal nerve (Fig. 4.2).

Below and lateral to the levator ani muscle on each side, and between it and the lateral pelvic wall, is the ischiorectal fossa filled with fatty connective tissue. Above and medially is the pelvic fascia, with the urethra, vagina and anal canal passing downwards between the muscles in the midline.

The pelvic fascia and ligaments

The pelvic fascia is the connective tissue lying between and above the levator ani muscles and below the pelvic peritoneum. It envelops on each side the vagina and cervix (where it is called the parametrium) and the bladder neck in front. It is condensed radially to form distinct supports for the pelvic organs. The most important are the transverse cervical or cardinal ligaments, but there are also the pubocervical ligaments that pass anteroposteriorly on each side of the bladder neck and the uterosacral ligaments that pass from the uterine isthmus (between the cervix and uterine body) backwards around the sides of the rectum.

The pelvic fascia extends thinly and loosely upwards between the peritoneal folds of the broad ligament running laterally from each side of the uterus. This ligament is wrongly named because it has no supportive function, being merely peritoneum draped over the round ligament, fallopian tubes and ovarian ligaments which pass laterally from the uterine horns (Fig. 4.4). The infundibulopelvic ligaments (Fig. 4.4) are, similarly, non-supportive continuations of the broad ligaments to the pelvic brim posterolaterally, carrying the ovarian blood vessels. Within the pelvic fascia pass all the branches of the internal iliac arteries with the veins and lymphatics to or from the pelvic organs (e.g. the uterine artery; Fig. 4.4).

The ovarian ligaments and round ligaments

These are conveniently described here (Fig. 4.4) but are not part of the pelvic fascia. The two, being continuous via the uterine horn, are analogous with the gubernaculum testis. Thus the round ligaments curve forwards to the internal inguinal ring and thence pass to the labia majora. The ovarian ligaments suspend the ovaries. The round ligaments have little supportive function but tend to keep the uterine body pulled forwards in its usual anteverted attitude.

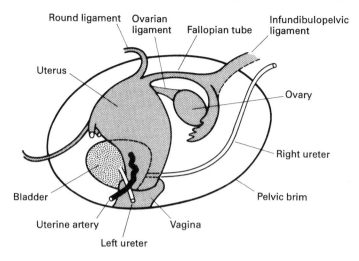

Fig. 4.4   The pelvic organs viewed obliquely through the pelvic brim from above, left and behind.

The ureters

The ureters (Fig. 4.4), after entering the true pelvis beneath the infundibulopelvic ligament on each side, pass vertically down the pelvic side wall to the ischial spine and turn forwards and medially in the pelvic fascia beneath the uterine artery in the base of the broad ligament to reach the bladder. They pass close by the sides of the cervix, just above the lateral vaginal fornices, where they are crossed by the uterine arteries. The ureters are prone to damage when dividing the uterine arteries at hysterectomy, by irradiation of or invasion by cervical carcinoma, by operations on densely adherent inflammatory swellings near the base of the broad ligaments, and when dividing the ovarian vessels in the infundibulopelvic ligaments.

THE PELVIC ORGANS

The vagina

This is an elastic, fibromuscular tube lined by non-keratinized squamous epithelium that is raised in transverse ridges or folds called rugae. The vagina passes upwards and backwards from the introitus at the vulva. It is about 10 cm long, variably distensible, and is normally closed by apposition of its anterior and posterior walls. It is held in a slight S-shape (Fig. 4.3a) by the tone of the levator ani muscles acting through the perineal body, which can be used voluntarily (and involuntarily, sometimes out of fear) to close the vagina forcibly. The cervix protrudes into its upper anterior wall, dividing the vaginal vault into anterior, posterior and lateral fornices.

Its anterior wall is related to the urethra and bladder neck, to which it is connected by dense connective tissue, and to the cervix. Posteriorly it is related to the perineal body and rectum. Its vault is directly adjacent to the deepest part of the uterorectal peritoneal pouch (pouch of Douglas), through which pelvic structures can be palpated (Fig. 4.3a), and to the ureters and uterine blood vessels on each side (Fig. 4.4). Laterally the vagina is separated from the levator ani muscles by pelvic fascia in which run the vaginal branches of the uterine arteries and accompanying venous plexuses.

The squamous epithelium has no special structures, unlike skin, but exudation through it keeps the vagina moist. The degree of exudate depends on the vascularity of the vaginal wall, which is determined by oestrogen. The normal vaginal contents appear creamy, being a mixture of tissue exudate, exfoliated cells and cervical mucus. Full maturation of the epithelium depends on oestrogen, while the addition of progesterone induces minor superficial cytological changes. Under the influence of oestrogen the mature (superficial) cells contain glycogen which is metabolized to lactic acid by lactobacilli, which are normal commensals in the vagina. Thus the vagina is normally acidic (pH 4–5) in women of reproductive age, especially in pregnancy. However, there is a pH gradient due to the alkaline cervical mucus, and during menstruation the vagina is almost neutral.

The uterus

The uterus consists of a body and a cervix. The body is pear-shaped and flattened anteroposteriorly, but the muscular side walls are disproportionately thickened, giving its cavity a flattened triangular or T shape. It connects with the fallopian tube at each horn (cornu) and the domed top of the uterine body, between its horns, is called the fundus. The cervix is a canal about 2.5 cm long, being narrowest at its internal os where it joins the uterine body. This junctional region is called the isthmus, although it is not anatomically distinct. The length of the uterine cavity including the cervix is about 6 cm in nulliparous women and up to 8 cm in parous women. The walls of the uterus are 1–1.5 cm thick and consist almost entirely of smooth muscle, the myometrium. The muscle fibres are arranged into three layers: inner and outer longitudinal fibres inserted into cervical connective tissue, and a much thicker middle circular layer. There are relatively few muscle fibres in the lower part of the cervix, which consists more of fibrous connective tissue. Thus it is the internal os that determines the competence of the cervix as a sphincter in pregnancy.

The endometrium is the mucosal lining of the uterine body and consists of tubular glands set in a highly cellular stroma. Under the influence of oestrogen and progesterone it undergoes distinct cyclical changes as described in Chapter 5, consequently varying in thickness from 1 to 5 mm.

The endocervix is the mucosal lining of the cervix. It is thrown into an arborescent pattern of folds, or crypts, and consists of a columnar surface epithelium and underlying loose cellular stroma, which is also very vascular, giving the endocervical mucosa a bright red colour. Its appearance remains constant through the ovarian cycle, but the amount and properties of its mucus secretion show distinct changes (see Chapter 5).

The ectocervix is the stratified squamous epithelium covering that part of the cervix projecting into the vagina and is continuous with the vaginal epithelium in the fornices. It is smooth and, being relatively thick, looks opaque and dull pink, in contrast to the bright, velvety endocervical mucosa with which it is continuous near the external cervical os. The line of demarcation between ecto- and endocervix is called the squamocolumnar junction. It is in this area that cervical epithelial dysplasia and carcinoma usually start and from which diagnostic cytology smears should therefore be taken. This junction often occurs far outside the external cervical os, and in pregnancy endocervical mucosa may cover much of the vaginal portion of the cervix. This appears to be the result of differential growth of the underlying cervical parenchyma, mediated by oestrogen, the mucosa being carried outwards. The junction may return to the external os (and even within it after the menopause), partly by involution of the underlying tissue but mainly by squamous change (metaplasia) in the mucosa due to physical exposure in the vagina.

The uterus is covered by closely adherent peritoneum (Fig. 4.3a) all over its posterior surface, including the supravaginal portion of the cervix, and over the anterior surface of the body. Anteriorly the peritoneum is reflected off the isthmus on to the bladder and laterally is reflected off the sides of the uterus in a vertical line to form the two layers of the broad ligaments.

The uterus is related anatomically over its peritoneal surface to intestinal loops and omentum. Anteriorly its isthmus is attached to the bladder by loose connective tissue which at caesarean section is easily divided to afford approach to the lower part (lower segment) of the uterus. Laterally (Fig. 4.4) it is related to its appendages (or adnexa) contained within the broad ligaments (fallopian tubes and ovaries, round and ovarian ligaments) and to the parametrium below and the structures passing through that tissue (ureters and uterine blood vessels).

The main uterine supports are the transverse cervical ligaments (see the section on pelvic fascia, above). The round ligaments tend to hold the uterus forwards (in anteversion) but are elastic.

The fallopian tubes (oviducts)

These are two, thin, muscular tubes connecting the uterine cavity via each uterine horn with the peritoneal cavity (Fig. 4.4). Each is about 10 cm long and consists of four parts: the intramural part (2 cm) traversing the uterine wall, the narrow isthmus (3 cm), the wider ampulla (5 cm) and the infundibulum (fimbriated opening). Each tube is contained within the upper border of the broad ligament, but the infundibulum and part of the ampulla are free and tend to curve around the ovary. The lumen of the tube is very narrow in the isthmus and intramural parts; in the ampulla it appears to widen but is filled by intricate folds of the mucosal lining (endosalpinx). The endosalpinx is a delicate columnar epithelium consisting of secretory and ciliated cells that help to support and propel both egg and sperms (see Chapter 5).

The fallopian tubes are related over their peritoneal surface to the ovaries and loops of intestine. At their inferior margin within the broad ligaments they are related to an arcade of anastomosing utero-ovarian blood vessels and to remnants of the mesonephric ducts (e.g. epoophoron) which sometimes develop cysts that can stretch the tubes greatly.

The ovaries

Their structure and function are described in Chapter 5. They are flattened ovoids 3–4 cm long suspended from the back of the broad ligament by a wide mesovarium that carries the ovarian blood vessels, lymphatics and nerves, and from the uterine horn by the narrow ovarian ligament (Fig. 4.4).

Blood supply

The uterine artery is a branch of the internal iliac artery and passes medially in the pelvic fascia, crossing above the ureter to reach the uterine isthmus (Fig. 4.4). Vaginal and cervical branches pass downwards, and the main uterine trunk passes tortuously up the side of the uterus to anastomose with the ovarian artery in the broad ligament.

The ovarian artery is a branch of the aorta on each side and enters the pelvis in the infundibulopelvic ligament (Fig. 4.4) from which it passes into the broad ligament beneath the fallopian tube. It supplies the ovaries and tubes and finally anastomoses with the uterine arteries.

The internal pudendal artery is the terminal branch of the posterior division of the internal iliac artery. Passing out of the pelvis through the greater sciatic foramen it curves around the ischial spine and proceeds forward in the ischiorectal fossa to supply the vulva, which is also supplied anteriorly by the superficial and deep external pudendal arteries, branches of the femoral artery (see the section on the vulva, above).

Correspondingly named veins accompany the arteries but are usually multiple or as plexuses, notably the pampiniform plexus in the broad ligament, which drains into the ovarian and uterine plexuses.

Lymphatic drainage

The main pathways, accompanying the major arteries, are outlined in Figure 4.5. The lower vagina drains, like the vulva (see above), into the inguinal nodes (shown as pathway 1). The cervix drains via lymphatics in the pelvic fascia (parametrium) to the internal iliac nodes (2) and to the external iliac nodes (3), including the obturator node (4). The ovaries drain along the course of the ovarian vessels (5) to the para-aortic nodes and also across the midline via the uterine fundus (6). The uterine body drains (7) as for both the ovaries and cervix and also via the round ligaments to the superficial inguinal nodes. Early metastasis of endometrial and ovarian carcinoma to relatively distant lymph nodes is one reason why lymphatic block excision or radiotherapy is usually unsuitable treatment for these conditions, unlike cervical carcinoma (see Chapter 24).

Innervation

The nerve supply of the vulva has been described above (see Fig. 4.2).

The uterine body and cervix are fairly insensitive except to distension, which causes not only severe pain but can also cause reflex vasovagal shock that is occasionally fatal. The nerve supply is entirely autonomic, both sympathetic (via the presacral plexus) and

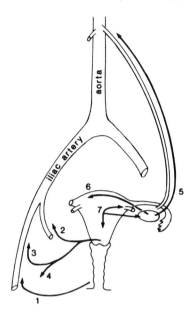

Fig. 4.5   The main lymphatic pathways draining the genital tract, numbered as described in the text.

parasympathetic (via the pelvic plexus), the cervix being innervated more than the uterine body. There are both sensory and motor nerves. Pain from the uterine body is referred to the lower abdomen and from the cervix to the sacral area. The myometrial response to catecholamines depends on the presence of both α-receptors (excitatory, mainly stimulated by noradrenaline) and β-receptors (inhibitory, by adrenalin). The balance of effect depends on hormones: oestrogens enhance α-adrenergic effect, and progesterone β-adrenergic. Some β-mimetic drugs can be used to inhibit labour when it occurs prematurely.

The ovaries and fallopian tubes are supplied by sympathetic and parasympathetic nerves accompanying the ovarian blood vessels from the preaortic plexus. The ovaries are sensitive only to compression, as on bimanual palpation, but the tubes are sensitive to all the usual stimuli.

The urinary bladder and urethra

These structures are important in gynaecology because urinary disorders including incontinence are commonly associated with genital disease, and they can be damaged at operations on the genital organs.

The bladder is a hollow muscular organ lined by transitional epithelium with an inverted pyramidal shape when empty. When full it is domed and has a capacity of at least 500 ml. The ureters enter the trigone of the bladder obliquely, thus affording valve-like protection against reflux of urine while being able to fill the bladder by peristaltic action.

The urethra is a muscular tube 3–4 cm long lined by transitional epithelium, except in its lower part where the epithelium is squamous and, like the vulva, is affected by oestrogen. The para-urethral glands open on to the posterior wall of the urethra and are commonly the site of chronic infection.

The muscle coat of the bladder is formed by a single meshwork layer of interlacing smooth-muscle bundles, called the detrusor muscle, now thought to have no continuity with urethral smooth muscle. The muscle coat of the urethra has an inner longitudinal layer of smooth muscle, and an outer layer of striated muscle thickest at the midpoint of the urethra and called the external urethral sphincter. There is no internal sphincter to the female urethra. Urethral resistance is aided by the levator ani muscles (specifically the pubococcygeus muscles) acting by pulling forwards and upwards on the posterior vaginal wall. The bladder muscle receives autonomic innervation from the pelvic plexus (S2–4) and hypogastric plexus (T10–L2). The urethral muscle layers both receive only parasympathetic nerve supply. The levator ani muscles are supplied by the pudendal nerve (S2–4).

Urinary continence is maintained as long as urethral pressure remains greater than vesical pressure. Urethral pressure is aided by the urethral muscle (both layers), the levator ani muscles, elastic tissue around the bladder neck, and by the intra-abdominal position of the proximal urethra. Raising intra-abdominal pressure, for example by straining or coughing, is transmitted equally to the proximal urethra and bladder. Further protection is afforded by reflex contraction of voluntary muscles: the levator ani muscles, which, acting through the perineal body, compress the urethra and bladder neck and accentuate the posterior urethrovesical angle (Fig. 4.3a); and the external urethral sphincter. Vesicle pressure is directly raised by elastic tension due to filling, and by activity of the detrusor muscle.

Micturition is mainly controlled by a parasympathetic nervous reflex via S3,4 which after infancy becomes conditioned at cerebrocortical level. Thus afferent impulses generated by bladder distension and weight on the trigone are normally inhibited unconsciously and, in response to rising stimulation, consciously.

The reflex can also be inhibited by painful stimuli, thus explaining the urinary retention which occurs so commonly after vaginal surgery or after perineal laceration at childbirth.

The mechanism of micturition involves in this order:

1 Reduction of cortical inhibition.
2 Voluntary relaxation of the pelvic floor, leading to lowering and funnelling of the bladder neck associated with straightening of the posterior urethrovesical angle.
3 Reflex contraction of the bladder detrusor.
4 Voluntary contraction of the pelvic floor and external urethral sphincter to squeeze the urethra dry again.
5 Reapplication of cortical inhibition.

Urinary incontinence is thus commonly caused by:

1 Loss of posterior urethrovesical support, often associated with vaginal prolapse.
2 Loss of urethral resistance, associated with ageing.
3 Detrusor irritability due to infection or psychological factors (see Chapter 22).

The rectum and anus

These structures are only important because their proximity to the genital tract exposes them to the risk of associated damage (see Fig. 4.3). The anal sphincter and canal can be lacerated during childbirth; the rectum can be damaged when repairing prolapse of the posterior vaginal wall and by radiotherapy for uterine cancer; and pelvic suppuration tracks down to the pouch of Douglas resulting in adhesions between the uterus and upper rectum which can endanger the upper rectum at hysterectomy.

ORIENTATION OF THE PELVIC ORGANS

The key to the orientation of the pelvic organs within the pelvis is the position of the cervix, which is situated in the very centre of the bony cavity of the true pelvis (see Fig. 4.3a), firmly suspended by the strong transverse cervical ligaments. The uterus can pivot about this point; it is usually angled forwards at 90° to the vagina (anteverted) as shown in Fig. 4.3a, but filling of the bladder rotates it backwards, while in some normal women the uterus may be usually thus retro-verted. The body of the uterus may also be angled (flexed) on the cervix; thus it is usually anteflexed (Fig. 4.3a) as well as anteverted, and when retroverted is occasionally also retroflexed (being then palpable in the pouch of Douglas and often painful on sexual intercourse). The position of the ovaries and Fallopian tubes depends of course on that of the uterus.

In pregnancy the uterine body rises into the abdomen, but the cervix remains supported in the centre of the pelvic cavity and the fetal head cannot descend until the cervix is dilated. When the head remains at a higher level, however, it cannot be due to the cervix but may be due to obstruction at the pelvic brim.

The key to the orientation of the pelvic organs with respect to the rest of the body is the angle of inclination of the pelvic brim. This is 55–60° from the horizontal in a standing woman as shown in Figure 4.3 (but steeper in black women). Thus the uterus is normally situated above the symphysis pubis; it is not palpable in the lower abdomen because it is far back. In early pregnancy the uterus grows forwards in the axis of the pelvic brim to come within reach at 10–12

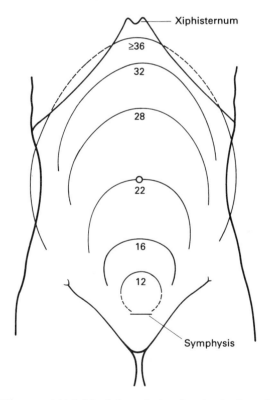

Fig. 4.6 The usual height of the uterine fundus in the abdomen at different stages (weeks) of gestation.

weeks' gestation. At this stage the uterus lies horizontally upon the empty bladder, but can be displaced upwards to misleadingly high levels when the bladder is full. The bladder should therefore be emptied before any attempt to assess uterine size. After 14 weeks' gestation the uterus grows vertically in the abdomen (Fig. 4.6). In late pregnancy the fetal head passes backwards to enter the pelvis in the axis of the pelvic brim (see later, Fig. 4.10). It does not move vertically downwards (i.e. towards the mother's feet) until it is just about to be delivered (as in Fig. 4.3b).

OBSTETRICAL ANATOMY

The uterus

In pregnancy the uterine body is distended by the gestation sac to a globular shape until 14 weeks' gestation, becoming elongated thereafter. With the cervix supported at its fixed level (see the section on orientation above), the fundus of the growing uterus moves forwards until it reaches the anterior abdominal wall where it can first be palpated at 10–12 weeks. After 12–14 weeks it moves vertically upwards within the abdomen, as shown in Figure 4.6. At 16 weeks the fundus has reached halfway from the symphysis pubis to umbilicus, at 22 weeks to the umbilicus and at 28 weeks halfway to the xiphisternum. After 32 weeks it expands mainly outwards. Thus assessment of gestational age by palpation of the uterus is best done by bimanual pelvic examination up to 14 weeks, by the fundal height until about 32 weeks and thereafter by the feel of the size of the fetus itself; after 36 weeks it is not possible to distinguish further.

The enlargement of the uterus stretches the round ligaments and ovarian attachments vertically, carrying the ovaries into the flanks. Because of disproportionate distension of the uterine fundus the round ligaments only reach halfway up the uterus at the end of pregnancy (term).

During pregnancy the uterus enlarges 20-fold in mass and its length reaches 30 cm at term. The myometrium grows mainly by hypertrophy of the individual fibres, which increase 10-fold in length; the total mass increases from about 50 to 1000 g but the thickness of the myometrium does not increase. The endometrium undergoes marked secretory change, becoming spongy (Chapter 5), and is called the decidua. The uterine isthmus expands with the uterine body to accommodate the pregnancy sac but remains below the sac and has to be dilated with the cervix in labour. The isthmus and cervix together constitute the lower segment of the uterus. The cervix becomes very vascular (hence its typical blue appearance) and oedematous. In the intercellular ground substance there is a vast increase in suspended water (i.e. as microdroplets) which loosens the collagen fibres and permits them to slide, enabling the remarkable dilatation that the cervix undergoes in labour. All the pelvic organs undergo marked increase in vascularity and the venous plexuses become greatly distended.

The bony pelvis

It is only the true pelvis (i.e. the part below the pelvic brim, or inlet) that is obstetrically important, being the rigid part of the birth canal. As shown later in Figure 4.10, from the inlet (A) to the outlet (C) its axis curves through about 50°. Also, its cross-sectional shape changes; Figure 4.7 shows that the normal (gynaecoid) brim is slightly wider in its transverse diameter than its anteroposterior diameter (the obstetric conjugate), whereas the outlet is wider in the anteroposterior diameter than the transverse. Note that the coccyx, whatever its angle, does not restrict the outlet because it is flexible. The mid-pelvis (level B, Fig. 4.10) is round in cross-section. The outlet may be restricted by the ischial spines in some cases. Normally, however, although the interspinous diameter is narrower than the others the spines are behind the centre of the outlet; although they appear prominent from above (Fig. 4.7a), viewed from below they are hidden by the sacrotuberous ligaments (Fig. 4.7b).

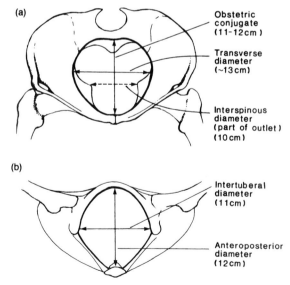

Fig. 4.7 Views demonstrating the main pelvic diameters. (a) Pelvic brim viewed perpendicularly to its axis from above; (b) pelvic outlet viewed from below.

The cross-sectional shape of the pelvis largely determines the position of the fetal head at each level (see Chapter 8 on mechanism of delivery). The inlet is the most restricting part of the pelvis because the outlet can be expanded in all directions by movement at the sacroiliac joints and symphysis pubis. Thus if the fetal head will pass through (or engage in) the pelvic brim, it will certainly pass through the outlet of a normally shaped pelvis. The lower normal limit of the obstetric conjugate is 10 cm. In general, if the sacral promontory cannot be reached on vaginal examination the obstetric conjugate must be greater than 10 cm. The actual diameter being measured digitally is from the lower border of the symphysis pubis to the sacral promontory and is known as the diagonal conjugate.

Abnormalities of pelvic shape are an uncommon problem now in this country thanks to relatively good nutrition. In any case there is no place now for the difficult labour and delivery that would have to be conducted to overcome the gross abnormalities commonly associated with rickets which were seen in the past. The most common abnormality now experienced is straightness, or even convexity, of the anterior surface of the sacrum in its upper part instead of its normal marked concavity. In such a pelvis the shortest anteroposterior diameter of the pelvic inlet (the obstetric conjugate) may lie below the pelvic brim. Previous fracture is an occasional cause of pelvic distortion.

The fetus

The widest part of the fetus is across the shoulders, but these can be angled through the mother's pelvis and rarely cause obstruction. Thus the biggest part in effect is the fetal head. It is fortunate that it usually presents first.

The fetal head is not quite spherical, and since some of its diameters in the sagittal plane (Fig. 4.8b) are greater than its maximal transverse diameter, the degree of flexion or extension of the head at the neck determines the ease (or difficulty) with which the head can negotiate the mother's pelvis. The important anatomical features are shown in Figure 4.8, which portrays the head almost fully flexed, the chin nearly on the chest; if the head as in Figure 4.8b is turned upside down and then viewed from below, as it would appear from the vagina, it would be seen as in Figure 4.8a. When the head presents with different degrees of flexion or extension the features to be found on vaginal examination are shown in Figure 4.9.

The particular sagittal diameter (Fig. 4.8b) that must negotiate the pelvis associated with each type of presentation (Fig. 4.9) is:

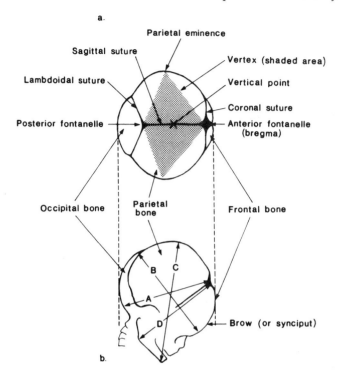

Fig. 4.8 Anatomical features of the fetal head looking (a) on to the vertex and (b) from the side. The particular diameters A, B, C, D, are described in the text.

Figure 4.9	*Figure 4.8b*	
Fully flexed vertex	A Suboccipitobregmatic	9.5 cm
Poorly flexed vertex	B Occipitofrontal	11.5 cm
Brow	C Mentovertical	13.5 cm
Face	D Submentobregmatic	9.5 cm

Thus the most favourable presentations of the head to negotiate the pelvis are when fully flexed or fully extended. The presenting shape is then almost exactly round, since the maximal transverse diameter (between the parietal eminences–biparietal diameter) also measures about 9.5 cm at term.

The brow at term presents such a large diameter that it is undeliverable vaginally. It is therefore very important to recognize a brow presentation as soon as possible. Unfortunately the diagnosis is difficult on abdominal palpation and is also commonly missed in

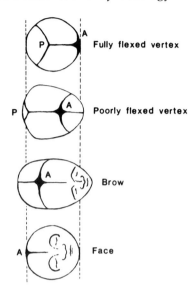

Fig. 4.9   The features of the fetal head presenting vaginally with different attitudes of the head. The fontanelles are marked A (anterior) and P (posterior).

labour until it is advanced. This is because at early dilatation of the cervix it may not be possible to identify more than the anterior fontanelle (recognized by its four radiating sutures), which is mistakenly assumed to indicate a poorly flexed vertex (compare with the brow in Figure 4.9). Never diagnose a vertex presentation until the posterior fontanelle (which is triradiate) has been identified on vaginal examination. The correct designation until then is cephalic, which keeps the mind alert to the uncertainty.

Cephalopelvic relationships

Position

When the fetal head presents as usual by the vertex, its relationship to the maternal pelvis is defined by the orientation of the sagittal suture and the occiput, which can be palpated vaginally. The head, as indicated by the sagittal suture, may occupy the transverse, the anteroposterior or an oblique diameter of the pelvis.

The exact position of the fetal head is defined by the orientation of the occiput, which is recognized on vaginal examination by the posterior fontanelle (see Figs. 4.8 and 4.9). Thus in each of the pelvic diameters just described the head may be in the left or right occipitolateral position; occipitoanterior or occipitoposterior; left occipitoanterior or right occipitoposterior; or right occipitoanterior or left occipitoposterior, respectively. The commonest position in which the head enters the pelvis is occipitolateral (curiously, more commonly with the occiput on the left rather than the right); the commonest position at delivery is occipitoanterior.

When the face presents, the positions are described in a similar manner but oriented to the chin; thus mentoanterior, etc. The positions of a brow presentation are not described in any particular way.

Level

Since the brim is usually the narrowest part of the pelvis the ability of the fetal head to negotiate it is of prime importance. When the greatest diameter of the head has passed through the brim it is said to be engaged. Since in general the head can be assumed to be

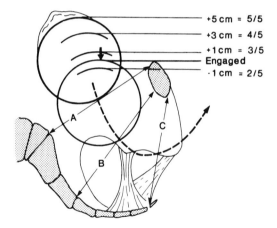

Fig. 4.10 Combined sagittal and internal views of the pelvis with the mother lying on her back. The anteroposterior diameters are shown of the pelvic inlet (A, obstetric conjugate), mid-cavity (B) and outlet (C) and the axis of the pelvis throughout (dotted line). The fetal head is shown as a sphere in the sagittal plane of the mother, the face being usually to one side. The relation of the level of the head to the pelvic brim (expressed as fifths of the head remaining above the brim) can be accurately derived in practice by relating the geometrically uppermost point of the head (arrowed here when at the level of being just engaged) to the horizontal plane of the anterior (palpable) point of the symphysis pubis (see text).

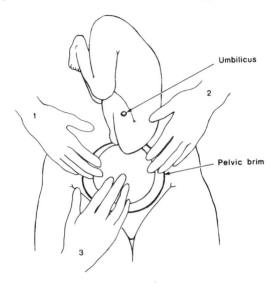

Umbilicus

Pelvic brim

Fig. 4.11 The surface markings on the maternal abdomen of the pelvic brim and fetus, in particular the fetal head, and the points to seek on palpation as described in the text. The index finger of the right hand shown in position 3 is seeking the point of the head arrowed in Figure 4.10. The overhanging fetal shoulder often gets in the way more than is shown and has to be pushed up out of the way, from below.

symmetrical it is engaged when at least halfway through the brim. On abdominal palpation, the level of the head is best described in terms of the proportion (conventionally in fifths) remaining above the pelvic brim (Fig. 4.10). Thus when the head is just engaged there is only between two-fifths and three-fifths above the brim, but five-fifths when wholly above.

The proportion of the fetal head which can be *felt* in the abdomen is not the same – a common mistake – as the proportion remaining above the pelvic brim, which can be accurately estimated as follows.

When examining the abdomen with the patient lying on her back (as in Fig. 4.10), the uppermost point of the head (arrowed in the figure) is in the same horizontal plane as the anterior border of the symphysis pubis when the head is engaged, assuming the usual angle of inclination of the pelvic brim. When the head is five-fifths above the pelvic brim the upper point of the head is 5 cm above this horizontal, the head at term being about 10 cm in diameter. This (arrowed) point is thus an accurate guide to the level of the head in relation to the pelvic brim. It is of course situated over the centre of the pelvic brim and can be palpated by backward pressure with the right hand halfway between symphysis pubis and umbilicus, as shown by position 3 in Figure 4.11. Inaccuracy in assessing the level of the head in relation to the pelvic brim occurs with the occipitoposterior position, in which the face projects forwards in the midline, and in black women, in whom the steep inclination of the brim projects the whole head forwards.

In practice, before assessing the level of the head it is necessary first to confirm the presentation, and this is done more easily with the two hands in positions 1 and 2 as shown in Figure 4.11. A rough idea of the depth of the head in the pelvis can also be obtained in this way.

The level of the head can be related clinically to the ischial spines on vaginal examination. The ischial spines being on either side, it is necessary to imagine a line joining them to which the lowermost part of the head can be related. As Figure 4.10 shows, the head is about 2 cm above the spines when just engaged in the brim. This assumes, however, that there is no moulding of the head; when this occurs, as in prolonged labour associated with cephalopelvic disproportion (when the head is too large for the pelvis), the head may be elongated to well below the spines yet remain unengaged. Thus the level of the head must never be assessed vaginally without assessing it abdominally also.

FURTHER READING

Dilly, N. (1989) Female pelvic anatomy. In: *Obstetrics*, edited by Turnbull, A. and Chamberlain, G. Churchill Livingstone, Edinburgh, pp. 9–24.

Vellacott, I. (1997) Pelvic anatomy. In: *Gynaecology*, 2nd edn, edited by Shaw, R.W., Soutter, W.P. and Stanton, S.L. Churchill Livingstone, Edinburgh, pp. 23–39.

5

Reproductive physiology

GAMETOGENESIS

Gametogenesis is the process of formation, development and maturation of the male and female gametes, the spermatozoa and ova, called respectively spermatogenesis and oogenesis.

It was described in Chapter 3 how primordial germ cells originating in the yolk sac entoderm multiply by mitosis and migrate to the urogenital ridge. They remain indifferent gametes until determined by specific gonadal development in response to the presence or absence of a Y chromosome in the somatic cells of the gonad. The gametes are now called spermatogonia and oogonia. They are committed to eventually becoming either spermatozoa or ova, and gonadal and gametal sex cannot be altered, as occurs in some species in response to environmental changes like temperature.

Oogenesis

Oogonia, like the primordial germ cells, continue to multiply enormously by mitosis and remain diploid (46,XX). Mitosis occurs mainly during the first half of fetal life and ceases before birth.

Primary oocytes become distinguished during fetal life by the onset of meiosis, but the process is arrested in prophase at the diplotene stage, the so-called resting dictyate stage. They remain at this stage throughout life until the time of ovulation. Otherwise they undergo atresia and the vast majority of primary oocytes are lost by degeneration in this way. A peak of over 5 million is reached by mid fetal life (mid-pregnancy) but the number falls sharply due to atresia to about 1–2 million at birth and 0.5 million at the onset of puberty. Only about 400 ever reach maturity and ovulation. Meanwhile the oocytes are susceptible to damaging agents, which have a permanent effect, and to age-related defects of chromosomal arrangement (such as lead to trisomy 21, which causes Down's syndrome).

The luteinizing hormone (LH) surge initiates resumption of meiosis of the oocyte, in a fully mature antral (Graafian) follicle, mediated by expansion of the surrounding cumulus of LH-receptive granulosa cells, and consequent disruption of their cytoplasmic connections through the zona pellucida which are thought to carry the maturation inhibitory factor to the oocyte. Prophase diakinesis is distinguishable by appearance of the germinal vesicle. This is followed by the **first meiotic division** resulting in unequal cell division into the **secondary oocyte** and **first polar body**. Both are still diploid, and the polar body remains within the zona pellucida.

The secondary oocyte is then arrested in the second meiotic division at metaphase (metaphase II) until after ovulation when penetrated by a spermatozoon. That is marked by evident lysozyme breakdown within the cytoplasm-releasing proteases, and the cortical granule reaction which releases signals somehow involved in blocking polyspermy. There are at least two blocks: the zona pellucida becomes impermeable and the oocyte (vitelline) membrane becomes unreceptive.

Sperm penetration of the oocyte induces resumption of the **second meiotic division**, which includes chromosomal reduction to the haploid **ovum** and **second polar body**. This final stage of oocyte maturation is immediately followed by appearance of the two pronuclei of the oocyte and sperm, and syngamy (of the pronuclei) to form the one-cell diploid zygote of the next generation within 24 hours of ovulation.

Folliculogenesis

Oocytes need protection by a surrounding layer of granulosa cells, which are derived from the primitive sex cord cells, which are in turn isolated from the mesenchyme (ovarian stroma and theca cells) by a basement membrane. Initially the granulosa cells form a barely complete single-cell layer, and the complex is called a **primordial follicle**. Groups of primordial follicles, at successive times, proceed to grow. The oocyte enlarges (the growing stage) from about 0.05 to 0.1 mm diameter – the single largest cell in the body – and the granulosa cell layer multiplies (Fig. 5.1). As the granulosa cells continue to multiply, a fluid-filled vesicle (antrum) forms in the granulosa cell layers (the early antral stage), prior to recruitment for final maturation, as described later.

Spermatogenesis

Spermatogonia, like the primordial germ cells, continue to multiply by mitosis and remain diploid (46,XY). Unlike oogonia, however,

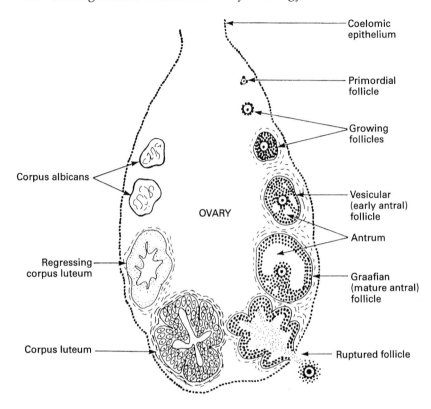

Fig. 5.1   The stages of ovarian follicular maturation and regression.

mitosis of spermatogonia virtually ceases in early fetal life, occurring mainly after puberty and then throughout life. Also by contrast with the ovary, development of the testicular cords ceases and cannulation to form the seminiferous tubules does not occur till puberty.

In adult life mitotic division of spermatogonia proceeds at a constant rate to meiotic division of spermatocytes (see below). However, some divided spermatogonia are retained as stem cells for further mitotic multiplication, which recommences at regular intervals.

Primary spermatocytes become distinguished by the onset of meiosis, which proceeds without interruption (unlike in oocytes) to **secondary spermatocytes**, which are haploid and also called spermatids.

Sperm maturation from the spermatid stage involves differentiation from a round cell with a large nucleus to condensation and flattening of the nucleus, development of the acrosome cap, flagellum and mitochondrial sheath of the mid-piece, and shedding of most of the cytoplasm, leaving only a cytoplasmic droplet attached to the origin of the flagellum.

This is the stage of the **spermatozoon**. It is released from its supporting Sertoli cell to which it was attached by its head. It is free to pass slowly from the seminiferous tubules via the efferent ductules into the epididymis, where final maturation occurs. This includes acquiring motility and fertilizing ability, and losing the cytoplasmic droplet.

The **duration of spermatogenesis** from spermatogonium, via nonfertile spermatozoon entering the epididymis to fully fertile state, lasts about 2½ months. The process occurs in regular waves starting every 16 days, though in different phases throughout the testis, ensuring constant availability of fertile sperm. The fertile sperm are stored for only a few days, in the tail of the epididymis and vas deferens. It is from those sites that they are ejaculated. The duration of storage of fertile sperm depends on frequency of ejaculation.

FOLLICULAR GROWTH IN THE ADULT

This is depicted in Figure 5.1 **Primordial follicles** grow initially by enlargement of the oocyte and the granulosa cells multiply to form a continuous layer of cuboidal cells around the oocyte, eventually a few layers thick, with a distinct basement membrane. The surrounding layer of stromal cells becomes vascularized to form the theca interna, but no blood vessels penetrate the granulosa membrane. Fluid collects in vesicular spaces (or antra) in the proliferating granulosa cell layers, and the growing antra eventually coalesce into one. Further enlargement of the **antral follicle** is associated in the final stage with isolation of the oocyte in a mound (cumulus) of granulosa cells, which becomes stalk-like. The oocyte becomes surrounded by a distinct layer of columnar granulosa cells (the corona radiata). The follicle, now called a **Graafian follicle**, forms a swelling on the surface of the ovary, ready for rupture. It takes 3 months for the follicle to grow and mature to ovulation: 2 months to reach an antral stage measuring 1 mm in diameter, 2 weeks to reach 5 mm, and another 2 weeks to reach 20–25 mm before ovulation. Thus follicular growth starts long before the final menstrual cycle.

Follicular rupture occurs by enzymatic erosion, not as a pressurized explosion. The oocyte, still surrounded by its corona radiata and mass of cumulus (granulosa) cells, is thus gently released and is immediately engulfed by tubal fimbria and transported rapidly by ciliary action into the fallopian tube. The collapsed follicle is quickly converted into the **corpus luteum** by enlargement and functional alteration (luteinization) of the granulosa cells, the layers of which are now for the first time penetrated by blood vessels from the theca interna.

The swollen granulosa cells now contain yellow pigment, which is why they are called lutein cells, but the term luteinizing is used to mean the functional change induced in the granulosa cells by the LH surge to secrete progesterone. The ability of the corpus luteum to secrete progesterone is limited by the number and maturity of the granulosa cells at the time of the LH surge because there is no further proliferation of granulosa cells, only the hypertrophy that typifies luteinization (Fig. 5.1). Thus progesterone levels in the blood secreted by the fully developed corpus luteum in the mid luteal phase are an accurate index of follicular maturation that occurred in the preovulatory phase, and mid luteal progesterone measurement is used in clinical practice as the simplest means of assessing ovulation, strictly follicular maturity.

The corpus luteum reaches its full development after about 4 days. If the oocyte is not fertilized the corpus luteum begins to wane after 8–10 days and ceases function after 12–14 days, and then slowly degenerates (so slowly that the remains of two or three such corpora lutea may be present in either ovary), ultimately becoming a fibrous structure, the corpus albicans. If fertilization and implantation occur the embryonic trophoblast secretes a gonadotrophin (human chorionic gonadotrophin, hCG) which maintains the corpus luteum.

The control of follicular growth and ovulation

Most follicles undergo atresia, at the primordial stage. There is, however, a steady progression of a small number of primordial follicles to the growing stage, and then to the early antral stage, the number at each stage being constant although declining with age, being in proportion to the number of primordial follicles still present. The mechanism controlling this steady recruitment of resting follicles to develop is not known, but basal amounts of gonadotrophin are required to stimulate the initial growth of the oocyte, which in turn probably stimulates the development of the surrounding granulosa membrane. Development to the early antral stage is probably also dependent on small amounts of gonadotrophins but the controlling mechanism is not known. Further maturation of antral follicles depends on the direct influence on granulosa cells of the cyclically increased secretion of follicle-stimulating hormone (FSH) that occurs after puberty. FSH in sufficient amount induces granulosa cell proliferation and induction of aromatizing enzymes, which enable oestrogen production by the granulosa cells. As Figure 5.3 (see page 61) shows, the ability of granulosa cells to produce oestrogen also depends on the supply of androgen precursors from the theca cells under the influence of LH, which is required in only small amounts.

Oestrogen production by the granulosa cells *was* considered important to enhance their maturation further, but this is now known not to be so in women, unlike in some other species. In women oestrogen is only important as a signal to prepare the genital tract to be receptive to coitus, sperm and implantation (Fig. 5.3).

The steady progression of primordial follicles to the growing stage, and then to the early antral stage, numbers about 20 at a time on average, although the number declines with age. Thus there are always about 20 antral follicles ready to respond to the rise in FSH that occurs at the end of the preceding menstrual cycle. Usually only one reaches full maturity, however, the others undergoing atresia. The control of this selectivity is probably explained by two mechanisms. Negative feedback by both oestrogen and inhibin (see later) from the developing follicles reduces circulating FSH levels, depriving the follicles of their potential stimulus, whilst the dominant follicle, which by chance and fitness has advanced more quickly than the rest, protects its FSH requirement by capturing the blood supply within the ovary and increasing it overall to that ovary. The blood supply is diverted and enhanced by the high local concentration of oestrogen. Thus, in what probably starts as an equal race (to develop), a small accidental advantage, which must inevitably occur, would rapidly become overwhelming. Whatever the mechanism, there is no doubt that the follicle itself plays an essential part in the control of its own development, ensuring its singular dominance and final signalling to the pituitary when fully receptive to the LH surge (see later). The LH surge induces the final maturation and rupture of the follicle, and the final maturation of the oocyte that is essential for fertilization to occur. It is clear that, although gonadotrophins stimulate the follicles in various ways, the follicles themselves control the whole process by negative and positive feedback on gonadotrophin release.

The number of antral follicles (usually one) that proceed to maturity and ovulation in any cycle depends on the magnitude and duration of the FSH stimulus. This is normally precisely balanced, but superovulation can be induced by excessive doses of exogenous FSH or stimulation of endogenous FSH secretion.

Although the atresia of all but one antral follicle in each cycle might be explained as suggested above, the mechanism whereby no antral follicle survives in the other ovary is less clear. It is likely to be due to reduction in FSH levels at a critical time due to the advancement of the dominant follicle and its increasing negative hormonal signals to the pituitary. It is also difficult to explain why atresia of very large numbers of primordial follicles occurs, although it is known to be influenced by gonadotrophins, which in rats accelerate the process, whereas oestrogen slows it. Why the corpus luteum, in the absence of conception, has such a remarkably constant life (13 days ± 1 (s.d.)) remains unknown, although it is clearly a controlled programmed event (apoptosis).

INSEMINATION, FERTILIZATION AND IMPLANTATION

The oocyte is carried along the ampullary part of the fallopian tube primarily by ciliary action. It has a life of about 24 hours but starts to deteriorate sooner, so there should ideally be spermatozoa already available in the ampulla for fertilization.

Insemination and sperm transport

Spermatozoa ejaculated near the cervix at coitus reach the tubal ampulla within 30 minutes. Although they swim through cervical mucus (at about 3 mm/min), the rapid transport to the tube is probably mainly due to uterine contractions induced by oxytocin and seminal prostaglandins (female orgasm is not essential). Of the many millions of sperm ejaculated, only about 0.1% penetrate the cervical mucus and only a few thousand reach the tubal ampulla. However, a steady stream is maintained, presumably by continuing uterine contractions, from a reservoir of sperm contained in cervical mucus and possibly in the tubal isthmus near the junction to the uterus. From the uterotubal junction the sperm are transported distally by countercurrents (eddies) in the tubal fluid caused by the cilia, which all beat towards the uterus and bear the oocyte in that direction. Sperm thus reach the oocyte, not by chemical attraction but by chance. They require a few hours in the female tract to be capacitated and then deteriorate after 24 hours. They may survive however in an uncapacitated state, in cervical mucus and perhaps attached to the tubal mucosa, for some days.

Allowing for the normal life of oocyte and sperm it is obviously best that insemination occurs at intervals no longer than 2 days to achieve fertilization if the exact time of ovulation is not known. Extremely (almost impossibly!) frequent ejaculation can deplete mature sperm critically, while abstinence for 10 days or more reduces sperm vitality. To achieve pregnancy, coitus every 1–2 days seems to be the optimum.

Cervical mucus serves an important function in receiving, selecting and storing sperm during the few days just before and at ovulation. Only normal sperm can penetrate mucus properly, thus selecting themselves. The receptiveness of preovulatory mucus is induced by the high levels of oestrogen at that time. The oestrogen stimulates greatly increased secretion of mucus, which also becomes thinner and its mucoprotein strands can slide, thus increasing its ductility (spinnbarkeit). It also contains salts which on drying can be seen to crystallize in typical fern-like pattern. It is important to note the presence of these features in clinical practice before drawing any conclusion when sperm in mucus examined microscopically are found to be absent or immobile. When there is little oestrogen present the mucus is scanty, viscid and cellular, and becomes so again soon after ovulation due to the antioestrogen effect of progesterone. It is then virtually impenetrable.

Despite its apparent semifluidity, mucus is a tissue, not a simple fluid. Electron microscopy shows that the mucoprotein strands form a mesh which is too dense for sperm passage except under the influence of preovulatory oestrogen levels. Then the mesh opens up, though the apertures are still barely wide enough to allow sperm through. Good progressive motility is required by the sperm to penetrate mucus. Sperm that appear to move normally in seminal fluid may nevertheless lack adequate penetrating ability, or may be immobilized in the mucus mesh by attachment of antibodies present in seminal plasma.

The high oestrogen levels that induce the changes in cervical mucus described above also stimulate increased libido in many women. However, the absent or muted cyclicity of libido in women compared with other mammals is largely due to the overriding effect of psychological factors in human sexuality. Nor are there any marked cyclical changes in the vagina or vulva that might particularly facilitate or stimulate coitus at the time of ovulation. The squamous epithelium is fully developed throughout the reproductive life of women, under the stimulus of oestrogen, and it is only the superficial cells that show cyclical change, microscopically.

Fertilization

As soon as a spermatozoon penetrates the oocyte, fertilization by any other sperm is immediately inhibited. Though the mechanisms are not fully understood it is clear that blocks to penetration occur both at the zona pellucida and vitelline membrane of the egg cell. Sperm penetration of the oocyte induces completion of the final meiotic division of the oocyte to the haploid stage (ovum) and the second polar body is extruded. That is followed immediately by appearance of the pronuclei of the ovum and spermatozoon (within 20 hours of meeting), and syngamy (of the pronuclei) to form the one-cell zygote. Cleavage marks the completion of fertilization and begins after 24 hours, reaching about four cells after 2 days.

Apart from the time-course of events to be observed during *in vitro* fertilization (IVF) treatment for infertility, there are few notable features of critical predictive value for fertilization. The oocyte must be fully mature, characterized by extrusion of the first polar body and full expansion (loosening) of the cumulus/granulosa cells. The spermatozoa must be capacitated, characterized by a change to 'whiplash' motility, and be capable of the acrosome reaction – breakdown of the acrosome membrane to release proteolytic enzymes to assist penetration of the zona pellucida. When IVF is attempted the sperm must be capacitated by incubation for a few hours in an appropriate medium. Development of the resulting zygote beyond the blastocyst stage requires implantation into the endometrium, which remains the main stage of failure at present.

The embryo and implantation

The fertilized, diploid egg is called a zygote or usually, when cell division commences, an embryo. The embryo is transported along the fallopian tube mainly by ciliary action, which is hormone-dependent, to the uterine cavity, which it reaches after about 3 days at the morula (still solid) stage. It implants after about 8 days at the blastocyst stage (Fig. 5.2).

The outer cell layer (trophoblast) of the blastocyst invades the endometrium (decidua) and grows rapidly as a syncytium engulfing endometrial glands and blood vessels. The blood vessels communicate with spaces (lacunae) which form in the syncytium and which become the future intervillous (maternal blood) spaces of the placenta.

Decidual reaction in the endometrium adjacent to the trophoblast is essential if the blastocyst is to be successfully implanted, and is induced by molecular signals as yet undefined from the blastocyst. The factors that make the endometrium receptive to the blastocyst are not fully known. They clearly include, however, priming of the endometrium with oestrogen to induce proliferation, followed for a few days by a predominance of progesterone to stop the proliferation and induce secretory changes. Progestogen contained in contraceptive preparations used from the start of the cycle

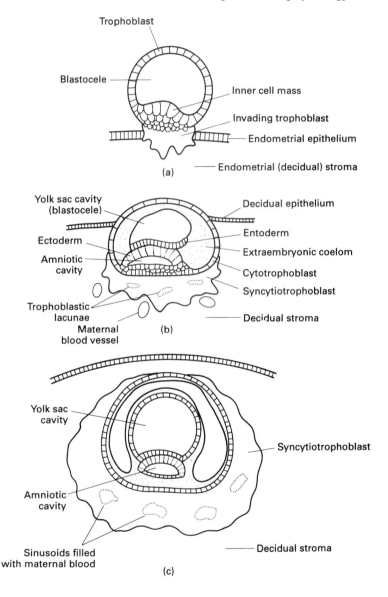

Fig. 5.2 Steps (a–c) in the implantation of the blastocyst. (a) Initial invasion of the trophoblast; (b) formation of trophoblastic lacunae; (c) invasion of maternal blood vessels and coalescence with lacunae (sinusoids), and associated differentiation of the embryo.

inhibits the preliminary endometrial proliferation required for implantation. After fertilization, excessive oestrogen would accelerate the passage of the embryo into the uterine cavity by increasing tubal peristalsis before the endometrium is receptive, and thus could cause failure of implantation. This is the presumed basis of the postcoital contraceptive method.

ENDOCRINE CONTROL OF REPRODUCTION

Ovarian hormones

Steroids of every sort are produced by the ovary, testis and adrenal cortex and by the trophoblast of the placenta. The steroid characteristic of each gland predominates on account of the particular balance of enzymes present. In these glands steroids are produced *de novo* from acetate via cholesterol or from blood-borne cholesterol in the form of low-density lipoprotein. Active steroids are also produced in other organs from steroid precursors which originate in the gonads or adrenal cortex. Thus androgen-sensitive hair follicles produce the active hormone dihydrotestosterone from testosterone, and subcutaneous adipose tissue produces oestrone from androstenedione, which is particularly important at the start of puberty and after the menopause.

Steroids are produced by all parts of the ovary: oestrogens (particularly oestradiol) and progesterone by granulosa cells; and androgens by thecal, stromal and hilar cells (hilar cells being analogous with the testicular Leydig cells). Note that the androgen-secreting elements all originate from the mesenchyme of the embryonic ovary (Chapter 3). The ovary produces similar amounts of testosterone and oestrogens but rather more of the weak androgens, dehydroepiandrosterone (DHA) and androstenedione. The adrenal cortex produces nearly as much androgens as the ovary. Progesterone is produced in relatively huge amounts by the corpus luteum – 100 times more than oestradiol. The one dominant follicle is responsible for virtually the entire output of oestradiol from the two ovaries in the few days leading up to ovulation, and of progesterone in the luteal phase.

Oestradiol is by far the most potent oestrogen. Its wide influence on reproduction has already been described, and is summarized in Figure 5.3. It is essential for growth of the uterus and vagina, stimulation of cervical mucus receptive to sperm, and initial development of the endometrium in preparation for implantation. It also has some influence on libido in mid-cycle (libido in Figure 5.3 being conveniently but perhaps not accurately located at the vulva!), although androgens and psychological factors generally play a

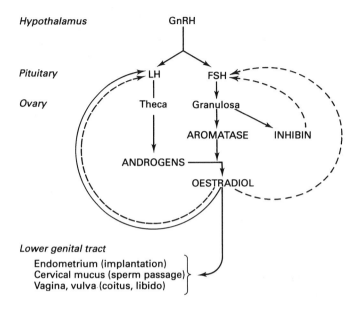

Fig. 5.3   The main pathways of control and end-organ effects of the reproductive hormones in the follicular phase of the ovarian cycle. Feedback effects are indicated as negative by broken lines, positive by unbroken lines. GnRH = gonadotrophin-releasing hormone (also referred to as luteinizing hormone-releasing hormone, LHRH). After luteinization the granulosa cells secrete mainly progesterone which initially, with oestradiol, exerts positive feedback on luteinizing hormone (LH) but thereafter has a negative feedback effect on both LH and follicle-stimulating hormone (FSH), via the pituitary.

bigger part. Oestrogens also contribute to breast growth (of ducts and alveoli), affect the pattern of musculoskeletal growth and subcutaneous fat distribution, and exert important controlling influences primarily via the pituitary on gonadotrophin release (called feedback, both negative and positive). These actions are mediated by the presence in all the target organs of specific oestradiol-binding (receptor) proteins within the cells. Furthermore, oestradiol stimulates the production by the liver of a specific globulin (sex hormone-binding globulin, SHBG) to which it is strongly bound in blood plasma, only a tiny fraction remaining free. In this way it is protected from metabolism but available to specific receptor proteins.

Progesterone is best known for its effect in maintaining pregnancy by inhibiting uterine activity, but it is also essential in the final preparation of the endometrium for implantation and it coordinates and slows the passage of the embryo along the fallopian tube. It has certain antioestrogen effects, notably on endometrial proliferation and cervical mucus. Like oestradiol (but less strongly) it exerts negative feedback on pituitary gonadotrophin release. It also exerts positive feedback but only after priming with oestrogen, in this way helping, *before* ovulation, to time the induction of the LH surge and amplify it. In the breast progesterone stimulates alveolar growth in combination with other essential hormones.

Inhibin is a non-steroidal hormone of large molecular size produced by the ovarian granulosa cells and testicular Sertoli cells, and has negative feedback, specifically on FSH release. Thus inhibin and oestradiol together exercise dual control of FSH secretion, though inhibin appears to exercise finer control than oestradiol (or other steroids) in the female. However, there are species differences of inhibin production and of consequent FSH levels, which seem to determine the number of oocytes released per cycle (and therefore litter size) typical of different species and breeds. Premenopausal cycles are associated with high FSH levels, despite normal steroid levels, presumably due to depletion of the cohort size of early antral follicles and thus inhibin. In normal circumstances inhibin may also have local paracrine or autocrine functions within the ovary. *In vitro* studies indicate that inhibin (from the granulosa cells) greatly enhances the effect of LH on theca cells to produce androgens – to be available to the granulosa cells for conversion to oestradiol – thus amplifying the responsiveness of the developing follicle.

Relaxin is a polypeptide hormone secreted by the placenta and decidua, having valuable effects on the myometrium and softening the cervix and pelvic ligaments in preparation for labour. It is also secreted by the corpus luteum and preovulatory follicle, and might facilitate follicular rupture.

Oxytocin is an octapeptide hormone secreted by the corpus luteum (apart from the posterior pituitary!) and may have a key role in luteolysis.

Growth factors are emerging as possible endocrine, paracrine or autocrine factors of importance in ovarian function and disorder. Insulin-like growth factor-1 (IGF-1), its receptor and binding proteins are all present within the follicle, and circulating or locally produced IGF-1 probably amplifies gonadotrophin action on theca and granulosa cell function. By contrast, epidermal growth factor (EGF) and its functional homologue, transforming growth factor α (TGF-α), which share the same receptor, inhibit granulosa cell function. The functional and clinical relevance of these actions remains unclear, but it may be particularly important that EGF mediates and enhances the effect of oestrogen on the endometrium. It could be another example of dual control by the ovary of key dependent functions. What is clear is that the ovarian actions of IGF-1 can be critically modulated in conditions of insulin hypersecretion, which suppresses hepatic production of the binding proteins of IGF-1, leading to ovarian hypersecretion of androgens (see Chapter 15).

The ovarian endocrine cycle

The ovarian endocrine cycle is of course closely related to the ovarian follicular cycle, which passes through follicular and luteal phases. Oestradiol and progesterone levels in peripheral blood reflect secretion rate by the dominant follicle. As shown in Figure 5.4, oestradiol (and to a lesser extent oestrone) levels increase

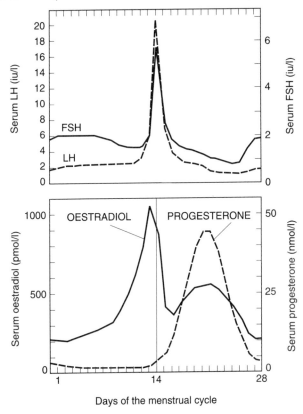

Fig. 5.4 Gonadotrophin and ovarian steroid cycles related to a typical 28-day menstrual cycle. The LH peak is on day 14 and ovulation would be on day 15. Note the different scales and molar values. Data drawn from Landgren *et al.* (1980) *Acta Endocrinol* **94**:89.

exponentially during the week before ovulation. Oestradiol reaches a peak a day or two before ovulation, then falls sharply (as the LH surge induces a switch to progesterone secretion). Oestradiol increases again due to secretion by the corpus luteum to reach a lower, flatter, secondary peak, before finally falling as the corpus luteum ceases to function (unless pregnancy occurs). The *average* levels of oestradiol are higher in the luteal than in the follicular phase.

Progesterone levels are low throughout the follicular phase but start to rise with (in fact just before) the LH surge shortly before ovulation, increasing steadily due to secretion by the corpus luteum to reach a wide peak, and falling again in a symmetrical pattern as the corpus luteum fails.

It is not practically feasible as a basic routine to look for the actual occurrence of ovulation, which requires daily ultrasonography, but functional maturity is more important and the steroid levels in blood provide an accurate guide to that. Mid luteal progesterone measurement is the best index (see Chapter 12). In the preovulatory phase it is ordinarily too difficult to catch the relatively sharp oestradiol peak. However, granulosa cell proliferation and maturation in the follicular phase determine the capacity of the resulting corpus luteum to secrete progesterone. Therefore the peak mid-luteal progesterone values are an accurate index of prior follicular development.

Genital changes dependent on ovarian hormones

The changes in the superficial cells of the vaginal epithelium, only recognized microscopically, and the more obvious changes in cervical mucus have already been mentioned. The most obvious event is the menstrual cycle, i.e. the cyclical shedding with bleeding of secretory endometrium when oestrogen and progesterone levels fall as the corpus luteum fails. The normal endometrial cycle consists of proliferative and secretory phases that correspond with the follicular and luteal phases of the ovarian cycle. The physical changes in the endometrium and the process of menstruation will be described in detail later.

Non-reproductive metabolic effects of ovarian hormones

Oestrogens affect nearly all other endocrine systems. By increasing their specific binding globulins in plasma, oestrogens cause an increase in the total circulating amounts of cortisol, thyroxine and progesterone, and also of iron and copper. Oestrogens also stimulate the secretion of cortisol and growth hormone, thus reducing carbohydrate tolerance despite enhancing the insulin response. Prolactin secretion is also stimulated, although without any obviously important consequence (except in pregnancy, due to the particularly large amounts of placental oestrogens). Oestrogens and progesterone have complex but generally opposing effects on fluid and electrolyte balance, oestrogens usually causing salt and water retention. Aldosterone secretion increases in the luteal phase, perhaps to counteract the salt-losing effect of progesterone despite the presence of large amounts of oestrogen. Renin is stimulated by oestrogen and plasma triglycerides rise. Biliary secretion and excretion tend to be reduced and blood coagulability increased. The widely varied effects mentioned, nearly all due to oestrogens, are small. Some have caused varying degrees of concern in relation to the long-term use of oral contraceptive preparations and postmenopausal hormone replacement. It now seems, however, that oestrogens tend to protect against arterial disease, and the adverse arterial effects of progestogens can be minimized by dosage and choice of non-androgenic compounds (see Chapters 11 and 23).

Gonadotrophins

The two gonadotrophins, FSH and LH, are glycoproteins, very similar in structure to thyroid stimulating hormone (TSH) and hCG. FSH and LH are produced by the anterior pituitary under the stimulus of gonadotrophin-releasing hormone (GnRH) from the hypothalamus. FSH and LH are also stored in the anterior pituitary and can be released suddenly in large amounts by a large dose of GnRH. Although gonadotrophins inhibit the secretion of GnRH by direct negative feedback on the hypothalamus, the main control of gonadotrophin secretion is by ovarian oestradiol and progesterone. Acting primarily on the pituitary they both usually exert negative feedback, but when oestradiol increases to high levels it exerts positive feedback, i.e. it induces a discharge of gonadotrophins, especially LH (the so-called LH surge). Progesterone also exerts positive feedback at first, but only after priming with oestrogen. Although there is only one form of GnRH, differential responses of FSH and LH occur according to the steroid environment of the pituitary.

That description of the control of gonadotrophin secretion applies to adult women after the neuroendocrine maturational changes at puberty. The patterns of gonadotrophin and sex steroid secretion at the various stages of life will be described later. In men, positive feedback never develops.

The adult gonadotrophin cycle

The adult gonadotrophin cycle is shown in Figure 5.4. As steroid levels in blood fall at the end of the luteal phase the FSH level rises due to release of negative feedback on the pituitary and hypothalamus. LH rises less, the release of LH being more sensitive to negative feedback. With the rising secretion of oestradiol and inhibin by the dominant follicle the FSH level falls again gradually. Although this fall occurs just when follicular maturation is accelerating, it seems that the dominant follicle secures its supply of FSH by diverting blood flow within the ovary to itself, presumably by its oestrogen output. Thus, both by reducing blood supply and FSH levels in blood, the dominant follicle secures its predominance totally over other antral follicles that started to respond to the earlier rise in FSH. The dominant follicle is probably first selected by being the one most ready, by chance, to respond to the prevailing gonadotrophin environment.

The primacy of the dominant follicle in controlling its own progress is further illustrated in its influence on the timing of the LH surge. As oestradiol levels in blood increase, so the LH level rises slightly due to increasing positive feedback, and finally there is a sudden, huge surge lasting about 48 hours. Though oestradiol primes the pituitary in readiness to release the LH surge, the actual trigger is the small rise in progesterone due to spontaneous slight luteinization by the fully mature preovulatory follicle. The LH surge stimulates the final maturation of the Graafian follicle and its rupture, and induces luteinization of the follicle. A small FSH surge accompanies the LH surge but does not seem to have any function.

Though the LH surge is usually illustrated as a peak, as in Figure 5.4, that is an artefact due to centring on the maximum value of once-daily measurements. The true peak lasts 24 hours, in a series of pulses, after a rise lasting 12 hours, and followed by a fall lasting 12 hours – total 48 hours. It is the onset of the LH surge, rather than any apparent peak, which is precisely related in time to subsequent follicular rupture, which occurs about 38 hours later. That knowledge is applied in the precise control of ovulation or egg collection in fertility treatments after an hCG injection to mimic the LH surge.

In the luteal phase, because of the high levels of both oestradiol and progesterone the LH and FSH levels fall sharply to lower levels than in the follicular phase.

In clinical practice FSH and LH can be readily assayed and their measurement is essential in distinguishing the causes of amenorrhoea and oligomenorrhoea (see Chapter 15), subfertility (Chapter 12) and recurrent miscarriage (Chapter 13). Human gonadotrophins can be used to induce follicular maturation in certain anovulatory conditions (see Chapters 12 and 15). And in some conditions endogenous gonadotrophin secretion can be stimulated by treatment to block negative feedback.

Gonadotrophin-releasing hormone

GnRH is also called FSH- and LH-releasing hormone and often abbreviated as FSH/LH-RH, LHRH or LRH. It is a simple decapeptide, secreted in pulses by the hypothalamus and transported via the hypophyseal portal blood vessels to stimulate production and release of FSH and LH in similar pulses by the anterior pituitary. The control of GnRH secretion is unclear. Feedback by oestradiol and progesterone, and by FSH and LH, plays an insignificant part normally. Administration of GnRH in appropriate pulses about every 90 minutes to women with primary hypothalamic failure (or to monkeys with an experimentally lesioned hypothalamus) leads to normal ovulatory cycles. This indicates that ovarian feedback control is essentially on the pituitary, and the hypothalamus exerts an obligatory but non-modulatory influence on the pituitary.

The assay of GnRH is irrelevant in the peripheral circulation. In clinical practice the distinction between hypothalamic and pituitary failure, which occurs rarely, can only be made by the difference in gonadotrophin response to injected synthetic GnRH. Synthetic GnRH can be administered in pulses by means of a portable battery-driven pump to induce ovulation in women with hypothalamic failure.

Prolactin

Prolactin is a polypeptide in the form of a single long chain, resembling growth hormone and human placental lactogen. There appear to be a few analogous forms in the human, which may account for occasional spurious results by radioimmunoassay. It is secreted by the anterior pituitary and controlled essentially by inhibition by dopamine secreted by the hypothalamus (its control is discussed more fully in Chapter 15). There is no significant variation in prolactin levels in blood through the menstrual cycle. Although prolactin seems to be essential for normal follicular steroidogenesis, particularly in the corpus luteum, very low levels in blood do not interfere with ovulation. Hyperprolactinaemia, however, inhibits ovarian function, by interfering with hypothalamic GnRH secretion, and is a common cause of amenorrhoea. It can be treated, to induce ovulation, with dopamine agonists to inhibit prolactin secretion by the pituitary.

Melatonin

Melatonin and related substances are secreted by the pineal body which is inhibited by light. Melatonin somehow acts via the brain to inhibit gonadal function and to influence various light-dependent cycles. It may thus play a part in the timing of puberty. Destruction of the pineal body, for instance by a tumour, can cause precocious puberty.

THE ENDOMETRIUM AND MENSTRUATION

The endometrium and endometrial cycle

The normal endometrial cycle (Fig. 5.5) consists of proliferative and secretory phases that correspond with the follicular and luteal phases of the ovarian cycle. Under the influence of oestrogen alone the endometrial glands and stroma both proliferate, mitoses being commonly seen on histology, the glands becoming longer as the endometrium thickens. The endometrial spiral arterioles (not shown in Fig. 5.5) become increasingly coiled, developing out of proportion to the needs of the endometrium but adapted to the future needs of expected trophoblast. Progesterone then blocks

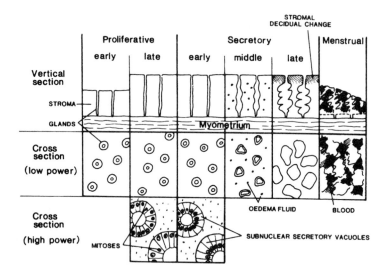

Fig. 5.5 Histological changes in the endometrium through the menstrual cycle (see text for description). Note the intact basal layer in the menstrual phase from which the endometrium regenerates and can proliferate, indicated by the dotted line.

endometrial proliferation and induces secretory changes, indicated initially by secretory vacuoles building up below the nuclei of the glandular epithelium. Later the secretion pushes past the nuclei into the glandular lumen, distending the glands, and the stroma becomes loose and oedematous. Finally the glands become grossly distended and tortuous, and near the endometrial surface the stromal cells become enlarged, pale and close-packed, rather like the much more marked decidual change that occurs when a blastocyst implants. The spiral arterioles are now at their peak development. In the absence of fertilization the fall in luteal steroid levels causes spasm of the spiral arterioles and necrosis and shedding of the endometrium (except for the basal layer, from which regeneration occurs under the influence of oestrogen in a new cycle). Between the dense basal layer of endometrium, which is relatively inactive, and the dense superficial layer due to stromal decidual change, the middle layer of distended glands appears to be spongy. It is particularly marked in pregnancy, and is called the decidua spongiosa.

Menstruation and the menstrual cycle

Menstruation is the shedding of secretory endometrium with bleeding which occurs at the end of each ovarian cycle if conception has not taken place. The shedding of non-secretory endometrium associated with anovulatory cycles or withdrawal of exogenous steroids like the contraceptive pill is not true menstruation, but this cannot be distinguished in practice.

Shortly before menstruation the endometrium (except its basal layer) shrinks and becomes disrupted due to the reduction in its ovarian endocrine support. At the same time the endometrial spiral arterioles undergo spasm leading to blanching of the endometrium, but this may be the result rather than the cause of the endometrial disruption, caused by the local release perhaps of catecholamines. The arteriolar spasm is then relaxed intermittently, leading to the main bleeding that occurs with menstruation. Thus the arterioles control the amount of bleeding, but as yet there is no effective therapeutic control of them. The total blood lost at each menstrual period is on average 40 ml, the normal range being 20–60 ml.

The menses thus consist mainly of blood and also the fragmented endometrium, including its secretions and tissue exudate. The menses are characteristically fluid, the blood unclotted. This is probably due to fibrinolysins released by the damaged tissue, which dissolve the initial clot. When clotting occurs it is usually because of excessive bleeding, presumably due to relative lack of local fibrinolysins. A rough guide to the amount of blood lost is the number of towels or tampons needed to contain it: normally no more than 12 are needed for the whole period.

The menstrual period lasts on average 4 days, the normal range being 2–6 days. The menstrual loss occurs with a distinct pattern during this time, starting suddenly and increasing to peak flow on usually the second day, then diminishing gradually to a watery loss as the endometrium regenerates.

The menstrual cycle, measured from the start of one menstrual period to the next, lasts on average 28 days, diminishing gradually from 30 days at 20 years of age to 27 days at 40 years. The normal range is 23–35 days. Individuals usually vary much less, by no more than 4 days, but most women have occasional aberration. The variation is much greater, with a particular tendency to long cycles, in the first 5 years after the menarche and the last 8 years before the menopause. The shortest possible fertile cycle, i.e. associated with ovulation, is 21 days, because it takes at least 8 days for follicular ripening and a normal luteal phase lasts for about 13 days.

The onset of menstruation is the easiest point of reference in practice, and the day menstruation starts is called day 1 of the cycle. In an average 28-day cycle ovulation thus occurs on day 15 (see Fig. 5.4).

Gonadotrophin and sex steroid cycles through life

FSH and LH are secreted by the fetal pituitary in response to pulsatile GnRH from the hypothalamus by 8 weeks of age (10 weeks' gestational age), but stimulation of gonadal hormone secretion is preceded by chorionic gonadotrophin. There are six distinct phases of pituitary–gonadal hormone secretion through life, depicted in Figures 5.6 and 5.7.

In pregnancy (Fig. 5.6), hCG levels in both mother and fetus peak at about 10 weeks' gestation and in males stimulate testosterone secretion by the interstitial (Leydig) cells of the developing testis. Testosterone secretion continues to be stimulated later by LH. Testosterone is critically important at this time to induce the male genital tract. By contrast, ovarian oestrogen is of no importance and in both sexes oestrogen comes mainly from the placenta and is neutral in its effect on the developing genital tracts (see Chapter 3).

In mid-pregnancy gonadotrophin levels are high because pituitary secretion is largely unconstrained. Negative feedback is acquired as sex steroid receptors develop in the GnRH neurones of the hypothalamus, and consequently FSH and LH levels fall, followed as a result by testosterone. Peak FSH and LH levels are slightly lower in males, presumably due to at least partially effective negative feedback by testosterone.

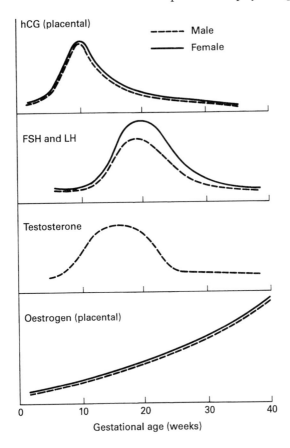

Fig. 5.6 Reproductive hormone levels during fetal life. Pituitary gonadotrophin levels are slightly lower in the male, probably because of partial negative feedback by testicular testosterone, which is initially stimulated by chorionic gonadotrophin. hCG = Human chorionic gonadotrophin; FSH = follicle-stimulating hormone; LH = luteinizing hormone.

After birth the sudden loss of placental oestrogen leads to release of negative feedback and a surge of FSH and LH secretion, and consequently of gonadal steroids for several months (Fig. 5.7).

During infancy, sensitivity to negative feedback increases and is maximal throughout childhood resulting in very low levels of gonadotrophins and gonadal steroids. The enhanced negative feedback appears to be due to a non-steroidal central nervous inhibitory

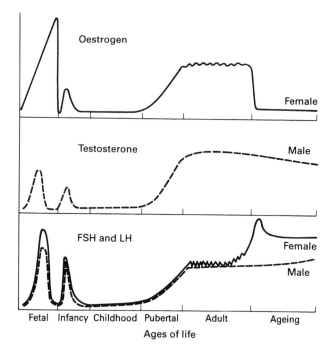

Fig. 5.7 Reproductive hormone levels through all stages of life. In fetal life oestrogen levels are as high in the male (not shown) as in the female due to placental origin. The fall after delivery leads to rebound increases in pituitary gonadotrophins and gonadal steroids, due to loss of negative feedback. That is followed by increased sensitivity to negative feedback which is maximal in childhood, until relaxed by neuroendocrine maturational changes at puberty. FSH = Follicle-stimulating hormone; LH = luteinizing hormone.

mechanism of unknown type. The neuroendocrine pathway appears to be via the posterior hypothalamus because compressive lesions in that area can lead to precocious puberty.

Pubertal – or strictly, prepubertal – maturation begins at about 8 years of age, indicated by gradually rising gonadotrophin and gonadal steroid secretion. This appears to be due to primary events in the central nervous system: loss of the non-steroid inhibitory mechanism, increased pituitary sensitivity to GnRH, and later, enhanced pulsatile secretion of GnRH linked with rapid eye movement (REM) sleep. Cyclical secretion of gonadotrophins and oestrogen governed by negative feedback effects leads to menstrual cycles.

Maturation of the central nervous control of pulsatile GnRH secretion is influenced by various genetic and environmental factors, including nutrition and body fat. Severe psychological factors can suppress pulsatile GnRH secretion, although usually occurring after puberty, thus reversing the process. Anorexia nervosa is a well-known example (see Chapter 15). During recovery from the illness, which is also associated with lack of REM sleep, there is return of pulsatile GnRH secretion, at first linked with REM sleep and later throughout the day and night.

In the adult, enhanced pulsatile GnRH secretion occurs throughout the day and night. The diminished sensitivity to negative feedback is accompanied in adolescent women by development of positive feedback and the cyclical LH surge which triggers ovulation.

The menopause marks ovarian exhaustion of follicles, and lack of negative feedback leads to very high gonadotrophin levels. Even before the menopause for several years there is a gradual rise in FSH levels (see Fig. 5.7) – but not LH – due to reduction of inhibin levels associated with diminishing cohort size of early antral follicles.

In ageing men testicular function wanes only slightly, indicated in endocrine terms by a slight reduction in serum testosterone and inhibin levels, and a consequent rise in gonadotrophin levels, although remaining within the normal limits for young men (Fig. 5.7). The primary change is in the function of the seminiferous tubules, in particular the Sertoli cells. Sperm numbers and quality gradually wane. Indeed, in men and women sperm and oocyte quality begin to wane as early as 30 years of age.

FURTHER READING

Austin, C.R. and Short, R.V. (1986) *Reproduction in Mammals*, 2nd edn. Cambridge University Press, Cambridge.

Hillier, S.G., Kitchener, H.C., Neilson, J.P. (eds) *Scientific Essentials of Reproductive Medicine*. W.B. Saunders, London.

Johnson, M. and Everitt, B. (1988) *Essential Reproduction*, 3rd edn. Blackwell, Oxford.

Shaw, R.W., Soutter, W.P. and Stanton, S.L. (eds) (1997) *Gynaecology*, 3rd edn. Churchill Livingstone, Edinburgh.

Speroff, L., Glass, R.H. and Kase, N.G. (1994) *Clinical Gynecologic Endocrinology and Infertility*, 5th edn. Williams and Wilkins, Baltimore.

6

Physiology of pregnancy, labour and lactation

Pregnancy produces alterations in the maternal physiology that extend well beyond the obvious changes in the genital tract. All the systems in the body undergo changes, many to produce physiological values totally outside the normal non-pregnant range. While most of these changes can be seen to be directed towards producing a successful fetal outcome, some introduce hazards to the mother, whether or not she starts the pregnancy in normal health. These physiological changes also alter our framework for assessing normal and abnormal organ function. The high steroid output from the ovary and placenta is directly responsible for the majority of the changes, although some of the effects are attributable to the non-steroidal hormones human chorionic gonadotrophin (hCG), human placental lactogen (hPL) and prolactin.

REPRODUCTIVE HORMONE CHANGES

hCG (Fig. 6.1)

hCG has similar actions to luteinizing hormone (LH) and has an identical α subunit but a distinct β subunit. It is produced by the developing trophoblast and is detectable by immunological methods specific to β-hCG from 8 days postovulation, and by routine urine pregnancy-testing kits by 35–39 days from the last period (assuming a regular 28-day cycle). Its principal site of action is on the corpus luteum, which is maintained throughout pregnancy and is essential for pregnancy survival until the placenta produces adequate oestrogen and progesterone levels at 7–8 weeks of pregnancy. hCG has an important effect on the male fetus's testicles and less well-understood actions on the fetal adrenal gland. In the male fetus it stimulates gonadal production of testosterone (in spite of very high oestrogen influence, which would probably otherwise suppress testicular activity) and this has the effect of producing male differentiation of the genital tract, hypothalamus and cerebral hemispheres.

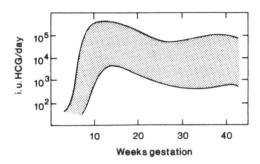

Fig. 6.1   Normal urinary human chorionic gonadotrophin (HCG) excretion.

Progesterone

Progesterone is the major pregnancy-conserving hormone. It inhibits the release of prostaglandins in the myometrium and decidua and consequently reduces myometrial activity. It also has a generalized smooth-muscle relaxant effect and numerous metabolic effects, to be outlined below. Until 10 weeks progesterone is mainly produced by the corpus luteum (the small peak in the progesterone curve; Fig. 6.2). Thereafter the large majority comes from the placenta. Similar considerations apply to oestrogen production.

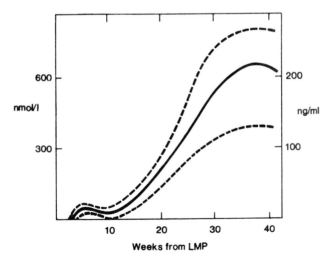

Fig. 6.2   Serum progesterone levels in normal pregnancy. LMP = Last menstrual period.

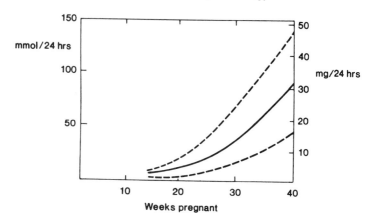

Fig. 6.3   Total urinary oestrogen output in normal pregnancy.

Oestrogens (Fig. 6.3)

In pregnancy the placenta produces greatly increased quantities of many oestrogens from fetal and maternal precursors. Oestrone, oestradiol and oestriol, the three main ones, are produced in similar amounts. Oestradiol is the most potent of these and is the major stimulus to growth of the uterus and breasts (although progesterone and other hormones are also important). Oestriol is interesting because it is almost entirely dependent on the fetal adrenal for its precursors. However, its function in pregnancy is unknown, and in

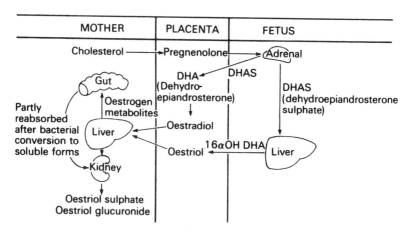

Fig. 6.4   Oestrogen metabolism in the fetoplacental unit.

rare instances a placental sulphatase deficiency leading to an inability to produce oestrogens in the placenta has been found to be compatible with a normal pregnancy but with a tendency to post-maturity, probably because of reduced production and release of prostaglandins secondary to the low oestrogen levels. Maternal metabolism (mainly in the liver and intestine) of the various oestrogens results in a high proportion in both blood and urine being conjugated oestriol. Oestrogen estimations have previously been fairly widely used in clinical practice as a guide to fetoplacental unit function but they have now been superseded by biophysical tests (Fig. 6.4).

hPL (Fig. 6.5)

hPL is produced by the placenta and is detectable from the fifth week of pregnancy. By late pregnancy it is being produced in very large quantities (up to 3 g/day). It has actions similar to prolactin and growth hormone, is important in the growth and development of the breasts, and may have other functions. It is probably partly responsible for the diabetogenic effect of pregnancy. Serum HPL estimation was previously also widely used clinically as a placental function test.

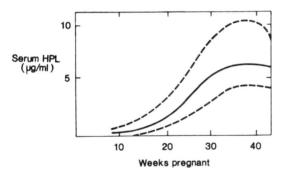

Fig. 6.5   Serum human placental lactogen (hPL) in normal pregnancy.

Prolactin

Oestrogen stimulates pituitary production of prolactin, and circulating prolactin levels increase progressively through pregnancy to about 20 times the non-pregnant level by term. Like hPL, prolactin encourages the growth and development of the breasts. Its effect in stimulating lactation is inhibited by the high oestrogen levels of pregnancy.

Relaxin

In pregnancy there is softening of connective tissue and relaxation of ligaments, particularly in the pelvic area. A hormone, relaxin, produced in the ovary and in decidua is responsible for these changes. In some animal species relaxin also has a role in cervical softening and the onset of labour, but the full extent of its function in the human is not yet clear. It is of some interest that women with ovarian failure who become pregnant with a donor egg and exogenous hormone support tend to fail to labour satisfactorily. It has been suggested that this may be due lack of relaxin.

GENERAL ENDOCRINE AND METABOLIC CHANGES

Thyroid

It is claimed that Egyptian tomb paintings show the use of a tight reed necklace to detect pregnancy thyroid enlargement – possibly the first recorded pregnancy test! Thyroid enlargement in pregnancy is common, particularly in areas with low iodine dietary intake. Otherwise women exhibit many of the features of hyperthyroidism, although remaining essentially euthyroid. The main features of pregnancy thyroid function are:

1 Basal metabolic rate – increased.
2 Protein bound iodine – increased.
3 Thyroxine binding globulin (TBG) – increased.
4 Total thyroxine and triiodothyronine – increased.
5 Free thyroxine index – normal.
6 Thyroid stimulating hormone (TSH) – normal.

The basal metabolic rate increase is due to the high metabolic activity of the fetoplacental unit and the increased maternal cardiac work rate. In common with other binding proteins, TBG increases in response to oestrogen, producing higher levels of the bound hormones. Because of this, free thyroxine or TSH levels are the best indices of thyroid function in pregnancy. There is very little passage of thyroid hormones between the fetal and maternal circulations.

Adrenal function

Corticosteroids

Blood levels and production rates of glucocorticoids increase considerably in pregnancy. Most of the increase in blood levels is in the protein bound portion (due to the increase in corticosterone binding globulin), but free cortisol is also somewhat increased, making the pregnant woman effectively mildly cushingoid. Corticosteroids, both natural and synthetic, can cross the placenta freely but adrenocorticotrophic hormone does not do so.

Aldosterone

Production and blood levels rise steadily throughout pregnancy to about four times non-pregnancy levels, the increase tending to counteract the sodium-losing effect of progesterone.

Carbohydrate metabolism

Pregnancy may be considered diabetogenic in a number of senses:

1 Some women with previously normal glucose tolerance will become chemical diabetics for the duration of the pregnancy.
2 Normal pregnant women on average produce slightly higher blood sugar levels in a standard glucose tolerance test (and also higher insulin levels).
3 Insulin requirements of diabetic patients generally increase appreciably in pregnancy.

This diabetogenic effect of pregnancy is attributed to hPL, and to the increased steroid output and the increased fat stores of pregnancy and largely disappears within 48 hours of delivery.

Fasting blood sugar levels are lowered by pregnancy, and the pregnant woman seems to withstand hypoglycaemia better than the non-pregnant woman.

The renal threshold for glycosuria is commonly lowered in pregnancy due to the large increase in glomerular filtration, and glycosuria correlates poorly with blood sugar levels. Low levels of glycosuria are consequently fairly common in pregnancy in women with normal glucose tolerance.

Carbohydrate metabolism in labour

In labour uterine activity produces increased glucose utilization, and gastric stasis commonly occurs, leading to a failure of absorption of water and carbohydrate. In this situation gluconeogenesis occurs with subsequent production of ketones. Thus ketosis and dehydration are common features of prolonged labour. They have the important side-effects of impairing uterine activity, and further prolonging the labour if not corrected, and of inducing acidosis in the fetus.

CARDIOVASCULAR SYSTEM

Cardiac output increases by an average of about 30% in early pregnancy, with no appreciable change thereafter. The increase is explained by proportionate increases in pulse rate (70–85 beats/min) and stroke volume, and the extra output which amounts to 1500 ml/min, goes mainly to the uterus (500 ml/min to the placenta and 250 ml/min to the myometrium), kidneys and skin.

Arterial blood pressure is slightly lowered in normal pregnancy, and peripheral vascular resistance is substantially lowered – partly by the low-resistance placental vascular bed and partly by a general peripheral vasodilatation – leading to a relatively large fall in diastolic pressure and an increased pulse pressure. The width of the heart increases radiologically and the apex beat and the axis of the heart are shifted slightly to the left. Systolic murmurs are common in pregnancy due to the increased output and alterations in the walls of the great vessels. Venous engorgement (e.g. piles and varicose veins) is common, partly because of smooth-muscle relaxation and partly because pressure is high in pelvic and leg veins, due to uterine obstruction of the inferior vena cava and increased blood flow from the uterus.

HAEMATOLOGICAL CHANGES

The major changes are as follows:

1 Blood volume increases about 30%.
2 Plasma volume increases about 45%.
3 Red cell mass increases about 45%.
4 Haemoglobin concentration usually falls slightly, although the mean corpuscular haemoglobin concentration and mean corpuscular haemoglobin remain unchanged.
5 White blood cell count increases to average $9000/mm^3$ (maximum $16\,000/mm^3$), with the increase mainly in neutrophils.
6 The erythrocyte sedimentation rate increases to 30–100 mm/h (but plasma viscosity remains normal).
7 Iron-binding capacity increases, due to the oestrogen-induced increase in transferrin.
8 Serum iron concentration falls.
9 Fibrinogen and factors VII, VIII and X increase substantially, making the pregnant woman's blood hypercoagulable.
10 Fibrinolytic activity decreases.

RESPIRATORY SYSTEM

The respiratory centre is affected by progesterone from early on in pregnancy and arterial partial pressure of carbon dioxide ($P\text{CO}_2$) is maintained at about 30–31 mmHg, a level which would result in apnoea in the non-pregnant. In addition the ventilatory response to small increases in $P\text{CO}_2$ is considerably increased, giving rise to the breathlessness of pregnancy. The reduction in $P\text{CO}_2$ is achieved by increased ventilation (40 per cent) which exceeds the increase in oxygen consumption (+20 per cent). Vital capacity is not affected by pregnancy, but respiration becomes more diaphragmatic than intercostal. The rib cage expands and the diaphragm rises appreciably.

RENAL FUNCTION AND WATER HANDLING

Renal blood flow and glomerular filtration rate increase by 50% in pregnancy. This results in higher clearance rates (normal creatinine clearance in pregnancy 140 ml/min) and diminished blood urea (normal pregnancy 0.4–2.2 nmol/l, 5–13 mg/dl).

The excretion of a water load and the renal handling of sodium are not appreciably altered.

Plasma osmolality is decreased in pregnancy as a result of the diminished $P\text{CO}_2$ and consequent lowering of electrolyte concentration. The resetting of the osmolality centre and subsequent alterations in antidiuretic hormone output may explain the polyuria and polydipsia of early pregnancy.

Water retention occurs in pregnancy over and above that needed for the increase in plasma volume and uterine contents. There is an increase in extracellular fluid, and oedema is common in normal as well as hypertensive pregnancy. It has been amply demonstrated that the presence of oedema in the absence of hypertension is a good sign associated with higher birth weights and decreased perinatal mortality.

There is considerable dilatation of ureters and renal calyces in pregnancy, due partly to ureteric obstruction and partly to a progesterone-relaxant effect. This dilatation, together with increased pregnancy glycosuria, leads to an increase in symptomatic urinary tract infection.

GASTROINTESTINAL SYSTEM

The gastrointestinal tract has not been much studied in pregnancy but there is a widely held belief that it suffers from a progesterone-induced relaxation producing a tendency to heartburn from pyloric and oesophageal reflux, and also gastric stasis in labour, constipation throughout pregnancy and a predisposition to gallstones.

Liver function

Most standard liver function tests show no change in pregnancy. The exceptions are the serum albumin level, which falls slightly, reducing the albumin/globulin ratio. However, these tests give a very poor indication of the complex total liver function. It is clear that many aspects of metabolism, depending at least partly on the liver, change radically in pregnancy (e.g. carbohydrate metabolism, clotting function).

Palmar erythema (liver palms) and spider naevi are often found in normal pregnancy and are confined to the parts drained by the superior vena cava. They are presumably related to high oestrogen levels and altered liver function.

IMMUNOLOGICAL CHANGES

Modifications in the immune response are necessary to stop the rejection of the placenta by the mother (and vice versa). Cell-mediated immunity is profoundly depressed in pregnancy. This is partly attributable to an oestrogen-induced increase in glycoproteins which coat the lymphocytes with a mucoid layer and partly to the effect of hPL and hCG in suppressing lymphocyte transformation.

Throughout pregnancy fragments of placental tissue (trophoblast emboli) break off into the maternal venous system and probably also play an important part in modifying the maternal immune response.

There is some suggestion that failure of this immune tolerance may produce pre-eclampsia and that failure of the initial immunological recognition of a pregnancy may be a cause of abortion. The depression of immune responses leads to an increased susceptibility to viral diseases and to malaria in pregnancy.

DIAGNOSIS OF PREGNANCY

Pregnancy may be suspected on the basis of symptoms:

1 Delayed menstruation.
2 Breast tenderness and fullness.

3 Polyuria.
4 Tiredness.
5 Nausea.

Symptoms 2–4 are often (but not always) experienced from the fifth week of pregnancy. Sickness usually appears a week or two later.

Pregnancy may be diagnosed on the basis of physical signs, but before 12 weeks this diagnosis is liable to error except in experienced hands. The signs are:

1 Uterine enlargement (apparent from 6 weeks).
2 Uterine softening.
3 Increased vascularity – detected by bluish colouring of vagina and cervix, or by arterial pulsation in vaginal fornices.
4 Breast changes (pigmentation of the areola and growth of Montgomery's tubercles) – unreliable.
5 Hegar's sign (softening and apparent disappearance to bimanual examination of the uterine isthmus) – unreliable and potentially damaging to elicit.

Diagnostic tests

The diagnostic tests currently in use depend on the immunological detection of hCG. With clean equipment and modest experience they are highly reliable. Standard pregnancy-testing methods rely on antibodies to the entire hCG molecule, which may cross-react to some extent with LH. Their sensitivity is therefore set above the level where interference from normal cycle LH production could occur. They should give a positive result within 25 days of conception (ovulation), but may give negative results after 20 weeks when hCG levels fall. Proprietary kits (Pregnosticon or Gravindex) are suitable for clinic, ward or general practice use.

More sensitive pregnancy testing systems depend on antibodies to β-hCG and these may be positive from 8 days postovulation (that is, 6 days before the period is due). Such methods of detecting β-hCG have important applications in confirming or excluding pregnancy in cases of suspected ectopic pregnancy, and in monitoring molar disease. In routine diagnosis of pregnancy, however, they are more nuisance than they are worth as a high proportion of pregnancies diagnosed before the first missed period never become established as a clinical pregnancy.

Ultrasonography, particularly with a vaginal probe, can detect a pregnancy sac from 5 weeks and a fetal heart beat from 6 weeks of pregnancy.

THE PLACENTA

The process of implantation consists essentially of the invasion of the decidual lining of the uterus by the trophoblast. The decidua is adapted not so much to facilitate this process as to limit it. (Experimentally, blastocysts can be made to implant in a large variety of tissues, e.g. eye, kidney or testis, and tend to display tumour-like invasiveness in sites other than the uterus.) In the uterus maternal blood vessels are eroded to form blood-filled spaces (choriodecidual spaces) in which the chorionic villi develop. Septa form more or less distinct compartments, into each of which a spiral artery opens, directing blood over a tuft of villi with the blood escaping through veins at the margin of the compartments. Very early in pregnancy the spiral arteries are invaded by trophoblast cells and become appreciably dilated as they approach the placental surface. A high-flow, low-resistance placental blood supply results so that the chorionic villi are completely bathed in blood with oxygen and carbon dioxide content very close to that of maternal arteries. Fetal and maternal blood do not mix. Gaseous and nutrient exchange take place through the walls of the chorionic villi.

The weight of the placenta increases at a different rate to that of the fetus, so that the placenta to fetus weight ratio changes from 4 : 1 at 10 weeks, to 1 : 2 at 20 weeks, 1 : 3.5 at 30 weeks and 1 : 5 at term.

The placenta has the following functions:

1 Production of the hormones hCG, hPL, oestrogens and progestogens.
2 Gas exchange (oxygen and carbon dioxide).
3 Nutrition of the fetus.
4 Excretion of fetal waste products.
5 Anchoring of the fetus.
6 Protection of the fetus from immunological attack (cellular immunity and immunoglobulin M (IgM), although the smaller IgG molecules can cross the placenta).
7 Heat transfer.

THE FETUS

The fetus reaches the size of a jelly baby at 9 weeks, and the size of a (1996!) Mars bar by about 15 weeks. Crown–rump lengths are shown in Figure 6.6. These can be measured by ultrasound and used for early pregnancy dating to within ± 4 days.

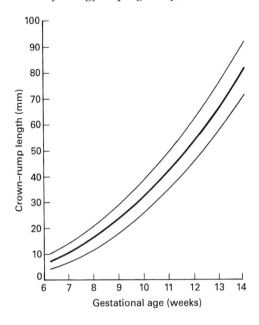

Fig. 6.6   Crown–rump length in early pregnancy: mean ± 2 s.d.

The normal range of biparietal diameters which are easier to measure and are used for dating later pregnancies is shown in Figure 6.7. It should be noted that the range of normal variation increases from mid-pregnancy and considerably after 28 weeks.

Fetal weight increases (in a sigmoid fashion) throughout pregnancy. It reaches 500 g at about 20 weeks and 1 kg at 28 weeks. Thereafter it increases about 200 g per week, to reach 3.4 kg at term (Fig. 6.8). The average male fetus weighs about 120 g more than the average female fetus at term.

Organogenesis

The major fetal organs (brain, heart, limbs, kidneys, gut, etc.) develop to something close to their final form between 4 and 9 weeks of pregnancy. Thereafter only minor changes occur in all systems, except the genitalia. Teratogenic substances acting before 4 weeks usually cause death of the embryo; between 4 and 9 weeks they are likely to produce major anatomical defects but after 9 weeks lesser anatomical abnormalities. Functional organ damage may be produced at any stage of pregnancy.

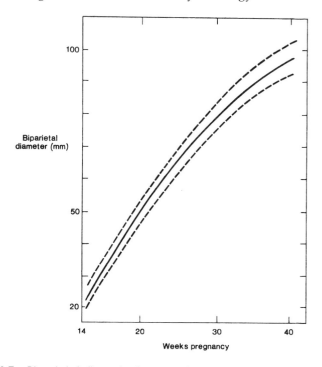

Fig. 6.7   Biparietal diameter in normal pregnancy.

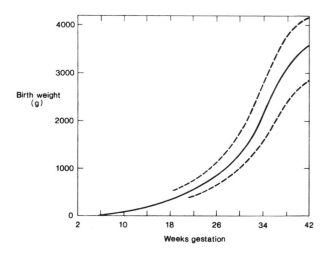

Fig. 6.8   Intrauterine fetal weight: mean and 10th and 90th percentiles.

Preparation for extrauterine life

Babies rarely survive with a birth weight below 500 g or maturity less than 24 weeks, although a baby of 283 g has survived to become a normal child. Typical survival rate of babies born alive, but prematurely, in a unit with first-class paediatric care is shown in Figure 6.9. Improvement in survival per week is considerable before 28 weeks but relatively modest after 28 weeks.

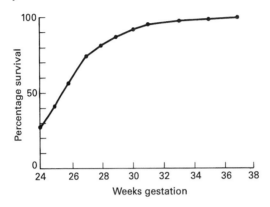

Fig. 6.9   Survival of babies born in Bristol 1994.

The premature baby may have considerable problems in many different physiological areas (notably breathing, temperature regulation, maintenance of blood sugar, bilirubin handling, combat of infection), but the most common cause of death is functional immaturity of the lungs. The pressure produced by the surface tension of water within the alveoli exceeds the maximum inspiratory effort of the baby and the alveoli cannot expand. To get over this problem, *surfactant*, a substance with detergent properties, is produced in the lungs and reduces surface tension approximately by a factor of 10. Surfactant is usually only produced in significant quantities towards the end of pregnancy, starting anywhere between 24 and 39 weeks.

Corticosteroids can induce surfactant production, and spontaneous labour is usually preceded by several weeks of increased corticosteroid output by the fetus, thus ensuring lung maturity before delivery. It is possible to measure in amniotic fluid (obtained by amniocentesis) the concentration of lecithin, which is the major component of surfactant. This can give an indication of the functional state of the fetal lung and hence of the likelihood of respiratory distress syndrome (RDS) if the fetus is delivered prematurely. Laboratories may measure the ratio between lecithin and sphyngomyelin (L/S ratio). Sphyngomyelin production in amniotic fluid is relatively constant during pregnancy so the L/S ratio gives comparable information to the lecithin concentration, and is less influenced by changes in amniotic fluid volume. An L/S ratio of over 2 is associated with a low risk of RDS.

Circulatory changes at birth

Within 2 minutes of birth, circulation through the umbilical cord ceases, with consequent increase in resistance to outflow from the left side of the heart. Blood is diverted into the pulmonary circulation, the expansion of the pulmonary vessels being encouraged by respiratory efforts. Both the foramen ovale and the ductus arteriosus close to some extent at this stage, but not totally for several days. This means that it may not be possible to diagnose congenital cardiac anomalies for a few days after birth.

AMNIOTIC FLUID

Amniotic fluid is produced partly by the amnion on the surface of the placenta, but fetal urine output makes a substantial contribution (about 0.5 l/day at the end of pregnancy). The fetus also swallows appreciable amounts (0.5 l/day at term), so that disturbances of fetal urine output or of swallowing can produce changes in amniotic fluid volume. There is a net increase in amniotic fluid volume of about 5 ml/day through most of pregnancy. Normal amniotic fluid volume reaches a maximum of about 1–1.5 litres at 36 weeks, diminishing slightly to term and more markedly postterm. In the early months of pregnancy the biochemical composition of amniotic fluid closely resembles fetal extracellular fluid, but in the second half of pregnancy it becomes more comparable to fetal urine.

GENITAL TRACT

The size of the uterus and the uterine blood supply increase progressively throughout pregnancy. The weight of the uterus increases from about 60 g (2 oz) in the non-pregnant woman to 900 g (2 lb) at term.

The uterus entirely fills the pelvis at 14 weeks and from this time tends to rise above the pelvic brim. In the early weeks of pregnancy the uterine cavity is almost circular and the position of the fetus is

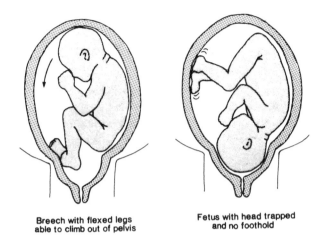

Breech with flexed legs
able to climb out of pelvis

Fetus with head trapped
and no foothold

Fig. 6.10   Head 'trapping' in the last trimester.

fairly random, constrained only by its tendency to face the placenta. In the middle months of pregnancy the uterus attains an elongated form and the fetus will usually lie with its long axis longitudinally. From about 30 weeks the large majority of fetuses adopt a head-down position (cephalic presentation). This is probably because the pelvis acts as a head trap. A fetus presenting as a breech with flexed legs can climb out of the lower uterus using the pelvis as a foothold, but this may be impossible with a cephalic presentation, or a breech presentation with extended knees (Figure. 6.10).

The uterus is divided into upper and lower segments, the lower segment starting at the point where the anterior uterine peritoneum is reflected on to the areolar tissue surrounding the bladder. Functionally the lower segment plays an inactive part in the contractions of labour, being passively stretched upwards and outwards over the presenting part of the fetus. The distinction is of practical importance in caesarean section operations. By the end of a prolonged labour the lower segment may so stretched that it is only a few millimetres thick.

The uterus contracts throughout pregnancy, infrequently early on but with increasing frequency and strength in the weeks preceding the clinical onset of labour. The mother will not usually be aware of these contractions unless she is concentrating. They start the process of thinning out and expanding (developing) the lower segment of the uterus.

Initiation of labour

The sensitivity of the uterus to oxytocic stimuli alters as term approaches. The factors determining this sensitivity are:

1 The degree of myometrial stretch (increased with twins or polyhydramnios).
2 The oestrogen/progesterone ratio (increased by oestrogen, decreased by progesterone).

The actual triggering of the onset of labour is brought about by an increase in fetal adrenal activity, probably in response to hypothalamic maturation. This adrenal activity results in increased oestrogen output from the placenta and increased prostaglandin synthesis and release from myometrium and decidua. The increased corticosteroid output also has an important effect in stimulating surfactant production in the fetal lungs. Once labour has started, the strength of contractions is augmented by oxytocin produced by the fetal pituitary and by prostaglandins released in response to cervical stretch and decidual trauma. (There is no significant increase in maternal output of oxytocin in pregnancy or labour.) Denervation of the uterus does not stop the normal onset of labour.

First stage of labour

Labour is usually assumed to have started when uterine contractions are occurring regularly every 10 minutes or less. The frequency, strength and duration of contractions (and hence the uterine work rate) increase over the first 3 hours or so of labour and then reach a stable state, when contractions will typically occur approximately every 3 minutes, last about a minute and produce an intrauterine pressure around 40 mmHg. Typical progress of cervical dilatation is shown in Figure 6.11.

In the early stages of labour the cervix becomes effaced or taken up, that is the tubular 'spout' disappears. Thereafter the cervix thins out and dilates progressively (Fig. 6.12).

As the cervix and lower segment thin out, the fetal head descends further into the pelvis. This is made easier by moulding of the fetal skull, a process entailing approximation and overlapping of the fetal skull bones, with subsequent diminution of presenting diameters (of more than 1 cm in extreme cases). The maternal pelvis can also mould to some extent, thereby increasing pelvic capacity, particularly in the lower pelvis. This is encouraged by the general relaxation of joints and ligaments in pregnancy and is brought about by the woman adopting a squatting or pushing position. The lower pelvis opens up like the petals of a tulip with increases of pelvic outlet diameters of 1 cm or more.

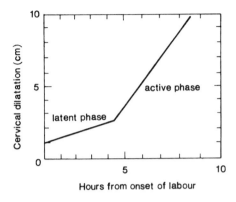

Fig. 6.11   Normal progress of cervical dilatation in labour.

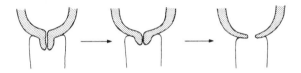

Fig. 6.12   Effacement of the cervix.

Second stage of labour

When the cervix is fully dilated, descent of the fetal head is more rapid. The mother experiences the urge to bear down (a reflex depending on sensory nerve endings on the pelvic floor and perineum). In the second stage the pelvic floor muscles and fascia surrounding the vagina are progressively dilated by the fetal head. For most women, and primigravidae especially, this entails a lot of hard work.

Contractions usually last over 1 minute at this stage and occur every 2 minutes. Placental blood flow is effectively stopped by contractions in late first stage and second stage and fetal blood oxygen levels and pH tend to fall progressively, making a prolonged second stage undesirable.

Third stage of labour

After the delivery of the baby the uterus continues to contract without any appreciable delay. With the first strong contraction the placenta separates from the uterine wall (if it has not already done so during the final expulsion of the baby) by a shearing effect at the level of the decidua spongiosa. The placenta is then gradually expelled from the uterus into the vagina. The placental bed vessels are constricted by the contracted myometrium. Uterine haemostasis is primarily due to this constriction, and the vessels only thrombose as a secondary phenomenon. Amniotic fluid at term is strongly thromboplastic and may have a role in triggering thrombosis in placental bed vessels following separation of the placenta. Clotting disorders will not usually produce excessive uterine blood loss as long as the uterus can contract efficiently and is undamaged.

Uterine contraction in the third stage returns approximately 500 ml of blood from the uterine vasculature into the general circulation, with temporary increase in venous return and central venous pressure. These changes are accentuated by the use of oxytocic drugs, and may be of importance in patients with serious cardiac disease. Ergometrine (but not oxytocin) also produces a degree of peripheral vasoconstriction with a rise in blood pressure of 10–20 mmHg in most patients, and a much larger rise in the occasional patient. For this reason ergometrine is better avoided in patients with serious hypertension.

LACTATION

During pregnancy the breasts increase substantially in size (average increase in volume is 250 ml per breast). Oestrogen produces growth of the duct system particularly and progesterone stimulates acinar growth. Prolactin, hPL, insulin, cortisol and thyroxine have also been shown experimentally to be necessary for optimal breast development. Prolactin is the stimulus to lactation but the effect of the high levels of prolactin produced in pregnancy is inhibited until delivery by the high oestrogen levels. Following delivery, rapidly falling oestrogen levels allow the onset of lactation. Suckling stimulates further release of prolactin and also stimulates the release of oxytocin which causes contraction of the myoepithelial cells surrounding the alveoli and 'let down' of the milk to the nipple. Basal prolactin levels gradually fall over the course of a few weeks and lactation is maintained by the episodic release of prolactin in response to suckling. Ovarian function is inhibited while high basal levels of prolactin are maintained, but ovulation may resume before lactation ceases, so that continued breast-feeding is not a reliable means of contraception.

FURTHER READING

Hillier, S.G., Kitchener, H.C., Neilson, J.P. (eds) (1996) *Scientific Essentials of Reproductive Medicine*. W.B. Saunders, London.
Hytten, F.E. and Chamberlain, G. (eds) (1980) *Clinical Physiology in Obstetrics*. Blackwell, Oxford.
Philipp, E.E., Barnes, J. and Newton, M. (1986) *Scientific Foundations of Obstetrics and Gynaecology*. Heinemann Medical Books, London.

7

Antenatal care

It has been estimated that at the time of Shakespeare 25 women died per every 1000 births in the City of London. The figure for England and Wales in 1890 was 6.5 per 1000 and in 1985–87 there were 8.5 deaths directly due to pregnancy and childbirth per 100 000 total births (see Chapter 10). Perinatal mortality shows the same trend in all developed countries, although their positions in the 'league table' are shifting; at the moment the UK is sliding down the table slightly, possibly due to the restrictions which recurrent financial crises have imposed on the maternity services. Much of this reduced loss of human life is due to generally improving social conditions and to advances in medicine such as blood transfusion and anti-biotics. However, there is no doubt that a significant proportion of maternal and perinatal mortality is directly related to the quality of obstetric care. If present trends continue, the obstetric practice of the next generation of general practitioners will, in most cases, be limited to a share of antenatal and postnatal care. There are many complications peculiar to pregnancy; in addition, pregnancy affects and is affected by numerous incidental diseases. A sound knowledge of the principles of antenatal care is, therefore, of importance to doctors in most branches of medicine. The fact that such knowledge is not universal, even in the UK, is emphasized by the presence of substandard care in the majority of the deaths reviewed in the *Maternal Mortality Report* for 1991–93, many of these representing failure of antenatal care.

The concept of antenatal care has a long and fascinating history, and although Ballantyne is usually credited with its initiation by his publication in 1901 of a *Plea for Pro-maternity Hospital*, its true origins probably go back much further, in particular to establishments that were primarily concerned with the provision of shelter for the unfortunate women of those days who were illegitimately pregnant. A classic example of such a hospital is the Hôtel Dieu in Paris, and an account of its work was published in 1788. Equal concern for the fetus as for the mother is a very recent development in obstetrics, now that caesarean section provides a safe alternative for the mother to the difficult and dangerous operative vaginal delivery of former times. The scope of antenatal care, and also its success in preventing mortality and morbidity has increased enormously in the last 10–20 years with the introduction of scanning techniques and prenatal diagnostic measures in particular. The ability to predict problems affecting the neonate is much greater, and this had led to much closer cooperation with neonatal paediatricians and the development of the concept of perinatal medicine.

OBJECTIVES OF ANTENATAL CARE

1 To prevent or detect and treat any abnormalities which threaten the life or well-being of the mother or fetus, by regular assessment throughout pregnancy.
2 To prepare her physically for the demands of labour and motherhood, by advice on diet, exercise and rest, with dietary supplements and drug treatment as necessary.
3 To prepare her psychologically and emotionally for child-bearing, developing her confidence in herself and her attendants by personal contact, mothercraft classes and relaxation techniques.
4 To provide opportunities for general health screening; for instance pregnancy provides an excellent chance to take cervical cytology smears from those most at risk (who are also those least likely to turn up to other cervical smear clinics).

Of these objectives, the avoidance of the considerable physical risk of pregnancy is clearly the most important. It is, however, essential not to lose sight of the other points, and the attainment of all these objectives together should not be impossible.

Place of delivery

There can be no doubt that the safest place for a woman to be delivered is a fully equipped modern maternity unit. The lower birth rate has meant that this is now possible for virtually all women, whereas 20 years ago patients had to be selected for hospital confinement on the basis of risk factors. General practitioner units attached to major hospitals share these advantages as well as allowing family–doctor relationships to flourish. Isolated general practitioner units, however, do not have the facilities to cope with serious emergencies, and their place is now limited to a few geographically isolated areas. When the confinement is normal and the mother and baby fit, early discharge home has much to recommend it, combining minimal disturbance of family life with maximum safety. When everything is normal, home confinement can be very satisfying for the family, but it is quite impossible to predict all abnormalities and home confinement entails small risks to the mother and fetus, even in cases which appear completely normal. Some women will choose to accept this slight increase in risk in exchange for the emotional benefits of avoiding hospital admission.

Shared antenatal care

Antenatal care can with advantage be shared between the hospital clinic and general practitioner working with the community midwife in cases where there are no serious complications (such as diabetes) which would demand constant hospital attendance. With shared care the patient usually has the minimum of travelling while still having access to the expertise and specialized equipment of the hospital, and the general practitioner is able to keep close contact with patients. Clearly the success of the scheme depends on there being a good working relationship between consultant and general practitioner and on there being adequate communication between the two. This is usually achieved with a personal card (cooperation card), or an entire set of notes, which the woman herself carries, and on which all important details of the antenatal care are recorded. She would normally be seen at the hospital for booking early in the pregnancy and then for review on one or more occasions between 32 weeks and term.

Midwife antenatal care

In selected low-risk cases antenatal care throughout the pregnancy can be provided by a midwife or a team of midwives. For this to work satisfactorily, there must be clear agreement between community and hospital midwifery services and the local obstetricians on criteria for acceptance for midwife care, access to back-up services such as ultrasound and arrangements for transfer of cases if complications arise.

Normal antenatal care

The normal pattern of antenatal care takes account of the tendency for the major complications of pregnancy (pre-eclampsia, placental failure and antepartum haemorrhage) to occur with increasing frequency as term approaches. Thus the woman is seen monthly until 28 weeks, fortnightly until 36 weeks and then weekly until delivered. Abnormalities in the patient's history or problems developing during the pregnancy may require modification of this scheme with more frequent visits. Some units are also separating out low-risk women for less frequent visits, particularly in the middle months of pregnancy.

Booking clinic

Ideally the woman should attend between 10 and 12 weeks of pregnancy as this allows sufficient time for organizing such measures as insertion of a cervical suture or chorionic villus sampling (CVS) should these be necessary. A full medical and family history is taken and also a detailed obstetric history. In the medical history heart disease, renal disease, tuberculosis, diabetes, gynaecological operations, drug usage and psychiatric illness are particularly important. Diabetes, tuberculosis and inheritable diseases are of particular consequence in the family history. The obstetric history is of greatest importance because many obstetric problems tend to recur in subsequent pregnancies and may be prevented if anticipated.

A general physical examination is carried out, including estimations of weight and blood pressure and urinalysis, and examination of cardiovascular and respiratory systems and the breasts. Abdominal and pelvic examinations may be carried out at this visit in order to assess the size of the uterus and to exclude any other abnormal masses. If an early pregnancy ultrasound scan is to be carried out then a pelvic examination may well be omitted. It is important to detect an ovarian cyst if present as this is quite likely to undergo torsion or suffer some other complication during the course of pregnancy (see Chapter 24). A speculum examination may also be done and a cervical smear taken, together with appropriate bacteriological swabs should any discharge be present. It is generally inappropriate to attempt to assess pelvic capacity at this stage of pregnancy as it is unpleasant for the patient and also less accurate than an assessment made in late pregnancy when there is a fetal head to act as a yardstick. Pelvic examination properly carried out is not a cause of abortion, but in cases of recurrent abortion it may worry the patient and should only be carried out for positive indications.

The following tests are carried out routinely at the booking clinic:

1 Haemoglobin estimation.
2 ABO and rhesus grouping.
3 Antibody screening of rhesus-negative patients.
4 Serological tests for syphilis Venereal Disease Research Laboratory (VDRL) or equivalent.

5 Rubella antibody titres. (Ninety per cent or more of women will be shown to be immune to rubella and consequently not at risk if exposed to rubella during pregnancy. The remaining patients will need to be investigated further if later exposed to rubella and in any case are usually offered vaccination following the pregnancy.)
6 Haemoglobin electrophoresis to look for haemoglobinopathies in Afro-Caribbean women and thalassaemia in those of Mediterranean descent.
7 A midstream urine culture or dip slide for bacteriuria.
8 Cervical cytology smear, if this has not been done within the previous 5 years.
9 Hepatitis and human immunodeficiency virus (HIV) screening should be offered to high-risk patients.

Maturity assessment

At the first visit a special effort should be made to establish maturity. The expected date of delivery (EDD) is calculated by adding 9 months and 7 days to the date of the first day of the last menstrual period (LMP), e.g. LMP 17.3.96 gives EDD 24.12.96. A note should also be made of:

1 How certain she is of the LMP.
2 Whether her cycle is regular.
3 Whether she was on oral contraceptives before LMP.

Uterine size is estimated critically to see whether it agrees with maturity calculated from the LMP. Many units arrange an ultrasound scan for all patients but it is particularly important if there appears to be any doubt about maturity. It is vital that a reliable EDD is arrived at in the first half of pregnancy to enable subsequent growth retardation to be detected (see p. 131). Early-pregnancy scanning will provide reliable dating where this service is available.

Investigations at subsequent visits

1 Normality screening. Most units now offer biochemical screening for spina bifida and Down's syndrome on a single blood sample taken at 16–18 weeks and tested for α-fetoprotein (AFP), human chorionic gonadotrophin (hCG) and possibly oestriol or other Down's markers. In addition most units now offer detailed anomaly scanning at 18 weeks (see p. 108)
2 Haemoglobin estimation. This is usually repeated at least twice during the pregnancy, at about 28 and 34 weeks.
3 Rhesus antibodies are checked in susceptible patients on two further occasions, usually at 28 and 34 weeks.

Clinical examination at subsequent visits

At each visit it is normal to test the urine for protein and glucose, measure blood pressure, look for signs of oedema and examine the abdomen.

The purpose of the abdominal palpation changes during pregnancy as it becomes possible to detect different features and as different abnormalities become important. The key points looked for are summarized here:

Uterine size

Throughout pregnancy one is concerned to measure the size of the uterus. If this is greater than expected the following possibilities should be considered:

1 Wrong dates.
2 Multiple pregnancy.
3 Hydatidiform mole (in first half of pregnancy).
4 Uterine fibroids.
5 Full bladder or rectum (in early pregnancy).
6 Polyhydramnios – excess amniotic fluid (often associated with fetal abnormality).

If the uterus is small for dates the possible explanations are:

1 Wrong dates.
2 Placental insufficiency.
3 Fetal abnormalities.

The size of the uterus should not simply be gauged by the fundal height. An attempt should also be made to assess the total volume of the uterus, or the actual size of the fetus in late pregnancy.

Fetal life

Fetal heart sounds may be heard with a stethoscope from about 22 weeks but can be detected with a Doppler ultrasound machine from 10 or 12 weeks of pregnancy and fetal heart movement may be detected by ultrasound from about 6 weeks. Fetal movements are usually first felt (quickening) by the primigravid patient between 18 and 22 weeks and by the multigravid patient between 16 and 18 weeks, although there is wide variation.

Fetal presentation

The presentation of a fetus refers to the part of the fetus (the presenting part) which is situated in or immediately over the maternal pelvis. Presentation is very variable until 30 weeks, but thereafter it would normally be the head (cephalic presentation), and it becomes important to detect breech presentation from 32 weeks onwards.

Fetal lie

The lie of a fetus refers to the direction of its long axis and is longitudinal, oblique or transverse. With a longitudinal lie the presenting part is either in or centrally above the pelvis. With an oblique lie the presenting part is in one or other iliac fossa, whereas with a transverse lie the long axis of the baby is directly transverse, with the baby's head and breech usually lying above the iliac crests. A baby which has its head in the pelvis and the breech under one costal margin would be considered to be lying longitudinally, in spite of having its spine in a slightly oblique position. It is not usually possible to detect fetal parts until about 22 weeks, and the fetal lie only becomes clearly definable from about 28 weeks. From 32 weeks the lie should normally be longitudinal and departures from this may merit investigation (see p. 126).

Multiple pregnancy

This may be suspected because of increased size of the uterus from 12 or 16 weeks, but by palpating multiple fetal parts it becomes detectable from about 28 weeks. With modern ultrasound scanning it has become extremely rare to miss multiple pregnancy.

Fetal abnormality

Fetal abnormalities that are not detected by early pregnancy screening may be picked up because of their associated polyhydramnios from 26 or 28 weeks onwards and sometimes because of the small size or abnormal feel of the fetus (for instance, difficulty in feeling a head) from 30 weeks onwards.

Engagement of the fetal head

Methods of assessing engagement are described on p. 47–9 and the implications of non-engagement are discussed on p. 47–9. It only becomes important in the last weeks of pregnancy.

Position of the fetal back

Apart from the detection of the occipitoposterior position, this has no practical value but interests mothers, midwives and occasionally examiners.

Advice in pregnancy

An important part of antenatal care is the advice given by the doctor and midwife on the subjects below. Booklets are widely available giving common-sense advice in terms that most patients will understand, and antenatal classes are organized at most hospital and some community clinics and by organizations such as the National Childbirth Trust (NCT). Nevertheless, the doctor should consider it part of his or her responsibility to talk to the patient on these subjects.

Diet

The pregnant woman should eat a well-balanced diet containing plenty of protein (meat, fish, cheese), calcium (milk) and fruit and vegetables to provide vitamins and to combat the tendency to constipation. She does not need to eat large extra quantities of carbohydrate foods. In the UK milk and vitamins are provided at no charge during pregnancy for women on income support.

Alcohol

Heavy alcohol consumption in pregnancy carries a high risk of fetal abnormality or growth retardation and mental retardation (the fetal alcohol syndrome). The evidence that modest alcohol consumption is harmful is equivocal but the soundest advice is to avoid all alcohol in pregnancy.

Smoking

Smoking in pregnancy is positively harmful, producing increased perinatal mortality (5 per 1000 excess, in the 1958 *Perinatal Mortality Survey*), growth retardation and diminished intelligence of surviving children. A number of studies have shown increased risks of childhood leukaemia associated with smoking in pregnancy. Strong efforts should be made to persuade the woman to give up smoking completely. As long as she does so in the first half of pregnancy the risk appears to revert to normal.

Work

Most women are able to work in their normal jobs during pregnancy until 28 weeks, although complications such as threatened abortion or hypertension may make this inadvisable. Some women work beyond 32 weeks and, as long as they remain well, we see no objection to this.

Rest and exercise

The pregnant woman should not overtire herself at any stage of pregnancy, but can continue to take a moderate amount of exercise throughout. Broadly she can continue to do whatever exercise she was enjoying before conceiving but is likely to need to slow down progressively through pregnancy. Walking, swimming and cycling can be encouraged, but the more violent forms of exercise should be discouraged, particularly in the later months. Water ski-ing (because of forceful entry of water into the vagina and possibly uterus) can be lethal during pregnancy. In the last trimester an extra few hours of rest in the day is beneficial.

Sex

Normal sexual relations may be continued throughout pregnancy unless complications (threatened abortion, antepartum haemorrhage) lead the doctor specifically to advise against it. It is no longer thought necessary to give up sex 4 weeks before delivery to avoid introducing bacteria into the vagina, but some couples give up at this stage anyway because of the mechanical problems involved.

Travel

Pregnant women should be able to drive throughout pregnancy as long as they are generally well. Seat belts should be worn, with the diagonal and lap straps above and below the 'bump'. Air travel in modern aircraft should be safe throughout pregnancy, but airlines will refuse to carry pregnant women in the later weeks of pregnancy because of the problems produced by a mid-air premature labour.

Dental care

Some degree of gingivitis occurs in about 50% of pregnant women, predisposing to caries. For this reason and as a general screening measure every pregnant woman should attend a dentist in pregnancy. Dental care is free during pregnancy and for 12 months afterwards.

Financial benefits

Those who have been in full-time work for 2 years or part-time work for 5 years should be eligible for statutory maternity pay, which consists of 90% of average weekly earnings for 6 weeks and then £52.50 weekly (rates as at March 1996). Otherwise the pregnant woman is entitled to an allowance of between £45.55 and £52.50 per week (rates as at March 1996) from 29 weeks for 18 weeks, as long as she has paid full National Insurance contributions for at least 26 weeks in the previous year. Some women also qualify for an earnings-related supplement. Some employers offer their own form of additional maternity allowance, or the woman may be able to take maternity leave with full pay if she intends to return to her work following delivery.

Those on income support, family credit or disability working allowance may be eligible for maternity payment (£100 per baby) from the social fund.

Pregnancy, labour and delivery

Most women are very interested in what is happening to their bodies during pregnancy, and what will happen to them during labour, what methods of pain relief are available and so on. A knowledge of these things allows the woman to face her pregnancy with greater confidence. Classes are organized in most centres to impart this type of information and also items such as mothercraft and relaxation techniques. The NCT also offers such classes in most large centres.

Mothercraft

It is helpful for the woman to be taught in advance the rudiments of mothercraft, and also to have sensible guidance about the sort of equipment and clothes she needs to buy for the baby.

Relaxation techniques

A number of relaxation techniques are used in the UK and other countries to diminish the pain or discomfort of labour. There can be no doubt that these techniques, if expertly taught, can be of great help to many of those who would have had fairly straightforward deliveries anyway. They cannot, however, overcome all mechanical problems, and there is a danger that some women will have a sense of personal failure to add to the experience of, say, a forceps delivery, if the impression is given that with these methods all women can expect normal pain-free deliveries.

Drugs in pregnancy

The thalidomide disaster has made the public well aware of the potential for drugs to produce fetal abnormalities. It has also led to the expectation that the medical profession will know which drugs are safe, and to the introduction of legislation allowing legal action to be taken on behalf of a child whose development *in utero* was impaired by drugs (or other medical action).

In general all drugs should be avoided if possible during the phase of organogenesis (roughly the first trimester; see p. 85). Otherwise only drugs known to be safe should be used, and if there is doubt the advice of a pharmacist should be sought. It is not possible to list all drugs problems here but some of the main ones are outlined.

Antiemetics

No adverse reactions are known to the preparations in common use such as Avomine, but a 1980 court decision in the USA accepted the possibility of Debendox being a rare cause of fetal abnormality. Debendox was previously the most widely used antiemetic in pregnancy. The metabolic disturbance associated with frequent vomiting seems a much more likely cause of fetal abnormality than any of the commonly used antiemetic drugs.

Antibiotics

Penicillins and cephalosporins are safe throughout pregnancy. Sulphonamides interfere with the bile-conjugating mechanism of the neonate and should be avoided if delivery is imminent. Tetracyclines should not be used at all in pregnancy as they stain developing bone and teeth in the fetus and have occasionally produced liver failure in the mother if given intramuscularly. Streptomycin can cause fetal eighth nerve damage. Trimethoprim is safe after the first trimester (but the sulphonamide warning above applies to the usual sulphonamide–trimethoprim combinations).

Hormones and related substances

Progestogens may affect fetal liver function and progestogens of the nortestosterone family (e.g. norethisterone, Primolut N) can cause masculinization of the female fetus. Stilboestrol has been linked to subsequent development of vaginal carcinoma and adenosis in teenagers whose mothers received this drug in pregnancy. Antithyroid drugs in excess can produce cretinism. Corticosteroids generally produce no overt problem, but have been linked with a slight increase in the incidence of cleft palate, and in animals produce some reduction in brain cell division. In very high doses they can initiate labour.

Anticoagulants

Heparin does not cross the placenta and has no fetal effects, although prolonged use has been shown to produce bone density loss in the mother. Oral anticoagulants do cross the placenta and have been associated with an increased abortion rate in the first trimester, and with fetal cerebral haemorrhage when given within a few days of vaginal delivery.

Sedatives

Phenothiazines, antihistamines and diazepam appear to be safe, but may cause neonatal depression.

Hypotensives

Methyldopa, hydralazine, labetalol and nifedipine can be used throughout pregnancy. β-Blockers in high dose may initiate premature labour.

Diuretics

Thiazide diuretics should not be used in pregnancy as they have several serious potential side-effects, including neonatal thrombocytopenia.

Cytotoxic drugs

Cancer chemotherapy drugs produce embryonic death or malformation when given in early pregnancy and are damaging to the fetus at any stage. Such treatment would usually either be accompanied by therapeutic abortion or delayed until after delivery.

Radiology in pregnancy

It is now clear that X-ray examination of the pregnant woman involves some risk to the fetus. The work of Dr Alice Stewart in Oxford demonstrated an excess of leukaemia or other malignant disease in childhood for those irradiated *in utero*. The magnitude of this risk is of the order of 1 in 30 000 for each abdominal film taken in the second or third trimester and some seven times higher in the first trimester. There is also probably a risk of genetic damage for future generations of comparable order. The recognition of these risks has inhibited the free use of radiology in pregnancy. The risks are, however, very small compared with the current perinatal mortality risk (about 6 per 1000; 1996), and if there is a sound clinical indication for an X-ray in pregnancy the benefit is likely to exceed the risk.

Ultrasound in the dose and frequency range employed diagnostically has not been found to produce any adverse effects in extensive studies.

While the number of X-rays done in pregnancy has dwindled, the number of ultrasound scans has increased enormously. Most major obstetric units now plan at least one scan for every patient with the following benefits:

1 Accurate dating of the pregnancy.
2 Early detection of multiple pregnancy.
3 Placental localization.
4 Detection of fetal abnormalities.

The first three objectives can be obtained by medical or nursing staff or radiographers with very little training. More extensive training and experience and more sophisticated equipment are needed to perform full anomaly scans and rule out such things as abnormalities of the heart and kidneys.

ANTENATAL COMPLICATIONS OF PREGNANCY

Miscarriage

This is dealt with in Chapter 13, but it is worth reminding the reader that patients with a history of middle-trimester miscarriage or of vaginal termination (particularly if past 10 weeks) should be considered for a cervical suture. This is best inserted at around 14 weeks under a general anaesthetic. A single suture of 5 mm nylon tape is inserted in a subserosal plane as high as possible around the substance of the cervix. The patient is usually kept in bed for a day afterwards to discourage abortion following the procedure (extremely rare). The suture is removed at 38 weeks, or sooner if labour occurs. If this is not done there is a risk of the cervix tearing or of the uterus rupturing in strong labour. It is usually possible to remove the stitch without a general anaesthetic.

Nausea and vomiting in pregnancy

Nausea is commonly experienced in early pregnancy, especially between 7 and 12 weeks. It is usually most marked in the morning and abates during the day. Simple dietary measures (such as dry biscuits or toast in bed in the morning, and avoiding fatty foods) allow most women to cope with the nausea without serious vomiting. However, a few patients vomit repeatedly and become ketotic, dehydrated and lose weight. This is called hyperemesis. In previous centuries when there was no effective treatment, such patients would quite probably die from the associated biochemical disturbance or liver failure. (This was the fate of Charlotte Brontë.) Effective treatment is now available, but the incidence of severe vomiting in early pregnancy is also much reduced, underlining the importance of psychological factors in its aetiology.

Patients with vomiting or marked nausea should be treated with antiemetics. A suitable preparation is Avomine tabs 1 t.d.s. If the vomiting gets worse in spite of these measures the patient should be admitted to hospital for intravenous therapy with saline or glucose saline and correction of any other demonstrable electrolyte imbalance. The nausea and vomiting are always controlled by intravenous therapy.

It is a wise psychological move to continue the therapy for at least a day longer than the patient feels is necessary. The patient can usually then be managed satisfactorily with oral antiemetics. Hyperemesis is more common with hydatidiform mole and multiple pregnancy and these should be looked for in every case.

Nausea and vomiting are also sometimes a problem in late pregnancy. It is then often associated with heartburn and reflux oesophagitis. Antacids (mist. mag. trisil. 10 ml or Gaviscon as required) will often control both the heartburn and nausea. Sometimes the symptoms are due to reflux of bile salts as a result of pyloric relaxation and do not respond to any treatment. Vomiting may also be associated with urinary tract infection, and rare incidental causes such as gut or cerebral tumours should be considered in intractable cases.

Fetal abnormalities

During the decade to 1990 the perinatal mortality halved in most major units in this country. A large part of this reduction is attributable to the progressive improvement in our ability to detect fetal abnormalities during the first half of pregnancy when termination may be offered. Some couples are clearly at increased risk because of history or age but all couples have some risk, whatever their age and regardless of history. Routine screening measures now pick up the majority of significant abnormalities in low-risk couples and the scope for helping high-risk couples is considerable and increasing.

Routine screening

1 A detailed anomaly scan at 18 weeks will pick up a high proportion of anatomical abnormalities such as neural tube defects, heart abnormalities, gut atresia, exomphalos, polycystic kidney, and may also detect markers of a number of chromosomal abnormalities.
2 Biochemical screening for spina bifida and Down's syndrome is now widely available. Spina bifida screening with serum AFP has been in use for many years but has been largely supplanted by detailed ultrasound scanning. Measurement of AFP, together with hCG, or hCG and oestriol at 16 weeks, gives a good prediction of the woman's individual risk for Down's syndrome. Those with a high risk (worse than 1 : 300, in Bristol) may then be offered amniocentesis. If offered to all women, this test detects about three-quarters of all Down's fetuses, with some other trisomies (Edwards' and Patau's syndrome).

Further screening tests suitable for all women will no doubt be developed in due course. Apart from this we depend on offering specific tests to those at high risk of particular abnormalities.

At-risk cases

Patients at risk of abnormalities are:

1 Those who have had an abnormal child in a previous pregnancy. (This does not include first-trimester miscarriage, virtually all of which are abnormal, as these do not appreciably affect the patient's chances of a subsequent normal term pregnancy.)
2 Patients in their late 30s onwards who are at increased risk of trisomies, particularly Down's syndrome. The risk of producing a Down's baby is about 1 : 1000 at age 25, about 1 : 100 at age 40 and 1 : 40 at age 45.
3 Those with a family history of inheritable disorders.

Ideally all at-risk patients should have received genetic counselling before the pregnancy and will have a clear idea of the risk of producing a fetal abnormality in this pregnancy, and also of the possibilities of early-pregnancy diagnosis of the abnormality concerned. Where appropriate these patients should be offered chorionic villus sampling or amniocentesis.

Chorionic villus sampling

CVS involves removing a small portion of placental tissue through a wide-bore needle inserted with ultrasound control either through the abdomen or the cervical canal. Its advantage is that it can be done between 10 and 12 weeks and give an answer within 2 days, because the biopsy material is actively growing. The main disadvantage is that it is associated with a miscarriage risk of around 2–5%.

Amniocentesis

Amniocentesis involves the insertion of a fine needle into the amniotic cavity to extract 10 ml of liquor. The exfoliated cells in the fluid can be made to grow in culture and can then be used for chromosome preparation. It is not generally performed before 16 weeks but carries a miscarriage risk of only 1 : 200. CVS has clear advantages in high-risk situations where any termination can still be performed vaginally, but in low-risk situations the low miscarriage risk of amniocentesis may be considered to be more important.

Scope of amniocentesis or CVS

1 *Chromosomal abnormalities*: After culture of amniotic fluid cells trisomies are detected and also other abnormalities such as Klinefelter's syndrome and translocations.
2 *Sex-linked conditions* (such as haemophilia and Duchenne muscular dystrophy): The sex of the fetus is fairly readily determined, thus revealing the risk of sex-linked conditions (usually no risk for females and 1 : 2 for males).
3 *Biochemical abnormalities*: (e.g. Niemann–Pick and Tay–Sachs disease). A number of biochemical abnormalities are detectable by appropriate tests on the cultured cells. The scope of these tests is expanding steadily and up-to-date information must be sought in such cases.
4 *Genetic disorders*: An increasing number of genetic disorders (e.g. cystic fibrosis) are directly detectable by DNA analysis.

Fetoscopy

It is possible to insert a small endoscope through the abdominal wall and through the uterine wall into the amniotic cavity to visualize the fetus directly in early pregnancy, and to obtain fetal blood from the placental surface. The risks of this procedure are appreciably greater than for amniocentesis, and as the indications are few it should only be performed in very few hospitals where experience will be concentrated. Its main application was for the detection of homozygous sickle-cell disease or thalassaemia. High-quality ultrasound is now tending to render fetoscopy unnecessary.

Cordocentesis

This involves the direct needling of the umbilical cord under ultrasound control. Fetal blood is thus obtained and can be tested for thalassaemia and other defects. The risk is less than for fetoscopy and the technique has largely replaced fetoscopy.

Fetal abnormalities in later pregnancy

A fetal abnormality should be suspected in the following situations:

1 Polyhydramnios.
2 Where the uterus is small-for-dates.
3 When the fetus feels abnormal, particularly if there is difficulty feeling a head.

If there is serious suspicion of fetal abnormality an ultrasound examination should be done. Biochemical tests are not generally helpful in establishing fetal abnormality in late pregnancy.

Where major fetal abnormalities are detected the obstetrician will normally elect to induce labour. Fetal abnormalities may present mechanical difficulties in labour, the most common problem being disproportion with a hydrocephalic fetus. In such instances the enlarged fetal head may have to be decompressed by introducing a catheter through the associated spina bifida with a breech presentation or by directly draining the head with a wide-bore needle. Fetuses with significant hydrocephalus always have grossly damaged brains and should not be considered salvageable. Such abnormalities would not normally escape a detailed 18-week anomaly scan but these scans are not universally available in this country, and only rarely available in the Third World.

Genetic counselling

Patients who have just had an abnormal fetus or who are at risk for other reasons should be offered counselling by specialist genetic counsellors who are available in most areas. Where such a service is not available an interested obstetrician can give appropriate advice. The essential basis for genetic counselling is an accurate diagnosis of the type of abnormality that has already occurred; therefore all abnormal fetuses should be subjected to postmortem examination.

For the most common major central nervous system abnormalities (anencephaly, spina bifida and hydrocephalus) the risk of recurrence is about 1 : 30, rising to 1 : 10 if two previous children have been affected. Folic acid taken before conception until 12 weeks of pregnancy will greatly reduce these risks. It is now advised that all women trying for a pregnancy should take folic acid 0.4 mg daily and any woman with a previous child with a neural tube defect should take 5 mg daily.

Multiple pregnancy

In the UK the incidence of twins is about 1 : 80, the incidence of triplets about $1 : 80^2$, of quadruplets $1 : 80^3$ and so on. The practice of induction of ovulation with gonadotrophins and with assisted reproduction techniques such as *in vitro* fertilization produces a significantly increased chance of multiple pregnancy, particularly of the high multiple pregnancies in association with gonadotrophin induction (see Chapter 12). The incidence of multiple pregnancy varies in other populations, being higher, for instance, in Nigerians and lower in the Chinese.

Twins may develop from the same ovum (then called uniovular, monozygotic or identical) or from two ova fertilized at the same time (binovular, dizygotic or non-identical). If they derive from the same ovum there is a possibility that they share the same placenta, chorion and amnion depending on the stage at which division occurs. Those sharing the same amnion are floating in the same amniotic sac and stand a great risk of cord entanglement. This situation is fortunately very rare, but it is relatively common to find identical twins sharing the same chorion. Non-identical twins never share the amnion, chorion or placenta, although fusion of two separate placentae is common. Examination of the placenta and membranes only gives a certain guide to the zygosity of twins of the same sex when the membranes are monochorionic (Fig. 7.1).

Some mixing of the placental circulation is also common with identical twins sharing the same placenta and this will occasionally lead to unequal blood flow, with one infant becoming plethoric and the other grossly anaemic and undernourished, sometimes dying *in utero*. There is also the risk of exsanguination of the second twin during delivery if the cord of the first twin is allowed to bleed.

Higher multiple pregnancies are usually derived from multiple ovulation, but sometimes one or more of the siblings is identical.

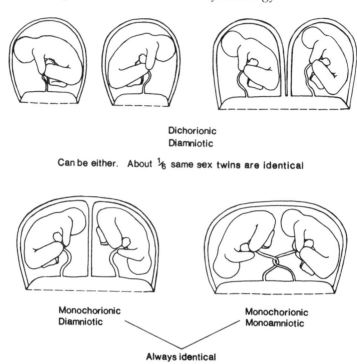

Dichorionic
Diamniotic

Can be either.   About ⅛ same sex twins are identical

Monochorionic   Monochorionic
Diamniotic   Monoamniotic

Always identical

Fig. 7.1   Placental arrangements in twin pregnancy.

Diagnosis

Very few multiple pregnancies should be missed by modern ultra-sound scanning, but doctors will inevitably find themselves some-times looking after patients who have not been scanned. For this reason (and to pass your exams!) it is still important to recognize the clinical features of multiple pregnancy.

There should be increased suspicion of multiple pregnancy when there is a family history of twins, a history of induced ovulation or of hyperemesis, although usually none of these factors is present. Clinical signs are more helpful, and the most important of these is the finding of increased uterine size or growth rate. The palpation of multiple fetal parts is also a fairly reliable sign later in pregnancy. Multiple pregnancy can rarely be diagnosed with certainty on the basis of clinical signs alone, and whenever it is suspected an ultra-sound scan should be arranged.

Complications of multiple pregnancy

Almost every complication of pregnancy is more common with twins and the risks increase with higher numbers of fetuses. Prematurity is so common that multiple pregnancy accounts for 15% of all premature deliveries. Placental insufficiency is another serious hazard; twins tend to be small-for-dates and triplets more so. The 1958 *Perinatal Mortality Survey* showed that 3.5% of all twins died of intrauterine asphyxia (mostly associated with placental failure). Because of greater requirements, deficiencies of iron, calcium and folic acid are common unless supplements are given. Acute pyelonephritis, pre-eclampsia, polyhydramnios and mal-presentation are also more common. The greater placental area means that placenta praevia is more likely. The minor problems of pregnancy such as backache, piles, varicose veins and dyspepsia are more common and troublesome.

Management

The most important part of management is the early diagnosis of multiple pregnancy. Iron and folic acid supplements should be given and frequent checks made on haemoglobin levels. The patient should be advised to make special efforts to get adequate rest and will normally be seen more frequently at the antenatal clinic. Some units routinely admit such patients between 28 and 32 weeks for hospital bed rest in the hope of reducing the incidence of pre-maturity, but there is no evidence that this is effective. Serial ultra-sound scanning from 28 weeks allows the early detection of growth retardation. Early admission in cases of suspected premature labour may allow prolongation of the pregnancy (see p. 129). Minor departures from normality (particularly in blood pressure) will be treated seriously and usually result in hospital admission. Many obstetricians feel that twins should not be allowed to go past 38 weeks because of the danger of placental insufficiency and all are agreed that they should not go past term. The patient should, of course, be booked for delivery in a specialist obstetric unit because of the increased likelihood of intrapartum difficulties (see Chapter 8).

Breech presentation

Breech presentation is abnormal after 32 weeks. About 25% of fetuses present by the breech at 30 weeks but most undergo sponta-neous version, leaving only about 2% as breech presentations by 36 weeks. The main aetiological factors in persistent breech presenta-tion are as follows:

1 Fetal legs extended at the knees.
2 Multiple pregnancy.
3 Uterine abnormalities.
4 Fetal abnormalities, particularly hydrocephalus and spina bifida.
5 Polyhydramnios.
6 Oligohydramnios.

The terms used to describe the various positions of the fetal legs are illustrated in Figure 7.2. The extended breech is especially common in the primigravida and is associated with a somewhat longer first and second stage of labour. The flexed breech is associated with a shorter labour but a higher incidence of cord prolapse. The overall risk to the fetus is not appreciably different with either type of breech and there is no justification for treating one form of breech differently from the other. (In the past some obstetricians have been more inclined to do elective caesarean sections for flexed breeches.) The fetus presenting by the breech is at increased risk for two main reasons:

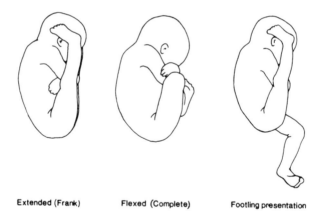

Extended (Frank)   Flexed (Complete)   Footling presentation

Fig. 7.2 Terms used to describe the position of the legs in breech presentation.

1 The fetal head does not pass through the pelvis until the body has been delivered so that no time is allowed for moulding and there is no opportunity to opt for caesarean section if the head proves to be too big to go safely through the pelvis.
2 Intrauterine asphyxia is more common because of cord problems (partly cord prolapse but also cord compression and entanglement as the thighs are compressed against the abdomen in the

first stage of labour), and partly due to cord compression and impairment of placental blood flow in the minutes between the delivery of the umbilicus and the delivery of the head.

Because of the lack of time for moulding to occur an appreciably larger pelvis is needed to deliver a baby safely as a breech than as a vertex. A good-shaped pelvis with an obstetric conjugate of over 11.7 cm is needed to deliver safely the average-sized term baby.

About a third of term breech fetuses have an unusually elongated head shape. The occipitofrontal diameter (OFD) is increased and the biparietal diameter (BPD) decreased, with the OFD/BPD ratio being as much as 1.5 (usually 1.2–1.3). This means that the BPD alone is an unreliable index of head size in breech presentation. The head shape returns to normal within months of delivery.

With modern management methods the perinatal mortality for vaginal breech delivery should be less than 0.5% (for mature normal babies).

Management of breech presentation

After 32 weeks it is essential positively to identify the head at each examination. If this is not possible on abdominal examination, a vaginal examination should be made to feel for a deeply engaged head, and if the head is still not found an ultrasound scan is indicated, as breech presentation is likely in such circumstances. Consideration should be given to attempting external cephalic version on breech presentations at 34 weeks. The risks of external version are:

1 Bruising of the uterus or premature rupture of membranes leading to premature labour.
2 Traumatic detachment of the placenta (abruption).
3 Cord entanglement leading to fetal distress.
4 Fetomaternal bleeding, leading to sensitization of rhesus-negative mothers.

External version is contraindicated in:

1 The hypertensive patient (risk of abruption).
2 Any antepartum haemorrhage.
3 Multiple pregnancy.
4 Previous caesarean section.
5 Any situation where the patient is destined to have a caesarean section in any case.

Provided that case selection is good and no undue force is used, and the patient is not anaesthetized, the overall risk of external version is minimal. However, if the risk of breech delivery continues to lessen, it is likely that the risks of version will exceed the difference between that of breech and vertex delivery and hence version will become unjustifiable.

When a breech presentation persists after 36 weeks and where reasons for caesarean section do not already exist, a pelvic assessment should be made. This is done partly by vaginal examination and partly by lateral X-ray pelvimetry. It is also a help to assess the size of the fetus by ultrasound. If these procedures show that there is ample room for the fetus then a vaginal breech delivery should be aimed for; otherwise an elective caesarean section should be planned.

Some obstetricians advocate induction of labour at 38 weeks for breech presentation to limit the size of the baby, but the place of this is debatable. Breech delivery is described in Chapter 8.

Malpresentations other than breech

Brow and face presentations are rarely diagnosed in the antenatal period and are dealt with in Chapter 8.

Pre-eclampsia and eclampsia

Pre-eclampsia was traditionally defined as a disease process occurring in pregnancy where two out of the three cardinal signs of hypertension, proteinuria and oedema are found. This is not a satisfactory definition, and a better one would be a disease process arising usually in the second half of pregnancy, characterized by hypertension and in all except mild cases by proteinuria and usually, but not always, by oedema. There is still some uncertainty about the aetiology of pre-eclampsia, although recent work has thrown much interesting light on this. There can be no doubt that most of the pathology of pre-eclampsia is due to intravascular coagulation, and there is some suggestion that failure of immune tolerance between the mother and fetus may play some part in its aetiology (see Further reading, below). Pre-eclampsia is more common:

1 In primigravidae.
2 In multiple pregnancy.
3 In cases of essential hypertension.
4 In diabetes.
5 In cases of hydatidiform mole.

This last condition is the only situation in which pre-eclampsia occurs in the first half of pregnancy.

The course of pre-eclampsia varies appreciably from case to case. Some patients maintain a mild elevation of blood pressure over a number of weeks without developing albuminuria, whereas others rapidly develop albuminuria and worsening hypertension and go on to eclampsia if not treated promptly. In general, the earlier the onset of pre-eclampsia in the pregnancy, the more serious is the outlook. Albuminuric pre-eclampsia produces serious impairment of placental function, leading to growth retardation or intrauterine death, and a five- to sixfold increase in perinatal mortality. Non-albuminuric pre-eclampsia only marginally increases the risk to the fetus. Some authorities refer to non-proteinuric pre-eclampsia as pregnancy-induced hypertension or gestational hypertension.

Eclampsia is the occurrence of fits in a pre-eclamptic patient. It is virtually confined to albuminuric cases. The tendency to fit is not clearly related to the degree of hypertension and is probably caused by local cerebral anoxia produced by plugging of small cerebral vessels with fibrin. Eclampsia and severe pre-eclampsia are often associated with:

1 Impaired liver function, sometimes with subcapsular haemorrhage.
2 Impaired renal function, often with oliguria and sometimes anuria.
3 Intravascular coagulation, occasionally sufficient to cause coagulation disorders (disseminated intravascular coagulation, DIC).
4 Impaired lung function.
5 Generalized oedema, including glottal oedema, sometimes leading to difficulty in anaesthetizing such patients.

Eclampsia due to untreated pre-eclampsia was probably the major cause of maternal mortality in the past, but it should now be considered a preventable disease. However, a considerable proportion of perinatal mortality is still attributable to pre-eclampsia. Diagnosis is usually easy as long as the patient is seen regularly and blood-pressure recording and urinalysis are carried out at each visit. Most failures of modern management occur because of failure to act at the first sign of pre-eclampsia rather than failure to elicit these signs.

Management

There is no cure for pre-eclampsia apart from termination of the pregnancy (with the attendant risk to the fetus of premature delivery). The essential part of management of the condition is close observation of the patient to determine whether intervention is necessary in the interests of mother or fetus, or whether the pregnancy can be allowed to proceed. It is usual to admit patients with pre-eclampsia to hospital for this observation. Safe management of significant pre-eclampsia at home is not really possible. There is some evidence that bed rest improves placental function and hence adds to fetal safety, but this is not the primary object of hospital admission. Observation includes frequent blood-pressure measurements, estimation of proteinuria, tests of fetal well-being and, in moderate or severe pre-eclampsia estimation of renal function, particularly by serum uric acid levels, liver function tests, platelet counts and clotting profiles. If there is serious deterioration of the condition of the mother or the fetus, she must be delivered. Hypotensive agents, diuretics and sedatives have no effect on the underlying disease process and indeed may increase the risk to the fetus by reducing placental perfusion. Thus they have little place in the long-term management of pre-eclampsia. They do, however, have an important role in the short-term emergency treatment of eclampsia or severe pre-eclampsia.

Emergency treatment of eclampsia or severe pre-eclampsia

The emergency treatment of eclampsia is similar to that of severe pre-eclampsia once the decision to terminate the pregnancy has been taken. It is essential in the first instance to control the fits or fitting tendency. This is effectively done by intravenous injection of diazepam 10–20 mg, followed by slow intravenous infusion of diazepam 40 mg in 1 litre of glucose saline. Phenytoin or magnesium sulphate offer alternatives. To control the blood pressure, hydralazine 40 mg/l may be added to the same infusion bottle. It has been traditional to nurse the eclamptic patient in a darkened, quiet room but the diazepam–hydralazine regimen makes normal labour ward conditions acceptable. Once established on this regimen the patient would normally be delivered without further delay. If the situation is particularly favourable for vaginal delivery this might be achieved by induction of labour, but in most instances the delivery method of choice would be caesarean section.

A close watch is kept on urinary output. If this falls, intravenous frusemide or mannitol may be needed. If the woman is allowed to labour, very close observation of her condition and that of the fetus is necessary. She should not be allowed to push in the second stage of labour, the baby being delivered electively by forceps or ventouse. Ergometrine should be avoided following delivery because of its tendency to induce hypertension. Syntocinon 5 units i.m. is a safe alternative.

The eclamptic regimen should be continued for 24 hours following delivery and a reduced level of sedation should then be used for several further days. Following delivery of the placenta the patient's condition tends to improve with a diminution of blood pressure and a tendency to diuresis. The blood pressure may not, however, return entirely to normal for several weeks or even months following delivery.

Treatment of eclampsia occurring at home

If possible the patient should be restrained during the fit so that she does not hurt herself by hitting hard objects. She should be turned on to her side and her airway checked. The fit should be stopped with an injection of diazepam 10–20 mg intravenously if this is available (intramuscularly if an intravenous injection is not possible). Other anticonvulsants can be used if diazepam is not available. The obstetric flying squad or emergency ambulance should be called to the patient's home. This is safer for her than sending her to hospital. She should not be left unattended while waiting for the flying squad.

Prognosis for future pregnancies

The patient with pre-eclampsia in her first pregnancy has approximately a one in three chance of having pre-eclampsia in her next pregnancy. It is probable, however, that the pre-eclampsia will be less severe and later in onset. This means that the outlook for subsequent pregnancies is generally quite good, even when the woman has lost her first baby because of pre-eclampsia arising very early in pregnancy. Virtually all women with recurrent pre-eclampsia are destined to become chronic hypertensives.

Antepartum haemorrhage

This used to be defined as bleeding from the genital tract between 28 weeks of pregnancy and delivery, with bleeding before 28 weeks being classed as a threatened abortion. However, the causes and treatment of bleeding between week 20 and week 28 are broadly similar to those of bleeding after 28 weeks, so a better definition of antepartum haemorrhage (APH) is bleeding from the genital tract between 20 weeks and delivery. APH may be due to:

1 Placenta praevia.

2 Placental abruption or accidental haemorrhage (premature separation of a normally situated placenta).
3 Bleeding from other parts of the genital tract.
4 Vasa praevia.

Clinical features

Placenta praevia (Fig. 7.3a)
Bleeding from a placenta praevia is typically painless, recurrent and usually unprovoked (although it may occasionally follow intercourse). The amount lost may vary between a few spots and several pints. If the patient is shocked the degree of shock is proportional to the visible blood loss. The uterus is usually well-relaxed and the fetal parts readily palpable, with the presenting part usually not engaged and sometimes deviated to one side. Except in the most severe cases, where there is marked maternal shock, the fetal heart is present.

Placental abruption–accidental haemorrhage
In abruption the bleeding may be partly or totally concealed as blood accumulates in the fundus of the uterus before tracking down to the cervix (Fig. 7.3b). In minor cases there may be no features to

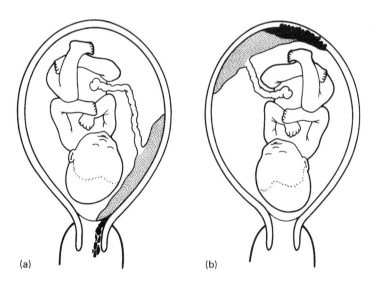

Fig. 7.3 Bleeding from placenta praevia and abruption. (a) Placenta praevia – blood readily escapes through the cervix; (b) placental abruption – blood is confined in the upper uterus, tracking laterally and into the uterine wall.

distinguish the bleeding from that of placenta praevia, but in moderate or severe cases there is typically pain with or preceding the bleeding. In some instances the patient presents with severe pain and shock before there is any visible bleeding, and the patient may be shocked out of proportion to the external blood loss. Typically the uterus is tense and tender and it may be impossible to feel fetal parts. In all except minor cases the fetal heart is often already absent when the patient is seen. When the patient is examined under anaesthesia it is often found that the fetal head is deep in the pelvis, and the cervix is appreciably dilated. In more severe cases a consumption coagulopathy may develop with hypofibrino-genaemia and sometimes also excessive fibrinolysis. Placental abruption may be caused by trauma (e.g. road accidents or external version) and is more common with severe hypertensives but in most cases there is no clear aetiology. Folic acid deficiency has been suggested as a cause but the evidence is unconvincing.

Other genital tract bleeding
Antepartum haemorrhage may also arise from a cervical polyp, a cervical carcinoma, a circumvallate placenta or trauma (possibly self-induced). A cervical erosion may also occasionally bleed slightly following intercourse or instrumentation. A careful speculum examination should reveal most of these sources of bleeding, but it is not safe to assume that a polyp or erosion is a source of bleeding until the more serious possible causes have been excluded.

Vasa praevia
Very rarely, bleeding may occur from an abnormal fetal vessel attached to the membranes over the internal os (called velamentous insertion of the cord; Fig. 7.4). Such bleeding virtually only occurs following artificial rupture of the membranes or during labour. It is often associated with fetal tachycardia and intrauterine death if delivery is not carried out immediately.

Management of antepartum haemorrhage

Unless there is clear clinical evidence of placental abruption, the bleeding should be assumed to be coming from a placenta praevia until proved otherwise. There is no place for vaginal examination until the fetus is sufficiently mature and circumstances are suitable for immediate delivery by caesarean section should such an examination reveal a placenta praevia, as it may provoke heavy bleeding. All cases of antepartum haemorrhage should be transferred at once to a major obstetrical unit. Unless the bleeding is minimal the flying squad should be called. Once in hospital a cardiotocograph is

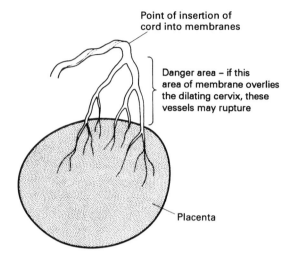

Point of insertion of
cord into membranes

Danger area – if this
area of membrane overlies
the dilating cervix, these
vessels may rupture

Placenta

Fig. 7.4   Velamentous insertion of the cord.

carried out. If fetal distress is present or if there is continued heavy
bleeding, immediate caesarean section is performed. Otherwise it is
usual to carry out a gentle speculum examination to visualize (but
not touch) the cervix to see whether the blood is coming through the
os (that is to say, from the placenta) or whether it arises from a
source in the cervix or vagina. One should not wait until the
bleeding has ceased, because even if a cervical lesion is found, one
cannot then be certain that it was the actual source of bleeding.

Further management consists of bed rest with ultrasound localization of the placenta and clotting screen. With a minor bleed which
settles, and with an upper-segment placenta and negative
Kleihauer, the patient may be allowed home after a day or two.
Rhesus-negative women should be given anti-D after any APH.

If placenta praevia is established, the initial bleed was a substantial one, or the bleeding recurs, the patient should remain in hospital
until delivered. In the case of repeated or heavy bleeding it may
be necessary to deliver the fetus by caesarean section immediately,
but otherwise it is normal to aim to deliver the patient at 38 weeks
(appropriate steps having been taken to confirm fetal maturity). It
should be noted that in the presence of a placenta praevia caesarean
section may be an extremely vascular, difficult and hazardous
operation and should only be undertaken by experienced obstetric
staff.

In conclusion, it should be re-emphasized that the complaint of

APH must be taken very seriously and the patient transferred at once, by flying squad or emergency ambulance if necessary, for proper investigation and treatment without any pelvic examination having been carried out at home. There is no place for waiting to see whether it happens again. Disaster may be only a blood clot away.

Management of placental abruption

Minor degrees of placental abruption cannot usually be diagnosed and their management is as outlined above for APH in general. However, major degrees of abruption are usually readily diagnosed and have their own form of management. The flying squad or emergency ambulance should be called and the patient transferred to a major obstetric unit unless, of course, she is already there.

An intravenous infusion should be started and at least 4 units of blood cross-matched. A central venous pressure line is invaluable in managing severe abruption, and without one most such patients will be undertransfused. When the patient is first seen, blood should be taken for clotting function tests, particularly fibrinogen concentration. This can be done formally in the laboratory if a suitable service is available, but information which is almost as valuable can be gained from observing clot formation in a plain glass tube at the bedside. If a firm clot has not formed within 10 minutes of taking blood it is reasonable to assume that the patient has hypofibrinogenaemia. If a clot forms and subsequently becomes friable, it is likely that she has excessive fibrinolytic activity. Such clotting function tests should be repeated at intervals until after the patient has been delivered.

The patient is best transfused with fresh blood (if it is available) in order to replenish depleted clotting factors. It is probably unnecessary to treat hypofibrinogenaemia or excessive fibrinolysis specifically unless the patient is actively bleeding, but if there is appreciable active loss then fibrinogen may be replaced with a pure fibrinogen solution or with fresh frozen plasma. Excessive fibrinolysis may be treated with ε-aminocaproic acid (Epsikapron).

Once the patient's condition has been assessed and a transfusion has been started, labour is induced by rupturing the membranes and starting a Syntocinon infusion if necessary. Rupturing the membranes allows a more ready drainage of blood from the uterine cavity and discourages further tracking of blood into the myometrium with release of thromboplastic substances into the circulation. Most patients with severe abruption labour readily and deliver without undue delay. If the fetus is alive it should be monitored closely. There is a very serious risk of postpartum haemorrhage in these cases and many of the deaths associated with placental abruption are attributable to postpartum haemorrhage occurring in patients already hypovolaemic from APH. The uterus may be badly bruised by blood tracking out from the retroplacental space into the myometrium, and this bruising interferes with uterine contraction in the third stage of labour. If, in addition, there is clotting dysfunction, then the scene is set for a brisk postpartum haemorrhage which is difficult to control and may readily prove fatal. In such circumstances the delivery must not be left to inexperienced junior staff. Intravenous ergometrine will be given and Syntocinon added to the drip. Haemorrhage may have to be controlled by bimanual compression of the uterus and any clotting abnormality should be corrected at this stage.

Acute renal failure and pituitary necrosis leading to Sheehan's syndrome are both possible complications of severe placental abruption, but careful attention to blood volume replacement aided by central venous pressure measurement should avoid these complications.

Polyhydramnios

Polyhydramnios (often abbreviated to hydramnios) is the presence of excess amniotic fluid in the uterine cavity. Volumes of amniotic fluid up to 1.5 litres are normal in the last trimester. However, it is not easy to measure amniotic fluid volume, so the diagnosis of polyhydramnios is generally a clinical one based on the following features:

1 A uterus which is large-for-dates and tense.
2 Difficulty in palpating fetal parts.
3 A fluid thrill.
4 Unstable lie.

Acute and chronic forms of hydramnios are described. The relatively rare acute polyhydramnios is typically associated with fetal abnormality or uniovular twins. There is often a rapid onset of uterine distension in the late second trimester or early third trimester with abdominal discomfort, and a high incidence of premature labour. The patient is best admitted to hospital, and an ultrasound scan arranged to look for fetal abnormalities, as well as a glucose tolerance test. If the fetus appears normal, steps should be taken to prevent premature labour but are likely to be unsuccessful.

The more common chronic polyhydramnios is associated with fetal abnormality (particularly gut atresia or anencephaly), maternal diabetes and multiple pregnancy and rarely tumours of the cord or placenta, but often no cause is found. It generally presents slightly later in pregnancy and is not very commonly associated with maternal discomfort or premature labour. Ultrasound examination and a glucose tolerance test will generally be performed. However, with the lesser degrees of hydramnios the patient need not be admitted to hospital until the onset of labour, but she should be warned to come into hospital early in labour or immediately the membranes rupture. Polyhydramnios presents the following dangers in pregnancy and labour:

1 Premature labour.
2 Possible unstable lie with malpresentation.
3 Rupture of membranes with cord prolapse.
4 Placental abruption due to the sudden reduction in uterine size following drainage of large volumes of liquor.

A close watch should be kept on the presentation in such cases. If the membranes are ruptured artificially this should be done in a controlled fashion to release the liquor slowly over the course of several minutes. Control can be achieved partly by pressing down the fetal head into the brim and partly by obstructing the vagina with the examining fingers. When an apparently normal baby is delivered to a woman with polyhydramnios a stomach tube should be passed without delay to exclude the possibility of oesophageal atresia as there is a serious danger that the baby will drown in its first feed if the oesophageal atresia is not detected.

Oligohydramnios

Oligohydramnios is the term used to describe a substantially reduced liquor volume. It is associated with failing placental function, with postmaturity with chronic leakage or amniotic fluid and with the rare cases of fetal genitourinary abnormalities preventing urine output (particularly renal agenesis). Severe prolonged oligohydramnios will lead to fetal pulmonary hypoplasia, postural limb abnormalities and squashed facial appearance – a syndrome known as Potter's syndrome when associated with renal agenesis. The diagnosis is suggested by the clinical impression that the uterine wall is wrapped closely around the baby with no intervening liquor, a feeling reminiscent of a freezer chicken where the polythene bag is stuck solidly on to the chicken. If the membranes are intact, this finding should lead one to suspect that the placenta is failing and to institute urgent investigations (see pp. 133–5). Ultrasound examination of the fetal bladder and kidneys is also indicated.

Unstable lie (variable lie)

It is normal for the fetal lie to be longitudinal from 32 weeks onwards. An unstable (or variable) lie is only of clinical importance in the last few weeks of pregnancy. The causes are:

1 High parity, with associated lax uterine and abdominal muscles.
2 Hydramnios.
3 Uterine abnormalities.
4 Rarely, pelvic 'tumours' such as placenta praevia, cervical fibroids or an ovarian cyst incarcerated in the pelvis.

With an unstable lie there is a danger that labour will start, or that the membranes will rupture while the fetus is lying transversely, which may lead to cord prolapse with the possibility of fetal death, or to the prolapse of an arm which fixes the fetus in an undeliverable position. It is advisable to admit the patient with an unstable lie from 38 weeks onwards to hospital to await the onset of labour. At the first sign of labour the patient is examined and, if possible, the presentation corrected to cephalic. Should the membranes rupture while the lie is unstable, a vaginal examination should be performed to exclude cord prolapse.

Abnormal lie

Some patients will be found to have a persistently abnormal lie in which the fetus lies in the same abnormal position without change. The causes of this are rather different from those of the truly unstable lie. Pelvic 'tumours' and more marked degrees of uterine abnormality are the more likely causes. The management is broadly similar to that of other forms of unstable lie, but should it prove impossible to correct the lie at the onset of labour then a caesarean section will be necessary. Caesarean section for a transverse lie may have to be done through a classical incision rather than a lower-segment incision but should only be undertaken by an experienced operator.

Disproportion

Disproportion exists when some part of the fetus is too big to pass through the maternal pelvis. The fetal head is usually the largest part of the fetus in cross-section, and disproportion usually refers to cephalopelvic disproportion. In a few instances, however, the shoulders may be larger than the fetal head, and shoulder dystocia (which is difficulty in delivering the shoulders after the head has delivered) is a special form of disproportion.

Disproportion was a common and very serious obstetric problem in previous centuries, accounting for much maternal mortality and morbidity. With women living in poverty, rickets was common; this frequently caused gross distortion and contraction of the pelvic inlet with obstetric conjugates sometimes as little as 5 cm, making delivery of any normal-sized baby impossible. In such circumstances, the woman would be likely to die a biochemical death after some days in labour, or alternatively might rupture her uterus and die more swiftly from blood loss. Those with lesser degrees of pelvic contraction might eventually manage to deliver a dead and partly collapsed fetus and then suffer total urinary or faecal incontinence because of pressure necrosis of the vaginal wall and bladder or rectum. Before the introduction of caesarean section as a moderately safe procedure at the end of the last century, a wide range of gruesome instruments were used to destroy the fetus and deliver it piecemeal in order to save the mother. Even in the most skilled hands the mortality and morbidity of these destructive operations were still high.

The virtual disappearance of malnutrition has meant that disproportion is uncommon and it now occurs in fewer than 1% of deliveries. Nowadays disproportion is only likely in cases where the pelvis is distorted due to bony disease such as lumbar kyphoscoliosis or a displaced fracture of the pelvic brim or outlet from a road traffic accident, or alternatively where the fetus is unduly large (as with poorly controlled diabetes or hydrocephalus). In the absence of such abnormalities disproportion is rare in women over 5 ft 1 in (1.54 m) and it is very rare in women who have previously had normal vaginal deliveries (although not totally unknown). In the past, much time and effort have been spent trying to predict disproportion in primigravidae by both clinical and radiological methods. However, the variable degree of moulding of the fetal skull and maternal pelvis, the variable resistance of the maternal soft parts and the variable efficiency of uterine action make prediction of disproportion unreliable except in gross cases. There is a growing tendency to allow all primigravidae to attempt vaginal delivery unless there is evidence of gross bony or fetal disease which would clearly prevent this.

There is now no place for assessment of pelvic capacity in early pregnancy. If the fetal head is engaged or can be made to engage in the pelvis at 36 weeks the likelihood of disproportion can be ruled out. The head will not be engaged at 36 weeks in almost a third of primigravidae and the majority of these will subsequently have normal deliveries. The reasons for a non-engaged head at 36 weeks are set out below, the first three being by far the commonest:

1 Full rectum.
2 Occipitoposterior position.
3 Resistance from maternal soft parts (pelvic floor muscles and ligaments or thick lower uterine segment).
4 Cephalopelvic disproportion.
5 Placenta praevia.
6 Increased pelvic tilt (high inclination brim) in African women.
7 Polyhydramnios.
8 Hydrocephalus.
9 Brow presentation.
10 Pelvic tumours.

If the head is deviated to one side and cannot be made to fit even partly into the pelvis, the likelihood of placenta praevia is increased, and an ultrasound scan for placental localization should be arranged forthwith. A scan will also demonstrate the position and normality of the fetal head in case of doubt. Otherwise it is reasonable for an experienced obstetrician to do a pelvic examination at this stage to exclude pelvic tumours and to make an assessment of the pelvic capacity. Unless a pelvic tumour is found or the size of the pelvis is clearly grossly reduced, no further action is necessary until the onset of labour. If the head is still not engaged at the onset of labour, the labour is managed as a trial of labour.

Trial of labour

A trial of labour is an attempt to achieve vaginal delivery in a case in which it is suspected that disproportion may exist. The patient is closely observed and is allowed to proceed in labour as long as good progress is maintained and no fetal distress develops, but otherwise caesarean section is performed. Such labours should only be conducted in a major unit where caesarean section is possible without delay. The conduct of trial of labour is described more fully in Chapter 8.

If on pelvic assessment at 36 weeks the obstetrician feels there is appreciable contraction, he or she may order an X-ray pelvimetry. This is nowadays usually confined to a single erect lateral view or a computed tomographic (CT) scan if available because of the known risks to the fetus of antenatal radiography. On the basis of this pelvimetry the obstetrician may decide to do an elective caesarean section, but in practice this is extremely rare. Following a caesarean section for a failed trial of labour, any subsequent delivery will be managed by elective caesarean section.

Premature labour

Any labour that occurs between 22 and 37 weeks should be considered a premature labour. Before 22 weeks there is no chance of the fetus surviving and after 37 weeks the risks are not significantly more than for a term fetus.

Causes of premature labour

These are:

1 Incompetent cervix.
2 Uterine abnormalities.
3 Multiple pregnancy.
4 Polyhydramnios.
5 Premature rupture of membranes.
6 Placental insufficiency.
7 Fetal abnormalities.
8 APH.
9 Intrauterine death.
10 Uterine trauma.
11 Maternal pyrexia or ill health (e.g. generalized infections or appendicitis).
12 Premature labour is significantly more common in those of low socioeconomic class.
13 Often there is no demonstrable cause.

Management of premature labour

The patient should be admitted as quickly as possible to a major unit that has neonatal special care facilities. The baby is safer being transferred *in utero* than being delivered peripherally and then transferred in an incubator. If there is any possibility of imminent delivery a doctor or midwife should accompany the patient to hospital.

If the patient is seen early enough it may be possible to stop labour. It is generally advisable to try to do so unless the patient is beyond 34 weeks, but individual circumstances (for instance, the occurrence of haemorrhage or the suggestion of placental failure) will influence this decision. Labour may be arrested with the following types of drugs:

1 β-Sympathomimetics.
2 Prostaglandin antagonists.

The drugs most widely used at present are the β-sympath-omimetic agents ritodrine and salbutamol. These are given as an intravenous infusion, starting at a slow rate and increasing until the contractions stop or unacceptable side-effects are produced. A major side-effect with this treatment is maternal and fetal tachycardia. The maternal pulse should not be allowed to exceed 140 beats/min. Additional side-effects that may be produced are hypotension, palpitations, tremor, anxiety and even panic attacks. A rare but possibly fatal complication is pulmonary oedema, the risk of which is increased by fluid overload. With these drugs 80% of premature labour can be arrested if the initial cervical dilatation is no more than 2 cm. When this intravenous regimen is successful, long-term arrest may sometimes be achieved with oral β-sympath-omimetic drugs.

There is now considerable evidence that surfactant production and functional lung maturity may be stimulated by high-dose steroid administration. A short course of dexamethasone given to the mother (6 mg/12-hourly for 48 hours) substantially reduces the likelihood of respiratory distress syndrome in the neonate. These dose levels of steroids should not be exceeded as there is some danger of actually encouraging premature labour.

Premature rupture of membranes

This is defined as rupture of the membranes before the onset of labour. It may occur at any stage of pregnancy up to or beyond term. Either the membranes lying over the internal cervical os may rupture (forewater rupture) or more commonly the leak occurs from the membranes higher up in the uterus (hindwater rupture). Forewater rupture is often due to an incompetent cervix which leaves an area of membrane unsupported and devitalized. With hindwater rupture a cause is rarely discovered. The risks of prema-ture rupture of membranes are:

1 Initiation of premature labour.
2 Ascending infection (risk to mother as well as fetus).
3 Cord prolapse (in labour, but rare before).

In addition, if delivery does not ensue and there is long-term leakage of liquor there is risk of producing fetal postural deformities (such as talipes) and pulmonary hypoplasia. Of the first three risks, cord prolapse is by far the rarest. In fact it is almost unknown before the onset of labour. The relative importance of the other two risks varies with the stage of pregnancy, but with modern management more babies are probably lost from prematurity than intrauterine infection.

Management of premature rupture of membranes

In cases of doubt the diagnosis can usually be readily established by inserting a sterile vaginal speculum to see whether liquor is leaking through the cervix. This examination is important because many alleged premature ruptures of the membranes are in fact examples of urinary loss or imagination and patients may be unnecessarily admitted, or even worse, stimulated to deliver.

Before 34 weeks aim to prolong the pregnancy.

1 Admit the patient to hospital for bed rest.
2 Avoid all vaginal examinations other than sterile speculum examinations to limit the risk of ascending infection.
3 Carry out infection screening – low vaginal swabs and white blood cell count.
4 Arrest premature labour if it occurs.
5 Consider elective delivery if the patient gets as far as 34 weeks or if there are any signs of ascending infection.
6 Antibiotics are not normally helpful unless there is evidence of infection.

After 34 weeks, if the patient is in a unit with good neonatal facilities, the balance of risks is probably in favour of delivery, and labour may be induced with Syntocinon after a 48-hour delay.

Placental insufficiency – intrauterine growth retardation

Placental insufficiency is a major cause of perinatal death. Placental insufficiency leads to fetal growth retardation in the early stages and fetal hypoxia and death in more advanced stages. The main causes of placental insufficiency are as follows:

1 Idiopathic.
2 Multiple pregnancy.
3 Smoking.
4 Postmaturity.
5 APH.
6 Essential hypertension or pre-eclampsia.
7 Other maternal illness (especially chronic urinary tract infection).
8 Maternal malnutrition.
9 It is also more common in women who have had previous small-for-dates babies, those of low socioeconomic class, primigravidae and women over 35 years of age.
10 It is important to realize that intrauterine growth retardation may relate to purely fetal factors such as chromosomal abnor-

malities (e.g. trisomies), damaged growth potential from infections (e.g. rubella, syphilis, cytomegalovirus) or the fetal alcohol syndrome.

Detection of placental insufficiency

Placental insufficiency should be anticipated in any of the abnormal situations listed above, but in a considerable proportion of cases there are no alerting factors in the woman's history. There are, however, clinical features of early placental failure which may be picked up by careful antenatal care as follows:

Uterine size
With placental insufficiency the uterus appears small-for-dates. This is due partly to the fetus being small-for-dates and also to a considerably diminished volume of liquor (oligohydramnios). A small-for-dates uterus could also be due to wrong dates or fetal abnormality. Whenever the uterus is found to be small-for-dates, appropriate investigations should be instituted to determine which of these three factors is the cause. One of the most important functions of anyone undertaking antenatal care is to ask critically: 'Is this uterus the right size for her dates?'

Fetal activity
Fetal activity will generally diminish when there is significant placental insufficiency. A number of units employ fetal activity charts (kick charts, or count-to-10 charts), based on work from Cardiff. The woman is asked to note the time it takes for the fetus to move 10 times. This varies widely (from a few minutes to 12 hours), but anything over 12 hours is abnormal. These kick counts can be done from 28 weeks on a twice-weekly or a daily basis with minimal expense and inconvenience. They appear to offer a method of picking up a fair proportion of those with placental failure while there is still time to intervene.

Maternal weight
Maternal weight should rise progressively through pregnancy, and failure to gain weight or loss of weight is frequently associated with placental failure. However, maternal weight is influenced by so many factors (e.g. sickness, oedema, diet) that it is not a very reliable sign.

If any of these risk factors or clinical features suggest the possibility of placental failure, tests must be arranged, and usually the patient will be admitted.

Tests of fetal well-being

Almost all obstetrical pathology carries with it a threat to the well-being of the fetus with the possibility of insufficient supply of nutrients or oxygen leading to fetal damage or intrauterine death. Our ability to intervene to prevent damage to the fetus depends on the availability of tests of fetal well-being. Much effort and money was spent in the 1960s–80s on the development and use of biochemical tests of placental function. Measurements of urinary oestriol or blood human placental lactogen (hPL) were used on a major scale around the world. Critical studies in the late 1980s failed to show any benefit of such tests in terms of reducing perinatal mortality and they have disappeared from practice. Although oestrogen or hPL output was generally much better with a healthy well-grown baby than with a small compromised baby, the variability of the results and the large overlap of normal and abnormal meant that they did not allow appropriate intervention. With a realization that fetal well-being relates to a complex of maternal, placental and fetal factors, has developed a tendency to rely on biophysical measures of fetal well-being for the most part directed at the fetus itself. The main measures are described below.

Fetal heart rate traces

The fetal heart rate may be recorded using a cardiotocograph (CTG) machine with an external ultrasound transducer. The interpretation of these traces is comparable to the detection of fetal distress in labour (see Chapter 8).

Cardiotocography offers the best way of assessing the current status of the fetus, but traces need to be repeated every 2 days to give continuous reassurance.

Ultrasound measurements

Serial ultrasound measurements of the fetal head and abdominal circumferences will give precise indications of fetal growth rate. With chronic placental insufficiency there is a tendency for abdominal measurements to be reduced substantially more than head measurements. This is referred to as asymmetrical growth retardation (Fig. 7.5). It arises because the abdominal circumference is largely determined by liver size, and the fetal liver of the well-nourished fetus contains large stores of glycogen, which are depleted early on in the process of growth retardation. The amount of liquor can also be determined approximately, usually in terms of the diameter of the largest pool of liquor. Ultrasound measurements give a relatively long-term view of fetal well-being (particularly fetal

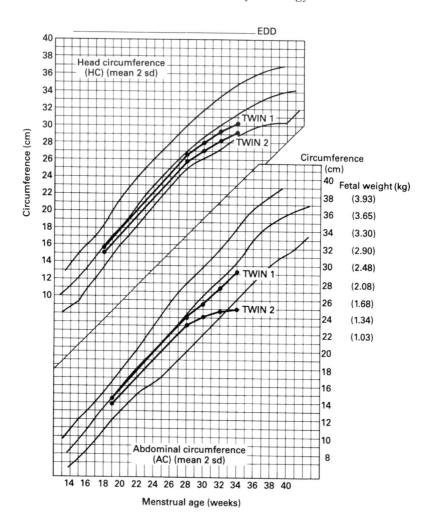

Fig. 7.5 Serial ultrasound scan results for a twin pregnancy, with twin 2 showing asymmetrical growth retardation. EDD = Estimated date of delivery.

nutrition). They clearly do not give any indication of the possibility of acute change in placental function such as that associated with a placental abruption. In view of the inaccuracy of measurements and the normal fetal growth rate, it is generally not worth repeating ultrasound measurements more often than every 10–14 days.

Doppler studies
Doppler ultrasound studies of blood-flow patterns in uterine arteries or cord vessels are becoming established as a reasonably acute and predictive indication of placental function and fetal well-being.

Biophysical profiles
Various attempts have been made to link a number of biophysical observations (usually CTGs, ultrasound measurements of the fetal head and abdomen, ultrasound assessment of fetal breathing movements and liquor pool size), giving a collective score.

Quite which mixture of biophysical observations will prove the ultimate best buy remains to be seen, but for the moment CTGs remain the main means of acute assessment of fetal well-being, with ultrasound measurements giving a good indication of longer-term placental function.

ANTENATAL CARE – OTHER HIGH-RISK SITUATIONS

The older primigravida

Women who are pregnant for the first time at the age of 35 or more have in the past been known as elderly primigravidae. This is a term (like senile vaginitis) which may be offensive to the patient herself and should be replaced by older primigravida.

The term is sometimes extended to those over 30 but there is no justification for this as the risks of pregnancy only increase appreciably over the age of 35. Age is a more important factor than nulliparity in determining the risk to the mother and fetus and indeed a 38-year-old woman having her fourth or fifth pregnancy is at greater risk than a 38-year-old primigravida. However, the older primigravida is considered a special case because the child is generally a particularly 'precious baby'. The woman will often have been infertile before conceiving and, even if not, her chances of conceiving again are less than those of a young woman. It is well worth noting that a 38-year-old today will probably be safer having a baby now than at any time in the past, as the age-related increase in risk is small compared with the massive decreases in maternal and perinatal mortality rates that have occurred over the last 20 years. Also, as general standards of antenatal and intrapartum care have improved, there is no longer such a contrast between normal care and the special care of the high-risk patient such as the older primigravida. However, most obstetricians agree that the older primigravida should:

1 Be delivered in a specialist unit.
2 Have the fetus closely monitored in labour.
3 Be delivered by caesarean section at the first sign of any problems.

The grand multipara

A woman having her fifth or subsequent baby is known as a grand multipara and is at increased risk of perinatal mortality and serious maternal problems. She will usually have had rapid, easy, normal deliveries previously. She is often of low socioeconomic class and reluctant to accept obstetric advice, particularly that she is likely to have any problems in this or subsequent pregnancies. The main problems of these women of high parity are:

1 Chronic anaemia and malnutrition.
2 Unstable lie, malpresentations and obstructed labour.
3 Late engagement of the fetal head with the possibility of cord prolapse when the membranes rupture.
4 Rapid labours, occasionally producing trauma to the baby by sudden compression and decompression of the head (precipitate labour).
5 Postpartum haemorrhage.

The grand multiparous patient should be booked for a specialist obstetric unit and should be followed closely in the antenatal period to detect the problems listed above. Following delivery she should be offered contraceptive advice in as subtle a way as possible, but she may well not accept it!

The obese patient

The obese patient is at high risk for a number of reasons:

1 She is at increased risk of hypertension, pre-eclampsia and diabetes.
2 Assessment of fetal, size, position and number is difficult or impossible.
3 Ultrasound examination is much more difficult as ultrasound is transmitted poorly through fat.
4 The fetus also tends to be obese, with increased risk of cephalopelvic disproportion and shoulder dystocia.
5 Anaesthesia and caesarean section and other operative interventions are more difficult and also carry considerably increased risks.

Ideally the patient should be persuaded to lose weight before becoming pregnant but this is rarely possible. If first seen when pregnant she should be persuaded to maintain a diet which will result in minimal weight increase during the pregnancy. She should be booked for a specialist unit and be followed closely in the antenatal period. A glucose tolerance test should be performed.

Rhesus disease (isoimmunization)

At the time of delivery or abortion (and occasionally at amniocentesis or external version) it is common for fetal blood cells to enter the maternal circulation. If the mother is rhesus-negative and the fetus rhesus-positive, these cells may sensitize her to produce anti-D rhesus antibodies. These antibodies are of the immunoglobulin G (IgG) series and in subsequent pregnancies can cross the placenta and affect the red cells of rhesus-positive fetuses. The red cells are haemolysed, producing fetal anaemia with increased bile pigment production. Most of this pigment is removed by the placenta (although some is excreted into the amniotic fluid) but following delivery the fetal liver is unable to cope with the increased haemolysis and jaundice develops rapidly, typically within a few hours of birth. The fetal anaemia may be severe enough to cause intrauterine death, which is usually preceded by the development in the fetus of gross oedema and ascites, a condition known as hydrops fetalis. In less severe cases the baby may be born alive, but then, if untreated, suffers deposits of bile pigment in the basal ganglia of the brain, a condition known as kernicterus, which can produce spasticity or death subsequently.

Nowadays rhesus disease is generally preventable, but previously about one-fifth of rhesus-negative women had developed rhesus antibodies by the end of their second pregnancy and about a third of rhesus-negative women eventually did so. The severity of the disease tends to increase in successive pregnancies, but at a very variable rate; some women develop severe disease in their second pregnancy, while others develop only mild disease in spite of many pregnancies.

Prevention of rhesus disease

If anti-D immunoglobulin is given to the mother within 48 hours of delivery it coats any rhesus-positive cells in the maternal circulation, masks their antigenic sites and prevents sensitization. It is now routine to give 100 µg intramuscularly following delivery of a rhesus-positive baby to an unsensitized rhesus-negative mother. (If the mother is already sensitized, such treatment has no value.) Maternal blood is also examined following delivery to judge the quantity of fetal cells in it, using the Kleihauer test. If large numbers of fetal cells are detected, the dose of anti-D is increased correspondingly. Anti-D should also be given to unsensitized rhesus-negative women following:

1 Miscarriage.
2 Termination of pregnancy.
3 Amniocentesis.
4 Chorionic villus biopsy.
5 External cephalic version.
6 APH.
7 Significant uterine trauma.
8 Mismatched rhesus-positive blood transfusion.

Recent research studies suggest that giving small doses of anti-D at 28 and 34 weeks to all rhesus-negative women protects the few who would otherwise become sensitized despite the standard anti-D-regimen.

If all these measures were employed universally, rhesus disease would become rare, but many women miscarry without knowing their blood group or without telling their doctor, so that rhesus disease will not disappear in the foreseeable future.

Detection of rhesus disease

Every woman should be blood-grouped before conception or as early as possible in pregnancy and rhesus-negative women have tests for rhesus antibodies at booking, 28 and 34 weeks.

Management of rhesus disease

Once rhesus antibodies are detected the woman is followed closely with regular antibody estimations (or titres). Low-level antibodies (less than 1.5 µg/ml) are generally associated with mild disease for which no active treatment is necessary, but higher serum antibody concentrations may be associated with moderate or severe disease, the actual severity being poorly related to the antibody level. Examination of amniotic fluid obtained by amniocentesis gives a clearer guide to severity of the disease. The optical density of the amniotic fluid is calculated at 450 nm (the wavelength of bile pigment), and the results plotted on a Liley chart (Fig. 7.6). This gives zones for mild, moderate and severe disease for different stages of pregnancy. With severe disease the fetus is likely to die

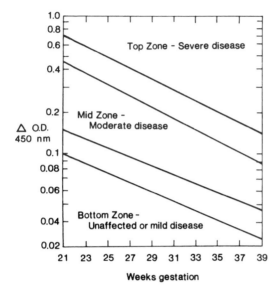

Fig. 7.6 Liley chart for prediction of severity of rhesus disease from amniotic fluid pigment values. OD = Optical density.

quickly *in utero* if not treated, whereas the fetus with moderate disease will generally survive until near term. Three forms of treatment are available antenatally – premature delivery, fetal transfusion and plasmapheresis.

Premature delivery
If the fetus is viable and the disease moderate to severe, this may be the only treatment necessary.

Fetal transfusion
The fetus may be transfused at intervals from 24 weeks with rhesus-negative cells, which will not be influenced by the maternal antibodies. This is achieved by directly needling the fetal cord under ultrasound control (cordocentesis) or by introducing a catheter through a needle inserted through the maternal abdomen and uterine wall into the fetal abdominal cavity. Red cells are absorbed intact and enter the fetal circulation. This treatment is appropriate to those who are likely to have an intrauterine death before 30 weeks, and the fetal salvage rate is about 50%.

Plasmapheresis

Repeated plasmapheresis can lower the maternal serum antibody concentration. This technique, used alone or in conjunction with intrauterine transfusion, has extended the possibility of treatment to those with very severe disease.

Outlook for future pregnancies

It can be expected that any future rhesus-positive fetus will be at least as badly affected as in the last pregnancy, and probably worse. Whether the fetus will inevitably be affected depends on the rhesus group and zygosity of the father, so paternal rhesus genotyping is normally carried out in cases of rhesus disease. If the father is heterozygous rhesus-positive (Dd), there is a 50% chance of his child being rhesus-negative, whereas a homozygous (DD) father can only produce rhesus-positive children.

MEDICAL ABNORMALITIES COMPLICATING PREGNANCY

The more important medical disorders of pregnancy will be considered here. For fuller accounts of this fascinating area of medicine the reader is referred to the Further Reading at the end of this chapter.

Non pre-eclamptic hypertension

Pregnancy presents a good opportunity for screening for chronic hypertensive states. Essential hypertension occurs in about 1% of pregnancies, and other forms of non pre-eclamptic hypertension very much more rarely. Patients with blood pressure of more than 150/100 mmHg in early pregnancy should be admitted for tests and observation. The patient should undergo a thorough general examination with palpation of femoral and radial pulses to exclude coarctation, auscultation of renal arteries to exclude renal artery stenosis and assessment of cardiac size and normality. The tests should include renal function tests, repeated midstream urine cultures and estimation of urinary catecholamines or vanillylmandelic acid to exclude a phaeochromocytoma. The observation of the trend in blood pressure over the course of a few days gives a good indication of its true level and of the prognosis for the pregnancy – a fall in blood pressure with rest is a good sign.

Essential hypertension approximately doubles the perinatal mortality overall, but minor degrees of essential hypertension with a diastolic pressure of less than 100 mmHg carry virtually no risk. With the more severe degrees the mother is also at risk of placental abruption, and of cerebrovascular accident, heart failure and possible permanent deterioration of her hypertension if there is superadded pre-eclampsia. The risk to mother and fetus is very much more if there is albuminuria present in the first half of pregnancy or if superadded pre-eclampsia develops later.

Essential hypertension of a more than minor degree is probably best managed in conjunction with a physician. If hypotensive treatment is necessary, this is ideally started before the patient embarks on the pregnancy. In pregnancy hypotensive treatment is probably beneficial if the average blood pressure exceeds 150/100 mmHg. The hypotensive agents most often used are methyldopa and nifedipine. Extra rest limits blood pressure rise and improves placental perfusion, and the more severe cases may need to be admitted to hospital for most of the pregnancy. A close watch on placental function and fetal well-being is necessary, and premature induction may well offer the best chance to the fetus. Ergometrine should be avoided at the time of delivery as it can cause a marked rise in blood pressure.

Phaeochromocytoma

This is a very rare but extremely serious complication of pregnancy. The maternal mortality rate of the published cases exceeds 50%, and was 100% where a hypertensive crisis occurred in labour. A phaeochromocytoma should be suspected if hypertension is severe or intermittent, and appropriate biochemical tests should be carried out. If a phaeochromocytoma is discovered it is best removed without delay and before delivery.

Diabetes in pregnancy

Diabetes has become a more common complication of pregnancy, as better control has led to improved fertility. Maternal diabetes carries very considerable potential hazards to both mother and fetus; great care is needed to detect all cases of diabetes in pregnancy, and great skill is needed to minimize those risks.

Effect of pregnancy on diabetes

1 Insulin requirements generally increase appreciably and control becomes more difficult.
2 Glycosuria is no longer a reliable indication of degree of diabetic control.
3 Some women who had normal glucose tolerance before pregnancy will develop impaired glucose tolerance or gestational diabetes (often reverting to normal after delivery).

Effect of diabetes in pregnancy

1 Without meticulous diabetic control the fetus grows abnormally rapidly, with increased fat deposition. This leads to an increased likelihood of mechanical problems at delivery.
2 Without meticulous control there is a high incidence of intrauterine death in the last months of pregnancy.
3 There is an increased incidence of polyhydramnios, especially if diabetic control is poor.
4 The incidence of fetal abnormality is increased.
5 The neonate is at increased risk of serious problems, including respiratory distress syndrome and hypoglycaemia.

Detection of diabetes in pregnancy

Glucose tolerance tests should be done in the first half of pregnancy in the following circumstances for women not previously known to be diabetic:

1 Close family history of diabetes.
2 Glycosuria on two occasions during pregnancy or heavy (2.0%) glycosuria on one occasion.
3 Any previous baby weighing over 4.5 kg (10 lb).
4 Previous unexplained stillbirth.
5 Marked obesity.

This screening of at-risk cases is particularly important since the risks run by an undiagnosed early diabetic far exceed those of a well-managed established diabetic. Some units now screen all antenatal patients for diabetes.

Management of diabetes in pregnancy

Management of the pregnant diabetic is difficult and is best carried out by teams with a particular interest in this field covering all the cases in the area. The key principles are summarized here:

1 Care should be shared between an obstetrician and a physician specializing in diabetes, preferably seeing the patient together.
2 Insulin requirements increase in pregnancy and most patients need a combination injection of both short- and long-acting insulins to maintain good control. If the patient is not already on this sort of regimen, it is usual to change to it at about 12 weeks.
3 Control is judged on the basis of blood sugar levels, and not on the degree of glycosuria.

4 Tight diabetic control reduces the incidence of pregnancy complications, so blood sugars should be kept within the normal non-
  diabetic range. A blood sugar run consisting of pre- and 2-hours
  postprandial samples is taken at weekly intervals during the
  pregnancy. These samples should all contain less than 5.5 mmol/l
  glucose.
5 Any obstetric complication or general ill health (particularly
  infections) is treated very seriously and generally merits admission.
6 Fetoplacental function is closely monitored in the last trimester.
7 The patient is delivered between 38 weeks and term, either by
  inducing labour if the obstetric situation is favourable or by elective caesarean section if there are any complications at all.
8 The fetus is monitored in labour, and early recourse is made to
  caesarean section if good progress is not maintained, or at any
  suspicion of fetal distress.
9 An experienced neonatal paediatrician should attend the delivery.

Heart disease in pregnancy

Heart disease in pregnancy is now relatively rare and is found in
only 1 or 2 per 1000 pregnancies, with congenital heart disease being
more common than rheumatic heart disease. The haemodynamic
changes of pregnancy and delivery throw extra strain on the heart
(Chapter 6) and result in increased risk to the cardiac patient. There
were 21 maternal deaths in the UK in the years 1988–90 attributed to
heart disease – almost equal to the number of deaths from haemorrhage. In the majority of cases, however, other factors were involved
and heart disease was not the direct cause of death.

The following are the main effects of pregnancy on the patient
with heart disease.

1 *Increased functional disability*: Pregnancy frequently results in a
  slight worsening of the functional disability.
2 *Risk of heart failure*: There is increased risk of both congestive
  failure and pulmonary oedema. Respiratory infection may
  precipitate congestive failure, and pulmonary oedema is particularly likely in patients with tight mitral stenosis and an efficient
  myocardium.
3 *Risk of endocarditis*: Bacterial endocarditis is a rare but definite
  complication of delivery.

Management of heart disease in pregnancy

1 Seek the advice of a cardiologist early in pregnancy and, unless

the disease is trivial, manage the patient jointly throughout pregnancy.

2 Termination is rarely indicated and must be avoided until failure is controlled. It may then be carried out for the usual (non-cardiac) reasons.

3 Advise extra rest. The more serious cases will be admitted to hospital for a period of rest before delivery, and any patient developing heart failure will need admission for the whole pregnancy.

4 Treat respiratory infection and anaemia vigorously.

5 Allow spontaneous labour and vaginal delivery unless there are obstetric contraindications.

6 Prescribe prophylactic antibiotics (ampicillin, gentamicin) during labour.

7 In the more serious cases perform elective forceps delivery.

8 Avoid ergometrine or other oxytocics in those at risk of pulmonary oedema.

Liver disease in pregnancy

Jaundice

Jaundice is a rare but potentially very serious complication of pregnancy. It may be classified as jaundice peculiar to pregnancy and jaundice incidental to pregnancy.

Jaundice peculiar to pregnancy

1 Acute fatty liver of pregnancy.

2 Recurrent intrahepatic cholestatic jaundice.

3 Jaundice complicating severe pre-eclampsia.

4 Jaundice complicating hyperemesis.

Acute fatty liver of pregnancy is a rare condition, usually occurring in the last weeks of pregnancy. It is characterized by rapidly progressive jaundice, abdominal pain and vomiting, clotting disorders, fetal death and usually maternal coma and death. Its aetiology is thought to be linked to the breakdown of protein synthesis in the liver under the increased demands of pregnancy, and of the reported cases in recent years, most have been associated with the use of parenteral tetracyclines. If the patient is to have any prospect of survival she is best treated in a specialist liver unit.

Recurrent intrahepatic cholestatic jaundice is relatively common. It is also known as benign idiopathic jaundice of pregnancy and gestational hepatosis. It is characterized by a mild jaundice occurring in late pregnancy, often associated with marked generalized pruritus. It tends to recur in subsequent pregnancies, and also possibly if the patient takes oral contraceptives. A raised alkaline phosphatase and a mildly raised bilirubin are the common biochemical findings. It has previously been thought that the condition does not affect the outcome of pregnancy, but recent reports suggest that there is a mild increase in perinatal mortality and postpartum haemorrhage.

Jaundice is a rare complication of severe pre-eclampsia, eclampsia or hyperemesis. The proper and prompt management of the underlying condition should, however, prevent either the development of jaundice or its progression.

Jaundice incidental to pregnancy

All forms of jaundice may occur in pregnancy: viral hepatitis and gallstones are the commonest causes. The viruses of both infectious hepatitis and serum hepatitis will cross the placenta, and special precautions are necessary in handling infected patients, particularly at the time of delivery, to avoid the transmission of infection to the obstetrician or midwife.

Pregnancy in a well-nourished woman in general has little effect on the course of incidental liver disease. The biochemical disturbances of liver disease do, however, seem to increase appreciably the risk of stillbirth, to interfere with uterine contractility and to lead to clotting failure, so that specialist medical and obstetric care is vital in all cases of liver disease in pregnancy.

Thyroid disease in pregnancy

The changes in thyroid physiology in pregnancy (see Chapter 6) make assessment of thyroid function somewhat more difficult in pregnancy. Binding proteins, including thyroid-binding globulin, increase in concentration in response to oestrogen, so that protein-bound iodine rises to well above non-pregnant levels. Also pulse rate and basal metabolic rate increase. However, the blood levels of the free hormones thyroxine, triiodothyronine and thyroid-stimulating hormone should remain unchanged, and departures from the normal range indicate thyroid disease.

Thyrotoxicosis

Untreated thyrotoxicosis tends to reduce fertility, and if it does occur in pregnancy it increases the rate of abortion, pre-eclampsia, premature labour and perinatal mortality. Thyrotoxicosis is generally treated medically during pregnancy with carbimazole. If the mother is maintained meticulously at euthyroid levels, there is probably no excess risk to the fetus, but accidental overdose with carbimazole (or any of the other antithyroid drugs, all of which cross the placenta) may render the fetus hypothyroid, with goitre formation or cretinism in extreme cases. Some physicians guard against this possibility by giving L-thyroxine 0.3 mg daily as well as carbimazole. Radioiodine should not be used either diagnostically or therapeutically in pregnancy because of the risk of long-term fetal thyroid damage.

Hypothyroidism

Hypothyroidism also impairs fertility and is rarely found in pregnancy. If untreated or inadequately treated, there is increased risk of abortion, fetal abnormality and stillbirth. Treatment with thyroxine should be instituted gradually, and should aim to render the patient euthyroid. Patients already being treated before pregnancy for hypothyroidism are likely to need increased doses of thyroxine.

Urinary tract disease in pregnancy

Asymptomatic bacteriuria

About 6% of pregnant women have asymptomatic bacteriuria, which is defined as more than 100 000 organisms per millilitre in freshly voided urine. The composition of the bacteriuric population is not constant, with some women spontaneously clearing their urinary tract of significant bacteriuria, while others have permanent bacteriuria often related to underlying renal infection. Bacteriuria has been associated with:

1 Increased likelihood of developing acute pyelonephritis in pregnancy.
2 Increased rate of premature delivery.
3 Decreased mean birth weight.
4 Anaemia.

Bacteriuria is more common in lower social classes, and this association may account for all the factors above, apart from the increased risk of pyelonephritis. It is a routine in most clinics now to screen at booking for asymptomatic bacteriuria. Those with positive tests are treated with a 7-day course of ampicillin or sulphonamides, which will cure about 75%. Those who get recurrent bacteriuria are treated again, and any who subsequently relapse merit full renal investigation following pregnancy as they are likely to have chronic pyelonephritis or serious renal tract abnormalities.

Acute pyelonephritis

Acute pyelonephritis is more common in pregnancy because of the relative stasis in the urinary tract brought about by the dilatation of ureters and renal calyces, and because of the increased sugar content of pregnancy urine. About half of acute pyelonephritis arises in those with asymptomatic bacteriuria. The disease may present in a mild form with little more than nausea and malaise, or in a severe form with high pyrexia, rigors, vomiting, loin pain and tenderness, and dysuria. The more serious forms may lead to premature labour and occasionally to intrauterine death of the fetus (due to the high pyrexia). Permanent renal damage may also follow if treatment is not promptly instituted. The diagnosis is usually made without difficulty and can be confirmed by urine examination. The causative organism is nearly always *Escherichia coli*. Treatment should be started without waiting for culture results. It is important to avoid high pyrexia by tepid sponging or by giving aspirin. Anaemia is a common sequel, presumably due to suppression of erythropoietin production from the kidney.

Chronic pyelonephritis and chronic nephritis

These two conditions often present in the same way in pregnancy with evidence of renal impairment, possibly with albuminuria or hypertension, but without clear evidence of infection or of a nephritic origin for the impaired renal function. They may only be distinguishable by renal biopsy, which is rarely used in pregnancy. They may have a serious effect on the course of pregnancy, increasing the likelihood of early and middle-trimester abortion, of intrauterine growth retardation and of superadded pre-eclampsia. The outlook is correspondingly worse where there is:

1 Albuminuria.
2 Hypertension.
3 Blood urea raised above 9 mmol/l (50 mg/100 ml).

Differentiation from pre-eclampsia may present some difficulty if the patient is not seen in the first half of pregnancy; otherwise investigation as outlined on pp. 140–1 for non pre-eclamptic hypertension will usually give a sufficiently clear diagnosis to allow the pregnancy to be managed satisfactorily. Consideration should be given to terminating the pregnancy in the more serious cases of renal impairment. In less severe cases, close antenatal care, treatment of infection, monitoring of fetal well-being and extra rest will generally allow a successful outcome.

Acute nephritis and renal tuberculosis

Both of these conditions are now very rare complications of pregnancy, and their general management is little affected by the pregnancy.

Anaemia in pregnancy

Some degree of anaemia is very common in pregnancy. The significant increase in maternal blood volume (+ 30%) and the ability of the placenta to extract iron from the maternal circulation to meet its own needs (150 mg) and those of the fetus (400–450 mg) mean that a considerable demand is put on the maternal iron stores. Many women, and particularly those in poor socioeconomic conditions, will have depleted iron stores at the beginning of pregnancy, and cannot expect to absorb the required quantity of iron (3 mg/day) from their normal diet. In such circumstances iron-deficiency anaemia develops. The 1958 *Perinatal Mortality Survey* showed that severe anaemia (haemoglobin below 8.9 g per 100 ml) was associated with a twofold increase in perinatal mortality. While it can be argued that some of the excess risk is related to the poor socioeconomic conditions which were responsible for the anaemia, there can be little doubt that severe anaemia directly increases the risk to both mother and fetus.

More recent studies in London suggest that a haemoglobin level in the range 10–12 g per 100 ml in the third trimester is optimal, being associated with bigger babies and lower perinatal mortality than higher haemoglobins. It has been a widespread routine in this and other countries to give the pregnant woman prophylactic iron and folic acid supplements from 12 weeks onwards. Iron should be avoided in early pregnancy because there is some evidence of a tendency to increased fetal abnormality rates. A single daily dose of one of the proprietary sustained-release preparations such as Pregaday, Fefol or Slow-Fe-Folic is suitable. Iron preparations tend to produce constipation and make the motions a very dark colour. It is acceptable to give iron only to those whose haemoglobin is initially below 12 g per 100 ml or falls significantly during pregnancy.

Much the most common cause of anaemia in this country is iron deficiency, generally related to failure to take iron supplements. Iron deficiency may, however, also be due to chronic infection (particularly urinary tract infection) and to chronic blood loss (piles, intestinal neoplasia, etc.). Haemoglobinopathies are common in Afro-Caribbean patients, and thalassaemias are common in those with Mediterranean ancestry. In immigrants, hookworm infestation, malaria and other parasites are possibilities. Folic acid deficiency is particularly likely with multiple pregnancy and epileptics.

Investigation and treatment of anaemia in pregnancy

Immigrant populations will normally be screened for abnormal haemoglobins at booking. Otherwise the initial investigation of anaemia will usually be a full blood count and film. If these show a picture of iron deficiency it is usually sufficient to treat the anaemia with oral iron and folic acid without further investigation. If the patient fails to respond to this treatment it is appropriate to do further investigations as follows:

1 Serum ferritin.
2 Serum folate concentration.
3 Serum vitamin B_{12} concentration.
4 Examination of stool for occult blood and parasites.
5 Urine culture.

If these investigations reveal nothing other than iron deficiency due to the patient's unwillingness or inability to take oral iron, it may be appropriate to treat her with parenteral iron. Neither intravenous nor intramuscular iron preparations should be used lightly as both can produce unpleasant side-effects – anaphylactic reactions with intravenous iron and very unsightly skin staining with intramuscular preparations. It is probably unnecessary to treat anaemia in this way unless the haemoglobin is below 9 g per 100 ml. Very occasionally with severe anaemia it may be advisable to transfuse blood before labour, and in extreme cases this should be done by exchange transfusions or by combining intravenous frusemide with transfusion to avoid the hazards of heart failure.

In cases of haemoglobinopathy iron stores may be overloaded in spite of anaemia, and increased iron administration may be unnecessary and even hazardous. The detailed management of haemoglobinopathies in pregnancy falls outside the scope of this book but detailed accounts of their management may be found in the books mentioned below.

FURTHER READING

Brudenell, M. and Wilds, P. L. (1984) *Medical and Surgical Problems in Obstetrics.* Wright, Bristol.
de Swiet, M. (1984) *Medical Disorders in Obstetric Practice.* Blackwell, Oxford.

8

Intrapartum care

The safe delivery of a healthy baby is every pregnant woman's goal, a wish intensified and reinforced as the months of pregnancy pass. Appreciation of the mother's and the family's intense emotions during labour and delivery is of paramount importance and a prerequisite to good care. This is well-understood by midwives but must also have the highest priority for medical staff, from consultant to medical student, who must never lose sight of those emotions.

Labour is the hurdle that has to be overcome to achieve the delivery goal, and is viewed with apprehension by many and with dread by some.

ANTENATAL CLASSES

Preparation classes for parenthood offer the opportunity for education about labour and delivery. Education about the onset, stages and mechanism of labour is as important to the mother as it is to the medical student and pupil midwife. Most pregnant women in the UK have access to such classes but the uptake is less than ideal in many areas. Classes aim to inspire confidence, provide accurate information and dispel myths.

They provide the opportunity for making friends and many classes continue as postnatal and breast-feeding support groups after delivery. Some classes are provided by the hospital midwifery staff, some at health centres by primary health care teams and some are organized by independent groups such as the National Childbirth Trust. Women and their partners should be encouraged to attend classes but more effort needs to be made by the providers to ensure that the classes are welcoming to the single, the shy, and the unsupported; that the timing of classes is convenient; that there is easy access; and that the information is correct, consistent and does not conflict with that being given in other parts of the hospital maternity unit, or with delivery suite politics and protocols.

A mother may choose where she is going to have her child, but the choice should be made in full knowledge of the facts. Delivery outside the major unit may be the appropriate choice for some women. Such a choice should be made after full discussion with the midwife and family practitioner and made with the knowledge that should a complication arise then transfer to the main unit will be advised. The establishment of good rapport, of good communication, of trust and understanding, and the sharing of decision-making responsibility together with appropriate selection are the cornerstones of successful home delivery. Good communication must exist too between the community care and the major unit teams.

Women may be delivered in the major unit by their community midwife and go home very shortly afterwards (domino delivery) and the community team may continue to look after the transferred problem cases together with the hospital team depending on the severity of the problem.

DELIVERY OPTIONS

Major obstetric unit

1 Consultant team.
2 Hospital midwife.
3 Domino.
4 General practitioner (GP).

GP unit

1 Midwife.
2 GP.

Home

1 Midwife.
2 Midwife and GP.

The expectant mother is encouraged to discuss her plans for the birth during the preparation classes and antenatal visits, to visit the delivery unit and to become familiar with the surroundings.

The sterile, hostile delivery rooms of old have been replaced in many units by rooms with attractive screens, pictures, radio and often television. Many units have some rooms furnished with floor mats to facilitate delivery in the squatting position, bean bags, rocking chairs and homely comforts. Also an increasing number of units have special bath rooms where the woman can relax in labour and deliver if she so wishes. With the humanizing of hospital and early discharge to home, increasing numbers of mothers are happy to have their babies in major obstetric units, appreciating the safety and the expertise available for both mother and infant should a problem occur. If she is confident in herself and her attendants and supported by her partner or chosen companion in familiar pleasant surroundings, a woman's labour can be a satisfying and rewarding experience. Attention to preparation for labour and delivery antenatally is vital for the woman who then anticipates eagerly possibly the most momentous event of her life.

The majority of women approaching labour are not patients in any real sense. They are fit healthy women experiencing a normal physiological event.

Management of labour must concern itself with care of the emotional as well as the physical state of the woman. The woman who had a dreadful experience with her first birth will be full of terror and dread about a similar time with her second. (For some women the first experience is so horrendous that they never allow themselves to become pregnant again – the ultimate failure of care.) In contrast, the primigravida who has a fulfilling experience with her first labour and delivery will be unlikely to be anxious or apprehensive about her second. A minority of women, who are usually identified antenatally, do have problems – specific disease, or pregnancy complications or other conditions – which mean that they are patients in the accepted sense and require specialist care; even so it is vital that the emotional aspect of care for these patients is not overlooked.

Antenatal preparation classes are the one time that the distinction between primigravidae and multigravidae is made very clearly, most groups holding separate refresher classes for multigravidae. Regrettably the distinction between primigravidae and multigravidae fails to be emphasized sufficiently in clinical practice.

PRIMIGRAVIDAE AND MULTIGRAVIDAE

There are anatomical, physiological and emotional differences between first-time labour and subsequent ones, and the basic management concept should be that if the first labour is successful, problems are rare in subsequent labours, but if problems occur in the first labour then they are likely to influence adversely the woman's whole future reproductive history. Indeed, it has been stated that the fundamental differences between a first and a later birth are so great that primigravidae and multigravidae behave like different biological species.

The main difference between the first and subsequent labours is the duration. The cervix, the vagina and the surrounding tissues of the pelvic floor have not been stretched before; the uterus has not contracted so strongly before. Inefficient uterine action, by far the most common complication of labour, is much more common in primigravidae than multigravidae. It is as though the uterus learns what contractions are for in the first labour and becomes efficient thereafter. Posterior position of the occiput, which is associated with inefficient uterine action, is also more common in primigravidae and is a further reason why labour is longer.

THE DIAGNOSIS OF LABOUR

The initial diagnosis of the onset of labour is made by the woman who then presents herself for admission to her place of confinement which for most women in the UK is a maternity hospital. Since occasional uterine contractions are noticed during the last few weeks of pregnancy, a frequency of one contraction every 10 minutes (1 in 10) is a practical guide to the actual start of labour. The difference between the contractions of late pregnancy and the contractions of labour is that the latter dilate the cervix. The onset of painful regular contractions may be preceded or accompanied by a 'show', that is the loss vaginally of the mucus plug in the cervix. This mucus is often streaked with blood. The membranes usually rupture fairly late in labour but occasionally may be the first sign of labour. They may cause a major flood and considerable inconvenience, or leak in a dribbling fashion.

In spite of these classic signs, the diagnosis of labour is none the less fraught with difficulties and it is therefore not surprising that the woman, especially is she is a primigravida, may be mistaken in her diagnosis. There is nothing more demoralizing for the pregnant woman than to be admitted believing she is in labour and then subsequently being told that she is not, and her attendants, both midwives and medical staff, must be aware of this. Rupture of the membranes may be confused with leakage of urine which occurs commonly in late pregnancy; rupture of the membranes may happen without contractions and labour occurring; a small antepartum haemorrhage may be confused with a heavy show. Braxton Hicks' contractions may be painful, strong and regular, without effecting cervical dilatation. Many of these difficulties in diagnosis may be resolved by the woman talking to her community midwife before coming to hospital.

On admission the crucial decision is whether to admit the woman to the delivery suite (confirm her diagnosis), keep her in hospital for observation (question her diagnosis) but have concern because of her symptoms; or send her home (discount her diagnosis) and reassure her all is well. The history and observations made on admission are therefore of paramount importance. It is also important that the woman understands that her diagnosis of labour may not be able to be confirmed immediately and that a period of observation to assess change in cervical dilatation may be necessary. Having decided that the woman is in labour – that the cervix is dilating – she is admitted to the delivery suite. There is no point in shaving the pubic hair unless a caesarean section is contemplated and then only the suprapubic hair need be shaved. The woman may prefer to do this herself or have her partner do it for her. An enema is unnecessary unless the woman is constipated, but a relaxing bath may be most welcome after the journey and assessment, and is usually offered. Remember not all women have easy access to or avail themselves of free bathing facilities.

MECHANISM OF LABOUR

This term is used to describe the movements of the fetal head and trunk through the maternal pelvis (Fig. 8.1). These have been outlined in Chapter 4. The head enters the true pelvis before or during labour and usually engages in the transverse diameter – the sagittal suture of the fetal skull is at right angles to the anteroposterior diameter of the maternal pelvis. With contractions the head descends and becomes more flexed. Thus the occiput becomes the lowest part of the head as a result of flexion and reaches the pelvic floor first. Here the levator ani muscles meet in the midline and form a gutter channelling downwards and forwards. The uterine contractions and tone in the levators act together on the head to produce internal rotation (that is, the occiput is rotated forwards so that it comes to lie beneath the symphysis pubis). Further descent occurs, the occiput escapes from under the pubic arch, and the head is born by extension. When the widest diameter comes through the introitus the head is said to crown (Fig. 8.1d). As the head is born, the shoulders enter the pelvis. They pass through the widest diameter of the pelvic inlet and rotate to accommodate themselves to the widest diameter of the outlet, that is the anteroposterior (AP) diameter. As the shoulders rotate into the AP diameter, the delivered head is carried round 90°. This external rotation (or restitution) is readily seen. The anterior shoulder escapes from under the symphysis and the trunk is born by lateral flexion.

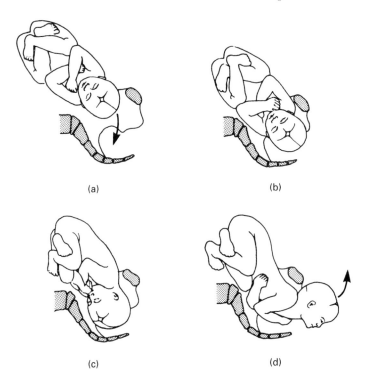

(a)　(b)

(c)　(d)

Fig. 8.1 Mechanism of normal labour. (a) Head enters the true pelvis, usually in occipitolateral position; (b) head descends to pelvic floor; (c) internal rotation; occiput comes to lie beneath symphysis pubis; (d) further descent; head is born by extension.

The stages of labour

Three stages of labour are recognized. Stage 1 is from the onset of labour to full dilatation (about 10 cm) of the cervical os. Progress is monitored by assessing cervical dilatation together with descent of the head through the pelvis, which is recorded on the partogram (Fig. 8.2). The first stage usually lasts between 8 and 10 hours in the primigravida and between 2 and 6 hours in the multigravida.

Stage 2 is from full dilatation to birth of the fetus. This usually lasts between 40 and 60 minutes in the primigravida and 10–15 minutes in the multigravida. The second stage may be divided into two phases. During the first phase the vagina dilates, allowing descent of the head to the pelvic floor where internal rotation occurs. With the second phase, further descent occurs, the occiput reaches the perineum and escapes from under the pubic arch and the head is born. This concept of two phases to the second stage originates from Dublin and is of particular relevance when considering forceps delivery (see below).

Stage 3 is from the birth of the fetus to the delivery of the placenta and membranes.

Management of normal labour

There are three areas of concern:

1 Maternal well-being
2 Fetal well-being
3 Progress of labour

Maternal well-being

The measures of maternal well-being involve the woman's physical condition and her emotional state and morale, and are interdependent on fetal well-being and the progress of labour.

The mother's physical condition is frequently assessed with particular attention to blood pressure, pulse, temperature and hydration. Free fluids are encouraged but food is avoided in case an anaesthetic is required. The woman is encouraged to empty her bladder at frequent intervals and the volume of each specimen is measured and recorded on the partogram (Fig. 8.2). Each specimen is tested for albumin, ketones and sugar.

During labour the woman should adopt whatever posture she desires (except the supine position). She should be encouraged to be as free as possible to walk, stand, sit or lie at will, but her wishes may be hampered by intravenous infusions, monitoring systems and the need to carry out observations. She should not lie flat on her back since pressure from the gravid uterus on the inferior vena cava will cause supine hypotension and diminished uterine and placental perfusion, occasionally causing profound fetal distress.

Pain relief
Psychological factors such as anxiety and fear influence the appreciation of pain and although psychoprophylaxis, hypnosis and acupuncture may prevent or relieve pain, the majority of women require analgesia of some sort. The type and timing of analgesia are crucial and individual labour is a painful process for the vast majority of women. Preparation and education antenatally, together with support in labour from her midwife and husband or birth partner, can influence the need for analgesia considerably but many

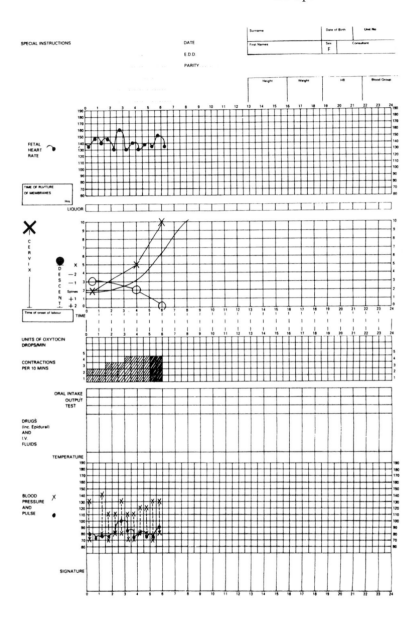

Fig. 8.2 A partogram recording all important observations.

women require some additional help. The following five measures are available in virtually all maternity units.

1 *Warm bath*: Relaxation in a warm bath may provide adequate analgesia for some considerable time in the early first stage.
2 *TENS*: Transcutaneous electrical nerve stimulation (TENS) is self-administered via electrodes placed on the mother's lower back, the intensity of the stimulus being adjusted by the woman herself. This gives satisfactory pain relief to many women. The efficacy is unpredictable however. Some women require no other form of analgesia while others find virtually no relief. The majority of TENS users obtain help for much of the early part of the first stage.
3 *Entonox*: Entonox (nitrous oxide 50%, oxygen 50%) is an inhalational analgesic which is especially effective at the end of the first stage and during the second stage since it is absorbed and expelled rapidly. Inhalation should begin just before the contraction starts and before the patient feels pain, as it takes 15–20 seconds to work. Timing the contractions is a prerequisite for this form of analgesia to be effective.
4 *Opiates*: Pethidine 50–100 mg intramuscularly is widely used in the first stage of labour. The midwife is allowed to prescribe up to two doses of 100 mg of pethidine. The dose should be given with thought to the patient's physique, and it should not be given within 4 hours of delivery – if such a judgement is possible – since it depresses the neonatal respiratory centre. It may cause vomiting. Mild analgesics like aspirin have no place since they are not effective. Strong analgesics like morphine and Omnopon cause such profound neonatal respiratory depression that they are generally avoided except in cases of intrauterine death. An antiemetic may be prescribed in conjunction with pethidine. If the baby is delivered within 4 hours of a pethidine injection then a respiratory-centre stimulant such as nalorphine may be required.
5 *Epidural anaesthesia*: This produces total pain relief without impairment of consciousness or fetal depression, but by relaxing levator tone interferes with the mechanism of labour, particularly at the stage of internal rotation, and makes maternal voluntary expulsive efforts difficult, thus increasing the incidence of malrotation and forceps delivery.

Fetal well-being

Labour is a hazardous time to any fetus since with each contraction blood flow through the intervillous space ceases and the oxygen supply to the fetus is reduced. A normal fetus can accommodate to these intermittent periods of hypoxia for some time, but an already hypoxic fetus is in jeopardy. The hypoxic fetus is at risk of intrapartum death from asphyxia. Consequently, careful monitoring of fetal well-being in labour is necessary.

The measures of fetal well-being are:

1 Fetal heart rate patterns.
2 Meconium.
3 Fetal blood pH.

Fetal distress is the term used when fetal hypoxia is suspected or confirmed, but gross abnormalities of the fetal heart rate and the presence of meconium suggesting fetal distress can occur without fetal hypoxia being confirmed.

Fetal heart rate
The fetal heart may be observed in various ways;

1 Auscultation with a Pinard fetal stethoscope through the mother's anterior abdominal wall is the most widely used method (originally described by Laennec of Brittany). It is most informative if auscultation is continued through and after a contraction so that alterations in rate can be appreciated. If no contractions occur then auscultation over 1 minute and during fetal movements is valuable.
2 Ultrasound: The alterations of blood flow in the fetal heart can be detected by the Doppler effect. This signal can be obtained through the mother's anterior abdominal wall.
3 Electrocardiography picks up the electrical activity of the fetal heart with a clip attached directly to the fetal scalp.

The terms used in the study of continuous fetal heart traces are shown in Figure 8.3.

The following fetal heart rate features are potential signs of fetal distress.

1 A baseline fetal heart rate above 160 or below 120 beats/min.
2 Lack of beat-to-beat variation (minor variations in heart rate which occur in response to autonomic reflex activity).
3 Slowing in heart rate occurring during or immediately after contractions. If the fetal heart rate slows at the onset of the contraction but returns to its basal rate immediately after the contraction ends, the deceleration is termed an early or type I deceleration or a V dip. If the fetal heart rate slows during a

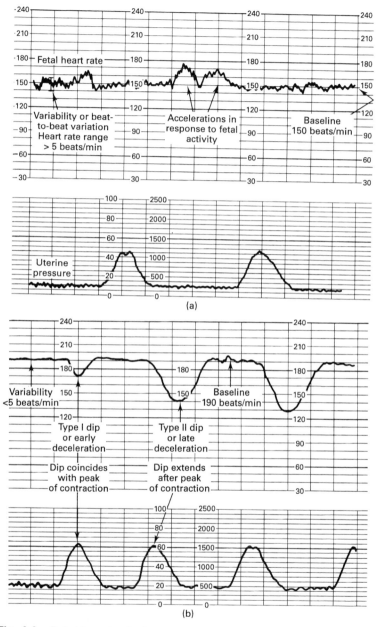

Fig. 8.3 Fetal heart rate traces – terms used in cardiotographs. (a) Healthy trace with normal baseline; good variability; accelerations; no decelerations. (b) Abnormal trace with poor variability; baseline tachycardia; type I and II decelerations.

contraction but is tardy in its return, returning to its baseline well after the end of the contraction, the deceleration is termed a late or type II or U dip. Variable decelerations may be a mixture of early and late and include other patterns. Fewer than 50% of cases with these heart rate changes will have true fetal distress.

Meconium

The fetal gut may contract and the anal sphincter relax under hypoxic conditions, releasing meconium into the amniotic fluid. The presence of meconium staining in the liquor is, however, an unreliable sign of fetal distress on its own. If the fetal heart rate is normal, then about 10% of patients with meconium-stained liquor have a distressed fetus, but if the fetal heart rate is abnormal the figure is about 20%. In order that this sign is not missed, amniotomy (rupture of the membranes) is frequently carried out once labour is established, that is the cervix is dilating at the rate of 1 cm or more per hour and is at least 3 cm dilated. Meconium staining occurs with nearly all breech deliveries.

Fetal blood pH

If hypoxia is present, carbon dioxide and lactic acid accumulate and the pH of the blood falls below 7.2. If hypoxia is suspected because of meconium or decelerations in the fetal heart rate, a fetal blood sample may be taken. In the majority of cases of suspected fetal hypoxia the blood sample will refute the suspicion. An amnioscope is passed through the cervix and the fetal skull visualized. The scalp is stabbed with a very short protected blade and blood is drawn up into a heparinized tube for pH analysis. The pH in the first stage falls but normally remains above 7.25. If the pH falls below 7.2 for whatever reason the fetus must be delivered at once as fetal death or permanent handicap is a significant risk.

Progress of labour

1 Dilatation of the cervix is assessed by vaginal examination and should occur at the rate of 1 cm/h once labour is well-established.
2 Descent of the presenting part may be judged on abdominal palpation in relation to the pelvic brim and it is customary to divide the head into fifths and assess the number of fifths remaining above the brim (see Chapter 4). Descent of the head can also be judged on vaginal examination by estimating the distance of the lowest part of the fetal head above or below the level of the ischial spines: for instance, if the head is 3 cm above the ischial spines, this is recorded as −3; if the head is palpable 2 cm below

the level of the ischial spines it is recorded as +2. As the head descends through the pelvis there is usually a degree of moulding, that is, the skull bones overlap. If there is any delay in descent, caput forms, that is the scalp becomes oedematous and thickened, making palpation of the sutures and fontanelles difficult. One must beware of considering caput as a reference point when defining the descent of the head since the thickened oedematous scalp may mislead one into thinking that the head is lower in the pelvis than it really is.

Uterine contractions of adequate strength and frequency are necessary for normal progress in labour. These are recorded by one of the following methods:

1 Palpation: This is a subjective and variable observation requiring experience for reliability but is of no inconvenience to the patient.
2 An external pressure transducer may be strapped to the anterior abdominal wall measuring contractions more accurately, although movement and anterior abdominal wall fat may make recording difficult. It is somewhat inhibiting for the patient since she has to remain attached to the recorder.
3 Internal uterine pressure can be measured via a catheter introduced into the uterus after rupture of the membranes. Although widely used in the past, this method is now rarely employed because of its intrusiveness.

The partogram

This is a visual display of the indices of maternal and fetal well-being mentioned above, together with progress displayed as cervical dilatation and descent of the head on abdominal palpation. Such charts have proved useful in the early detection of abnormal labour. Whether partograms are used or not, regular recordings of maternal and fetal well-being and progress are essential during labour (see Fig. 8.2).

Active management of labour

If labour is not progressing normally, i.e. the cervix is not dilating at the usual rate of 1 cm or more per hour, then in order to prevent a prolonged labour, with all its attendant maternal and fetal problems, steps are taken to normalize the rate of cervical dilatation.

1 Artificial rupture of the membranes (ARM).
2 Syntocinon infusion (synthetic oxytocin to stimulate contractions).

Rupture of the membranes will stimulate uterine contractions probably by releasing prostaglandins, and the contractions will improve cervical dilatation.

Syntocinon is the trade name for synthetic oxytocin which is given intravenously and improves the strength and frequency of uterine contractions, especially if the membranes are ruptured.

These two steps may be taken at the same time. A number of studies have found that the outcome of labour is improved by active management with fewer forceps deliveries and caesarean sections.

THE SECOND STAGE

Phase 1 of the second stage may go unheralded since during this time the patient has no desire to push. Although the cervix is fully dilated the vagina has to dilate and uterine contractions have to bring the head to the pelvic floor. When the head reaches the pelvic floor and internal rotation occurs, the patient usually has an over-whelming desire to push. Involuntary expulsive efforts are seen and there is evidence accruing that the patient should be encouraged to push as she feels the need to, rather than the traditional long-sustained pushing with each contraction. With each expulsive effort the head further descends, bulging the perineum and causing the anus to pout. Internal rotation may be seen to occur on the perineum. Inhalational analgesia, if analgesia is required, is ideal during the second stage and should be inhaled before the contrac-tion starts, as indicated previously.

The fetal heart rate must be recorded after each contraction if a continuous record is not available. The membranes should be ruptured if they are still intact.

Delivery usually takes place with the patient in a semi-sitting position, but the patient should be allowed to adopt whatever posi-tion she wishes provided that the attendant is able to control the delivery of the head to avoid tearing of the perineum and have access to the face, eyes, nose and mouth of the fetus at once. If it looks as though the perineum is going to tear, an episiotomy (see below) is carried out. The head is delivered slowly by extension. The baby's pharynx should be cleared with a mucus aspirator during restitution and before the delivery of the shoulders. The baby's head is then drawn towards the mother's sacrum, aiding the passage of the anterior shoulder under the symphysis. The head is then drawn up towards the symphysis and the posterior shoulder slides over the perineum. Gentle traction with one finger in the posterior axilla may be necessary.

As the trunk delivers, the baby is taken up on to the mother's abdomen so that she may see and feel and hold the baby at once. The cord is clamped and cut at least 5 cm from the umbilicus. The baby must not be allowed to get cold and must, therefore, be wrapped. The baby may need further mucus aspiration, but there is no reason why, if its condition is satisfactory, the wrapping and aspiration should not be done in the mother's arms.

The baby's condition is traditionally assessed using the Apgar score which rates each of five features – colour, tone, respiration, heart rate and reflex activity between 0 and 2 – at 1 and 5 minutes after birth.

THE THIRD STAGE

Active management of the third stage is now usual as it reduces the risk of postpartum haemorrhage – still a cause of maternal death. An oxytocic, usually Syntometrine 1 ampoule (containing ergometrine 0.5 mg and Syntocinon 5 units) is given intramuscularly as the anterior shoulder delivers. The oxytocic injection causes the uterus to contract strongly and the placenta to separate almost at once. Having ascertained that the uterus is contracted, the left hand is placed on the abdomen above the symphysis, holding the contracted uterus out of the pelvis. The right hand exerts steady firm downwards pressure on the cord. The active management of the third stage has reduced the overall blood loss at delivery and the number of cases of haemorrhage.

The placenta and membranes must be carefully examined for completeness, and the cord inspected to record the number of arteries. If one of the two arteries is absent, fetal abnormalities may be present. After delivery the uterus is frequently palpated and blood loss observed to detect excessive bleeding. The pulse and blood pressure are recorded. Any episiotomy or lacerations are sutured as soon after delivery as possible with further careful infiltration of additional local anaesthetic.

The baby should be put to the breast at the earliest moment before weighing, measuring and attending to the cord, all of which removes the baby from the mother. The mother and father should be offered the traditional cup of tea and then, with the mother in a comfortable bed, her baby in a cot beside her, with a firmly contracted uterus and no bleeding, she is encouraged to sleep.

EPISIOTOMY

This is an incision usually made with scissors in the perineum after

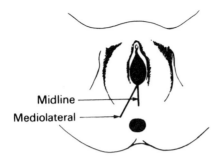

Fig. 8.4 Incisions for episiotomy.

infiltration with local anaesthetic (e.g. 10 ml of 0.5% lignocaine) along the line of the incision. The incision starts in the midline and is usually carried in a mediolateral direction to avoid the anal sphincter, although a midline incision is often made by experienced practitioners (Fig. 8.4). The exact line of the episiotomy may be dictated by vulval varices, which should be avoided, or previous episiotomy scars, which should be refashioned.

Indications

1 To prevent incipient tearing of the perineum.
2 To remove obstruction during delivery of the head of the premature infant and thus prevent rapid changes in intracranial pressure.
3 To facilitate intravaginal manoeuvres, i.e. forceps delivery, and give protection to maternal tissues.

Complications

1 The episiotomy may extend if it is too small or care is not taken at delivery, particularly of the posterior shoulder. The tear usually turns medially, tracking down towards the anal margin, and may involve the sphincter and even rectum. The vaginal part of the episiotomy may tear up the posterolateral vaginal wall.
2 Bleeding may be profuse, particularly if an intravaginal tear is not recognized.
3 Other complications are dealt with in the section on maternal trauma, later in this chapter.

INDUCTION OF LABOUR

Those attendant upon pregnant women throughout the ages have tried to induce labour for various reasons in various ways, from herbal potions to Indian braves on horseback leaping across the prostrate patient. For centuries before the advent of antibiotics, the risks of infection with its dire consequences to both mother and baby if the membranes were ruptured were recognized. Induction should never be undertaken lightly because failure leads to caesarean section and still occasionally to sepsis. It should only be carried out in a maternity unit fully equipped to proceed to caesarean section at a moment's notice.

The induction rate in most units is decreasing due mainly to more reliable measures of fetal well-being and also to more non-interventionist patterns of obstetric practice. However, there are still numerous indications for induction of labour and these are discussed in the relevant sections of the previous chapter. When considering whether to induce labour the balance or risks for both mother and fetus must be considered. The indications are briefly reviewed as follows:

Indications for induction

1 Pre-eclampsia/hypertension.
2 Prolonged pregnancy.
3 Antepartum bleeding.
4 Placental insufficiency.
5 Diabetes.
6 Rhesus haemolytic disease.
7 Fetal abnormality or death.
8 Multiple pregnancy.

Bishop's score

The Bishop's score is a way of expressing the factors relating to ease of induction or how readily the woman will go into labour after induction (Table 8.1). It is used in many units.

Methods of induction

The methods of induction are:

1 Amniotomy (ARM):
   a. Low (forewaters).
   b. High (hindwaters).

Table 8.1   Bishop's score – inducibility rating

	Score			
	0	*1*	*2*	*3*
Dilatation of cervix	0	1–2 cm	3–4 cm	5 cm
Station head	–3	–2	–1/0	+1
Length of cervix	3	2	1	0
Consistency of cervix	Firm	Medium	Soft	
Position of cervix	Posterior	Mid	Anterior	

Total score 0–5 = unfavourable; 6–13 = favourable.

2 Oxytocic agents:
   a. Intravenously.
   b. Orally (sublingual).
   c. Extra-/intra-amniotically.

Hindwater rupture and oral oxytocics are virtually never used in modern obstetrics. It is usual to ripen the cervix with prostaglandin given in the form of a vaginal pessary or gel before rupturing the membranes. The prostaglandin makes the cervix more favourable, improving the Bishop's score, and in many cases initiates labour. In these instances the membranes are then ruptured with the patient in established labour, greatly reducing the risk of infection and failed induction.

If the membranes are ruptured artificially but labour is not established after a few hours then an intravenous infusion of Syntocinon is set up.

The membranes ruptured are those below the presenting part, i.e. the forewaters (low amniotomy).

Procedure for ARM

1 Review the indication.
2 Reassess maturity.
   (An enema is only needed if the patient is constipated. Her pubic hair does not need shaving.)
3 Abdominal palpation confirms the fetal lie (which must be longitudinal) and the position of the presenting part, which should be in the pelvis (at least partly). The fetal heart is auscultated.
4 The woman is positioned so that a vaginal examination can be made to check pelvic capacity, the position and station of the presenting part and the state of the cervix. If there is no suspicion

of placenta praevia, one or two fingers are passed through the cervix and the membranes are swept off the lower segment and the cervix is stretched. This procedure alone often stimulates contractions, probably due to a release of prostaglandins. The forewaters are ruptured with an amniotomy hook, Kocher's forceps or a similar instrument.

5 The colour and amount of amniotic fluid are noted. If bleeding occurs, the blood should be analysed at once for fetal haemoglobin. Undetected rupture of vasa praevia may result in an exsanguinated fetus.

6 After ARM, prolapse of the cord should be excluded by vaginal examination. It is usual to monitor the fetal heart rate after ARM and abnormalities may indicate cord prolapse or, rarely, fetal bleeding from vasa praevia.

7 Dictated to some extent by the Bishop's score, an intravenous infusion of Syntocinon may be set up at the same time as ARM if the score is unfavourable or after a few hours if contractions have not started, even with a favourable score.

Sublingual tablets of oxytocin and prostaglandin may be used but absorption is variable and they are not widely used. Tetanic uterine contraction has occurred as a complication of oxytocics given by this route.

Intrauterine fetal death and mid-trimester abortion

Prostaglandins have proved especially useful in these distressing circumstances. Vaginal prostaglandin E_2 pessaries ripen the cervix and induce contractions without early rupture of the membranes and the consequent risks of sepsis. Prostaglandins may also be used intra- and extra-amniotically.

Dangers of oxcytocic administration

1 Hypertonic uterine contractions.
2 Uterine rupture.
3 Fetal hypoxia.

All of these complications are extremely rare if the course of labour is carefully monitored.

Dangers of induction

1 Failure to establish labour.
2 Long painful labour.

3 Increased incidence of forceps delivery and caesarean section.
4 Sepsis both fetal and maternal.
5 Prolapse of the cord.

Although induction of labour is usually successful, should labour fail to become established and the patient does not deliver within 24 hours she will require a caesarean section. Infection of the membranes (chorionitis or amnionitis), intrapartum fetal pneumonia and endometritis are all sequelae of prolonged rupture of the membranes (more than 24 hours), but infective complications have been recorded after much shorter times. If the presenting part is not in the pelvis the cord may prolapse. Any uncertainty about maturity may result in the delivery of a premature infant.

ABNORMAL LABOUR

Classically, problems with labour have been categorized as due to the power, the passenger or the passage – uterine contractions, the fetus or the birth canal.

Power problems

1 Abnormal uterine action.
2 Too weak: hypotonic incoordinate uterine action (links with occipitoposterior (OP) position).
3 Too strong, too frequent: hypertonic uterine action.

Passenger problems

1 Malposition of the head: OP (links with hypotonic uterine action), deep transverse arrest.
2 Malpresentation of the fetus – breech, face, brow, shoulder, cord.
3 Abnormality, e.g. hydrocephaly.
4 Too big in cephalopelvic disproportion.

Passage problems (rare)

1 Small pelvis – trauma, rickets.
2 Vaginal septum.
3 Pelvic tumours, e.g. fibroids, ovarian cyst.
4 Cervical dystocia - failure to dilate.

Power problems

Abnormal uterine activity

Hypotonic uterine action is by far the most important cause of abnormal labour particularly in the primigravida. Here the contractions are irregular, they may be infrequent and they are ineffectual. They vary in strength but usually cause considerable distress, especially as labour is prolonged. The woman knows that cervical dilatation is slow and that she 'isn't getting anywhere' and can become demoralized without support. Dehydration and ketosis are often causal or at least aggravating factors, and should be corrected if present.

Hypotonic uterine activity is associated with OP position of the fetus, the contractions being too weak to effect flexion and rotation of the fetal head. Adequate uterine action is achieved by active management in rupture of the membranes and intravenous Syntocinon infusion.

Hypertonic uterine action

Here the contractions are too frequent, there is a high resting tone in the uterus and the contractions are excessively painful. This situation causes maternal exhaustion, and the likelihood of fetal hypoxia is high. Caesarean section is sometimes necessary if fetal distress or maternal exhaustion develops. This situation can be iatrogenic following the use of Syntocinon. It is essential to monitor the strength of uterine contractions when a Syntocinon infusion is used because of the risk of hyperstimulation and titanic contractions leading to fetal hypoxia.

Passenger problems

Occipitoposterior position

The commonest malposition is the OP position (Fig. 8.5). This is the usual cause of a high head at term in the primigravida. The head is incompletely flexed and a larger than usual diameter, the occipitofrontal diameter, presents. At the onset of labour the head usually flexes and the malposition is corrected. The occiput may remain posterior after the onset of labour in about 20% of cases.

Diagnosis

Abdominal palpation reveals fetal limbs over the front of the uterus. The back is not felt in the flank and there is flattening of the abdomen below the umbilicus. On vaginal examination the anterior fontanelle is readily palpable anteriorly and the posterior fontanelle may be palpated in the posterior part of the pelvis.

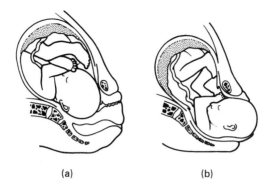

Fig. 8.5   Occipitoposterior position (a) in labour; (b) at delivery.

Causes of OP position
1 Incoordinate hypotonic uterine activity – fails to flex and rotate.
2 Android-shaped pelvis – inhibits rotation.
3 Anthropoid-shaped pelvis – big AP diameter, no need to rotate.
4 Epidural analgesia – lax pelvic floor inhibits rotation.

Mechanism of labour with OP
The occiput is frequently posterior at the onset of labour, but the uterine contractions cause flexion of the fetal head, which enters the pelvic brim with the sagittal suture in the transverse diameter. Contractions cause further flexion, which brings the occiput below the sinciput, making it the lowest part of the head, and it thus reaches the pelvic floor and rotates anteriorly.

If the contractions fail to bring about adequate flexion the head will enter the brim with the occiput in the posterior position, usually not a direct OP position but with the occiput lying in the right oblique diameter of the pelvis, i.e. a right occipitoposterior (ROP) position. As this means that a bigger presenting diameter is coming into the pelvis, it may take longer for the head to get into the pelvis; also, this less flexed head is a poor fit against the lower segment and therefore not such a good stimulator of contractions. It may be necessary for quite considerable moulding of the fetal head to take place for the head to be able to enter the pelvis and frequently caput forms. If the pelvis is big enough and in the presence of good uterine contractions, the head may reach the pelvic floor and the occiput may rotate the long way round the pelvis to an occipitoanterior position and the baby deliver by the normal mechanism. If the pelvis is roomy the head may rotate to a direct OP position and deliver as a persistent occipitoposterior (POP), with the baby's face delivering beneath the symphysis pubis (face to pubes).

Management of labour with OP

In either of these instances it can be seen that a longer than normal labour is anticipated and it is therefore important to maintain the woman's morale and ensure that she does not become dehydrated. Adequate analgesia is also necessary. In spite of the risk of producing poor levator tone and possible problems with rotation of the fetal head, epidural analgesia is especially helpful to women with an OP position. It is essential to ensure adequate uterine contractions and intravenous Syntocinon is often required, especially after epidural analgesia. Careful monitoring of the fetal heart rate and inspection of the amniotic fluid for the appearance of meconium are necessary as labour may be prolonged and fetal distress occur.

Delivery with OP position

1 Ninety per cent of labour where the initial position is left OP (LOP) or ROP will conclude with a normal delivery, the head having flexed and carried out a long internal rotation through 135° to deliver occipitoanterior (OA). Good uterine contractions are necessary for this to happen.

2 The head may remain in the OP position and deliver face to pubes. About 6% of OP positions deliver this way, usually where the mother has a capacious pelvic cavity. Because the occipitofrontal diameter, which measures 11 cm, presents to the vulva instead of the smaller 10 cm suboccipitobregmatic, perineal lacerations are more common, and a third-degree tear is not unknown.

3 POP with arrest: If spontaneous delivery does not occur, the situation must be assessed carefully. If after phase 1 of the second stage, when the vagina has dilated and the head has reached the perineum, the head has failed to rotate in spite of adequate contractions and an adequate outlet, it will have to be delivered operatively. There are four options:

   a. Manual rotation of the head may be followed by spontaneous delivery if the mother is not too exhausted, but it is more usually completed with obstetric forceps. Manual rotation is relatively safe for both mother and baby, but adequate analgesia – usually an epidural anaesthetic – is required. The head is often pushed up as the rotation is carried out and may slip back into a posterior position unless forceps are applied as soon as the rotation to OA has been done.

   b. Rotation of the head with Kjelland's forceps requires adequate analgesia (ideally a spinal or epidural block) and the services of an experienced obstetrician, one experienced in the use of Kjelland's forceps. In inexperienced hands fetal and maternal trauma may be caused by the use of Kjelland's forceps.

c. Vacuum extraction (ventouse): With the cervix fully dilated, the suction cap of the ventouse is applied over the occiput or as near to that as possible, so that when traction is applied flexion will be encouraged. With downwards and backwards traction the head flexes, the occiput rotates round anteriorly and delivery is achieved, or sometimes the head fails to rotate and delivers face to pubes.

d. Caesarean section: One of the commonest mistakes in obstetrics is to assume that because the cervix is fully dilated the baby is ready and can be delivered vaginally. Never is this truer than in the case of OP presentation, where caput and moulding may appear at the vulva, leading the unwary obstetrician to assume that all is ready for forceps delivery. In reality the head is above the pelvic floor, often still palpable abdominally and the patient should be delivered by caesarean section.

The risks of postpartum haemorrhage are increased since labour may have been prolonged and an operative delivery has occurred. There is an increased perinatal mortality and morbidity due to hypoxia and with trauma, and increased maternal morbidity due to trauma in many cases.

Deep transverse arrest

This is a separate entity. Here the head has entered the pelvic brim with the sagittal suture in the transverse diameter of the brim, but as the contractions cause less flexion than usual, the occiput and sinciput remain at the same level. The head remains in this position as it descends through the pelvis and fails to rotate either anteriorly or posteriorly, becoming arrested in the transverse position. When a deep transverse arrest is diagnosed its cause must be sought. Are uterine contractions adequate to help the head flex? Is there reasonable tone in the pelvic floor? Is the pelvis a normal shape? The criteria for delivery of the deep transverse arrest are exactly those for the OP position. If the head reaches the perineum in the second phase of the second stage then rotation may easily be effected manually and the head delivered with the occiput anterior with little risk to mother or baby. If the head remains in the transverse position at the level of the ischial spines in spite of full dilatation of the cervix, then operative delivery is likely to be hazardous for fetus and mother, and abdominal delivery should be undertaken.

Face presentation (Fig. 86)

The incidence of face presentation is 1 in 300. The commonest cause was anencephaly, but very few anencephalics now escape detection

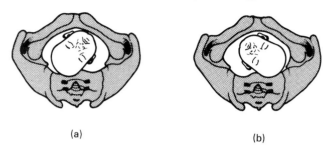

(a)

(b)

Fig. 8.6 Face presentation. (a) Left mentoanterior; (b) right mento-anterior.

in early pregnancy. Hypertonus in the extensor muscles of the fetal neck is said to be a cause of face presentation and the baby delivered as a face often lies in its cot with its neck extended for several days after birth. The cause of the hypertonus is unknown. Rarely a thyroid tumour or hypoglossal cyst may cause the head to be extended. A lax uterus or hydramnios may predispose to extension of the head and face presentation.

Diagnosis
This may not be made until the face appears at the vulva, or the diagnosis may be made on vaginal examination. Ultrasound examination may indicate face presentation.

Mechanism of labour and delivery
When the head is fully extended and the face presents the presenting diameter is the submentobregmatic (10 cm), the same as the suboccipitobregmatic which presents with the fully flexed head. To describe the mechanism of labour the mentum (chin) replaces the occiput, and extension and flexion are reversed. In a left mentoanterior (LMA) position the head descends with increased extension, the chin rotates anteriorly and the head is born by flexion. So a face presentation with the chin anterior can deliver vaginally. However, if the chin is posterior, vaginal delivery cannot occur because the head and shoulders get stuck at the pelvic brim and obstruction occurs.

Caesarean section is indicated if there is slow progress and excessive moulding, or if presentation is mentoposterior.

The baby's face will be very swollen and bruised due to caput formation. The mother must be warned about this before she sees the baby and reassured that it will disappear within a few days. The baby's neck may remain extended for several days.

Outcome
As long as the baby is normal and the position mentoanterior, the outcome is little different from a vertex presentation (bruising apart).

Brow presentation (Fig. 8.7)

Here the head is midway between extension and flexion. The largest diameter of the skull, the mentovertical, is the presenting diameter. Since in the normal-size term infant (i.e. 3.5 kg) this measures 13.5 cm, it is apparent that delivery is impossible. The incidence of a brow presentation is 1 : 1000 and its cause is unknown.

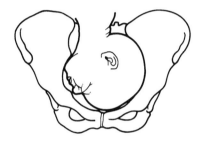

Fig. 8.7   Brow presentation.

Diagnosis of brow
On abdominal palpation the head feels big and is not engaged. On vaginal examination the anterior fontanelle is presenting and the supraorbital ridges can be felt. An X-ray or ultrasound scan confirms the diagnosis and is often requested to exclude hydrocephaly since this is the impression obtained on abdominal palpation. Since the presenting part does not fit the lower segment the membranes may rupture early and the cord prolapse.

Management
In early labour it is reasonable to wait an hour or two to see whether with adequate uterine contractions the brow converts to a face by increasing extension, or an OA position by increasing flexion, but this expectant attitude cannot be maintained for long, otherwise labour will become obstructed with eventually a risk of uterine rupture. If the brow persists then delivery is by caesarean section.

Outcome
Operative delivery will increase the maternal morbidity, but fetal mortality and morbidity should be low if caesarean section is carried out early.

Malpresentation

The commonest malpresentation is the breech and its diagnosis and antenatal management are discussed in Chapter 7. It is emphasized again here that the decision to allow the patient with a breech presentation to go into labour and attempt a vaginal delivery is only taken after careful antenatal assessment, together with constant assessment as to the progress of labour, particularly the rapidity of the descent of the breech. The woman having a baby by the breech must be delivered in a major obstetric unit, supervised by a senior experienced obstetrician and be attended by an anaesthetist and a paediatrician. If, in spite of full dilatation, the breech has not reached the perineum, the fetus should be delivered by caesarean section.

Management of breech delivery
Detailed discussion and explanation with the woman and her birth partner well beforehand with the use of visual aids is advisable so that they understand the management plan. Ideally this exercise should be undertaken by the doctor who will carry out the delivery but in practice this may not be possible. The main principles are as follows:

1 *Minimal interference*: Avoidance of interference for as long as possible provided the baby's condition is satisfactory should be the guiding principle in breech delivery.
2 *Exclude cord prolapse*: A vaginal examination should be made when the membranes rupture to exclude cord prolapse as this is more likely to occur in breech presentation.
3 *Close monitoring of fetal heart*: A breech is at increased risk of fetal distress due to cord compression or prolapse and should be monitored continuously in labour.
4 *Delay pushing*: Pushing is not encouraged until the breech is at the vulva.
5 *Controlled delivery of the head*: It is vital to ensure that the baby is not at risk of intracranial haemorrhage from too rapid delivery or hypoxia from too slow delivery.
6 *Position – lithotomy*: It is advisable to deliver the baby with the mother in the lithotomy position since this affords the best opportunity to control and assist the delivery of the head.

7 *Episiotomy*: At full distension of the perineum an episiotomy is usually made for the same reason, unless the perineum is deficient or very lax. The woman pushes with contractions. If the legs do not deliver spontaneously, gentle pressure in the popliteal fossa to flex the knee will enable the foot to be flipped over the perineum.

8 *Pelvic–sacral hold*: It is essential to help the back remain uppermost because if it slips round the head will also rotate, the chin will get caught on the symphysis pubis and the head will fail to deliver – a catastrophic situation. Although 'hands off' is a good guideline for breech delivery, in order to keep the back uppermost, the obstetrician may wrap a towel around the fetal pelvis (the baby is usually slippery) and hold it gently with thumbs lying along the back of the sacrum and fingers around the front of the pelvis and top of the legs. The baby must not be grasped around its abdominal cavity as this can cause trauma to the intra-abdominal organs, particularly the liver.

The sole purpose of this 'hands on' action is to maintain the back anteriorly. It is important that no traction is applied as traction can cause the arms to extend and become trapped alongside or behind the head (nuchal displacement of the arm).

The mother continues to bear down as the shoulders come into view. The arms may deliver spontaneously; if not, gentle pressure in the antecubital fossa to cause the arm to flex will allow the arm to be flipped out. The Løvset manoeuvre is useful for delivering extended arms, but extended arms rarely arise spontaneously and are usually produced as the result of injudicious traction on the fetus. The Løvset manoeuvre involves rotating the fetus through 180° to bring the erstwhile posterior shoulder anteriorly to lie directly under the symphysis pubis so that the arm may be brought down across the face and delivered; rotation in the opposite direction allows delivery of the other arm.

9 *Delivery of the head – options:*
   a. Forceps – most commonly used: Gravity and the mother's expulsive efforts should bring the head into the pelvis with the next contraction and the occiput will appear below the symphysis. When this is seen, the feet are held gently in the left hand and raised vertically and then held by an assistant. The head is delivered by forceps in a slow controlled manner to avoid damage.
   b. Mauriceau–Smellie–Veit manoeuvre (jaw shoulder traction): The baby's body is supported along the supinated left arm of the obstetrician, the middle finger of the left hand is introduced into the baby's mouth and the ring and index finger of the left hand are on the baby's lower jaw.

The obstetrician's right arm lies on top of the baby's body with the middle finger pushing on the occiput encouraging flexion and the index and ring fingers are on the shoulders. The head is delivered with the two hands exerting gentle traction and maintaining flexion. This method is useful if there is no time to apply the forceps or they are not available.

c. Burns–Marshall method: The feet are held in the left hand and raised gently vertically up above the baby's body. The right hand guards the perineum and slows the passage of the head as the occiput pivots on the back of the symphysis and the head is born by extension.

Breech delivery should not be hurried, but is it obvious that it should not be prolonged either, since the baby's oxygen supply via the placenta is increasingly reduced as delivery proceeds, and the baby is not able to take a breath until the face has been delivered. Delivery of a baby by the breech should take no more than 5–8 minutes at the very most, counting from the delivery of the legs.

Should any problem arise during labour, i.e. slow descent of the breech, inefficient uterine activity or any other abnormality, then the delivery should be by caesarean section.

Variable lie and shoulder presentation

During the latter weeks of pregnancy the fetal lie usually stabilizes with the breech or head presenting, the lie being longitudinal. In highly parous patients with lax anterior abdominal walls, patients with a space-occupying lesion of the lower segment or pelvis (e.g. placenta praevia or fibroids), the lie may be variable or persistently transverse. This may occur in the primigravida too but less commonly, and suggests an abnormally shaped uterus. Often no cause is found for the abnormal lie.

During pregnancy, management is expectant since the lie usually spontaneously becomes longitudinal by 38 weeks. If it does not, the woman is admitted to hospital at that time, since should the membranes rupture there is a very real danger that the cord may prolapse, and should contractions occur and the lie remain transverse, the shoulder will impact in the pelvis. The arm may prolapse and labour will become obstructed.

Before 38 weeks the woman is urged to report immediately should she suspect that her membranes have ruptured or that labour may have started. Expectant treatment continues in hospital. If the membranes rupture and the cord prolapses, immediate caesarean section should be carried out. If labour starts with a transverse or varying lie, caesarean section should be undertaken. In the majority of cases, however, the lie stabilizes spontaneously by 41 weeks and labour starts with a longitudinal lie. If the lie remains variable or transverse approaching 42 weeks, elective caesarean section is arranged, after confirming the maturity of the fetus. External cephalic version is rarely helpful since the abnormal lie usually recurs; but once contractions have started it is very difficult, and if the membranes have ruptured it is impossible to carry out successfully.

MULTIPLE PREGNANCY

Since twins are the commonest multiple they will be considered in detail. Triplets may be delivered vaginally but caesarean section is usually done for multiples greater than 2.

Diagnosed twins

During labour it is necessary to monitor the heart of both infants. A scalp clip may be applied to the presenting part of twin 1, and twin 2 may be monitored externally. It is important to anticipate the problems attendant on twin delivery.

Problems

Throughout labour both twins are at increased risk of fetal distress as placental function is usually suboptimal; otherwise most problems particularly affect twin 2.
   In the second stage there is a risk of:

1 Abnormal lie.
2 Abnormal presentation.
3 Intrauterine hypoxia.
4 Cord prolapse.
5 Placental abruption.

The problems associated with the third stage are:

1 Postpartum haemorrhage.
2 Uterine atony.

An intravenous infusion must be running before the second stage begins. The following personnel should be in attendance when the second stage begins:

1 An experienced obstetrician who can carry out intrauterine manipulations and a Caesarean section.
2 An anaesthetist.
3 At least one paediatrician and preferably two, as twins are often premature and may be small.

Twin 1

The delivery of the first twin is managed as it would be for a singleton with the same presentation. The cord must be cut between two clamps as usual. This is particularly important, as bleeding from the cut end of the cord leading to the placenta may cause exsanguination of twin 2 if there is an anastomotic connection between the fetal circulations in the placentae.

Twin 2

As soon as twin 1 has been delivered, abdominal palpation should be carried out to ascertain the lie and presentation of twin 2, and its heart auscultated. External manipulation will usually correct an oblique or transverse lie. The presenting part is guided into the pelvis and the membranes are ruptured with the next contraction and certainly within 5 minutes of the delivery of twin 1. The obstetrician carefully checks after rupture of the membranes to exclude cord prolapse. The patient is encouraged to bear down. Contractions may be stimulated with Syntocinon if they are slow to re-establish. The second twin is at ever-increasing risk from hypoxia and placental separation once twin 1 has delivered and the size of the uterus decreases. If there is any delay in descent then forceps may be applied to the head or the breech extracted by gentle traction on the legs.

A manoeuvre is permissible in relation to twin delivery that has no other place in modern obstetric practice – this is internal version and breech extraction. If the lie is transverse despite attempts at external version or the cord prolapses, then a hand can be introduced into the uterus, the fetal foot sought, and the leg brought down. The baby is then extracted by pulling on the leg which straightens out the lie and brings the breech down into the pelvis. This manoeuvre can only be done with any degree of safety to mother and baby in the case of twin 2, where the birth canal has been dilated by twin 1 and the membranes of the second sac only just ruptured. Uterine rupture and fetal death are the ultimate hazards of this manoeuvre in any other circumstances. Occasionally the second twin may need to be delivered by caesarean section.

Undiagnosed twins

Scans are so reliable now that undiagnosed twins have effectively disappeared from the scanned population. For those who have not been scanned, however, it remains a possibility. The usual scenario is that the second twin is found after the delivery of the first and after the oxytocic has been given. The abdomen should be palpated and the fetal lie made longitudinal; the membranes should be ruptured and twin 2 delivered as expeditiously as possible, with internal version and breech extraction if necessary.

PUDENDAL BLOCK

Blocking the pudendal nerve provides adequate perineal analgesia for mid- and low-cavity pelvic manipulations.

The pudendal nerve curves around the ischial spine and supplies the skin of the vulva. Infiltration of 10 ml of lignocaine 1% just beneath the ischial spine will produce introital analgesia. The infiltration may be made transvaginally or percutaneously using a long 10-cm needle. With the latter route a bleb of local anaesthetic is injected intradermally midway between the anus and the ischial tuberosity. The needle is passed through the bleb and directed to the ischial spine. With both routes a finger in the vagina directs the needle towards the ischial spine. It is desirable to infiltrate the perineum posteriorly, especially along the line of a proposed episiotomy.

FORCEPS DELIVERY

Obstetrical forceps were invented in the 17th century by the Chamberlen family and kept in secret use by members of the family for over 100 years. The instruments were covered in leather to prevent them making a noise and giving a clue about the Chamberlen's secret instrument.

There are two main types of modern forceps: those for applying traction and those for rotating and applying traction (Fig. 8.8).

Simple traction forceps

1 Long curved forceps (e.g. Neville Barnes) are for mid-cavity deliveries.
2 Short curved forceps (e.g. Wrigley's) are for low 'lift out' deliveries where the head is on the perineum.

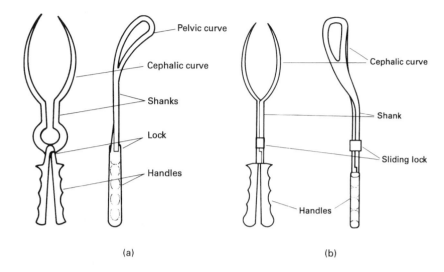

Fig. 8.8   Forceps in common use. (a) Neville Barnes; (b) Kjelland's

There is no place for high forceps delivery where the head is above the pelvic brim. The risk of trauma to mother and fetus is too great. Mid-cavity deliveries should be undertaken only after very careful assessment, as in many cases vaginal dilatation has not taken place and the head is still above the pelvic floor. The forceps consist of two parts, each part having a blade and a handle. The blade is curved to fit the fetal head and also to fit the pelvis. Each blade is applied separately (the left always first), care being taken that the blade is correctly positioned along the side of the fetal head. The handle is locked after correct application. The sagittal suture must be in the AP diameter of the pelvis or very close to it.

Rotational forceps

Kjelland's forceps

These forceps have a much flatter pelvic curve and are used for rotating the head from OP or occipitotransverse positions to OA positions. It is a powerful instrument, with the potential of great benefits but also of producing serious trauma. They are rarely used in the authors' obstetric practice, except by senior obstetricians. Rotation of these malpositions can also be accomplished by manual rotation with subsequent extraction using conventional forceps. The dangers to mother and baby have been emphasized above, and the use of Kjelland's forceps is consequently in decline.

Prerequisites for forceps delivery

1 The cervix must be fully dilated.
2 The head must be no more than two-fifths palpable per abdomen.
3 The occiput must be anterior (unless rotational forceps are being used).
4 The bladder should be empty.
5 The uterus must be contracting.
6 The membranes must be ruptured.
7 Analgesia should be adequate.
8 The operator must have the required skill.

Ideally the vagina should be dilated and the head on the pelvic floor.

Adequate uterine contractions must be present, using intravenous oxytocin if necessary. If the head is on the perineum and the occiput remains posterior at the outlet then it is possible to deliver the fetus face to pubis, but in the mid-cavity the occiput should be anterior before attempting forceps delivery. If the uterus is not contracting, serious postpartum haemorrhage is more likely.

Indications for forceps delivery

1 Delay in the second stage. This may be due to weak uterine contractions or poor maternal expulsive efforts. A rigid perineum may also cause delay. Fetal causes of delay include malposition of the fetal head, especially OP or occipitotransverse positions. Cephalopelvic disproportion may also cause delay and should be excluded before undertaking forceps delivery. Delay due to weak uterine action may be overcome using Syntocinon, and an episiotomy will relieve delay due to a rigid perineum.
2 Maternal distress or exhaustion at this stage is to be regarded as a failure of management, but occasionally the mother is in such a distressed state that she is unable to cooperate and push adequately.
3 Forceps delivery is also indicated when a short second stage is necessary (e.g. cardiac patients, those with severe hypertension or those who have had a previous caesarean section). It is important that the patient who is delivering a baby preterm should also have a short second stage, and delivery of the head should be controlled, as precipitate delivery (particularly of the premature head) may cause tentorial tears with subsequent damage or

death. Forceps may be applied to the head of the preterm infant to control its delivery, but it must be remembered that the premature head is more vulnerable than at term and the forceps themselves may cause damage. An adequate episiotomy will facilitate the delivery of the preterm head as safely as forceps.

4 Fetal distress may occur for the first time in the second stage and is usually due to hypoxia. It should be watched for carefully, especially if there is an underlying cause for fetal distress such as placental insufficiency. The distressed fetus may be more prone to cerebral trauma because hypercapnia produces cerebral vascular dilatation. Caesarean section may well be a safer alternative to a difficult and traumatic forceps delivery.

Dangers of forceps delivery

Most forceps deliveries are very straightforward but injudicious or unskilled use of any type of forceps may damage the mother or fetus. Vaginal and cervical lacerations and postpartum haemorrhage may all follow forceps delivery and the fetal skull may be fractured. Facial palsy results from inaccurate application of the blades. Cerebral irritation is sometimes seen, particularly after rotational forceps delivery, and cerebral damage resulting in long-term morbidity is not unknown. Many of these complications can happen after a spontaneous delivery or ventouse delivery and may relate to the indication for the forceps rather than the delivery itself. The use of forceps is under review and likely to decrease.

VENTOUSE

This instrument consists of a metal or silicone cup and chain, with a tube attached to a vacuum bottle (Fig. 8.9). The cup (which comes in three sizes) is placed on the fetal scalp and a negative pressure of 0.8 kg/cm^2 is established which sucks the scalp into the cup, forming a chignon. Traction may then be applied.

The ventouse may be used in place of forceps and the indications are the same. Excessive traction will simply pull the cup off, so it has a built-in safety feature. It is possible, but inadvisable, to apply the ventouse before the cervix is fully dilated where there is delay in the first stage, as maternal and fetal damage may follow. Since disproportion is a common cause for such delay, ventouse extraction is to be avoided, since gross fetal and maternal damage may result. Minor scalp damage and cephalhaematoma are occasional complications.

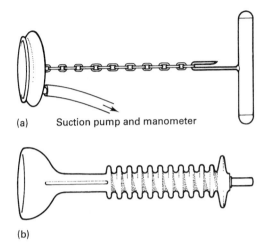

(a)   Suction pump and manometer

(b)

Fig. 8.9   The ventouse. (a) The original metal cup and handle; (b) the modern soft silicone cup.

CAESAREAN SECTION

Julius Caesar was not delivered by this operation, in spite of the name. Under Roman law (*lex Caesare*) dating from 670 BC, the fetus had to be taken from the body of a mother dying during pregnancy or labour and the operation thus became known as caesarean section. It was not until the late 19th century that the classical section was perfected and only in the early 20th century that the lower-segment operation was devised. Caesarean section did not become safe until the advent of blood transfusion and antibiotics, and even today is occasionally a direct cause of maternal death.

Indications

Caesarean section is undertaken for a variety of indications. The principal ones are:

Fetal indications

1 Fetal compromise before the onset of labour (e.g. growth retardation, hypoxic heart traces, severe rhesus disease).
2 Fetal distress in first stage.
3 Inadequate placental reserve, e.g. growth retardation.

Maternal indications

1 Previous caesarean section for recurrent cause.
2 Two or more previous caesarean sections.
3 Significant previous gynaecological surgery, e.g. repair of fistula, repair of prolapse.

Combined indications

1 Antepartum haemorrhage.
2 Cephalopelvic disproportion.
3 Malpresentation.
4 Malposition.
5 Hypertensive disorders.

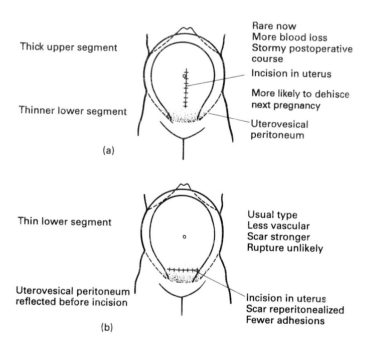

Fig. 8.10 Caesarean section. (a) Classical caesarean section; the skin incision is usually longitudinal too but may be transverse. (b) Lower-segment caesarean section; the skin section is usually transverse too but may be longitudinal.

Method

If caesarean section is the elective method of delivery then it is done about a week before term. More usually it is done as an emergency procedure in labour. General anaesthesia is commonly used, but epidural anaesthesia is gaining popularity and has the advantage that the mother may see and hold her baby almost immediately. A skilled obstetric anaesthetist should be available and blood should be grouped and saved. The lower-segment incision is now used almost universally because it is less vascular and the scar is less prone to rupture in a future pregnancy than the classical scar (risk 0.5% versus 3%). The sites of the incisions are illustrated in Figure 8.10. Classical caesarean section is only used for a transverse lie with ruptured membranes or occasionally for placenta praevia.

CAUSES OF POSTPARTUM HAEMORRHAGE

Primary postpartum haemorrhage (PPH) may be due to a placenta retained in the uterus after partial separation. Once the placenta is delivered, PPH is almost always due either to an atonic uterus or to trauma to the genital tract, with other causes being very rare.

Retained placenta

Partial separation of the placenta interferes with uterine contraction, and the maternal sinuses of the separated placenta are held open and bleed. If the placenta fails to separate at all, as in the very rare cases of morbid adherence (e.g. placenta accreta), there is no bleeding since the sinuses are not exposed. It is more usual for some separation to occur followed by haemorrhage. If the placenta separates completely but is retained in the lower segment due to contraction of the cervix, this too will interfere with contraction of the fundus and placental site and predispose to haemorrhage.

Uterine atony

If the uterus has been overdistended (for example, in polyhydramnios, multiple pregnancy or with a large baby), it may fail to contract after delivery. Atony is more likely after a long exhausting labour if dehydration or ketosis is present or if deep anaesthesia is used, but is a common cause of PPH.

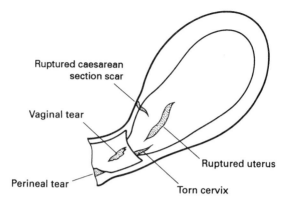

Fig. 8.11　Possible traumatic causes of postpartum haemorrhage.

Lacerations

Tears anywhere in the genital tract, from vulva and vagina through the cervix to the uterus, that are unrecognized or inadequately repaired may cause bleeding (Fig. 8.11). Operative vaginal delivery or intrauterine manipulations will increase the likelihood of trauma to the genital tract.

Other causes

Clotting defects rarely cause PPH because haemostasis relies primarily on uterine muscle contraction and retraction. Clotting failure may cause serious problems if associated with inefficient uterine action and may happen, for instance, with a severe placental abruption. Uterine fibroids may interfere with efficient contraction of the uterus and predispose to haemorrhage. Injudicious traction on the cord of the unseparated placenta may cause uterine inversion, although occasionally inversion occurs spontaneously.

Diagnosis

All blood loss at delivery is measured, but it is notoriously difficult for the collection to be complete. It has also been shown that estimates of blood loss are usually completely erroneous, the assessment often being far too little. The larger the volume lost, the more inaccurate is the assessment.

Management

1 Stop the bleeding.
2 Resuscitate the patient.

The first step is to give ergometrine 0.5 mg intravenously. The second is to rub up a uterine contraction. Blood for cross-matching (10 ml) is taken as an intravenous infusion is set up. If there are enough personnel these steps can be undertaken simultaneously and be in progress while the cause of the PPH is being sought. If the placenta is retained it must be removed. If the placenta is delivered it must be examined for completeness. In either event, if the uterus is atonic and full of blood clot, a contraction must be rubbed up and the clots expelled. If the uterus fails to remain contracted, a continuous intravenous infusion of Syntocinon is set up (20 units of Syntocinon in 500 ml of dextrose saline). Bimanual compression of the uterus is very effective and may be life-saving in situations where oxytocics and blood are not available. It is effective as long as the placenta is out.

A hand is inserted into the vagina as high as possible and the uterus is compressed on to the vaginal hand by placing the other hand suprapubically on the patient's abdomen, holding the fundus down and continuing to rub up a contraction. It is important to realize that this can be done without any form of anaesthetic. If significant bleeding continues, examination under anaesthesia must be performed. Tears will be repaired but sometimes internal iliac artery ligation or hysterectomy may be necessary. There is no place for hot douches or uterine packs. These are a waste of time, predispose to infection and may damage the uterus.

Removal of the retained placenta

With a retained placenta, even if bleeding is not a feature it may occur at any time and therefore an intravenous infusion should be set up and blood cross-matched. Manual removal should be carried out *under anaesthesia, since to put a hand into the uterus may provoke shock.*

Before anaesthesia is induced, the bladder is emptied and controlled cord traction is performed after ensuring that the uterus is contracted, since separation may have occurred in the meanwhile.

After anaesthesia is induced, and a hand slipped through the cervix following the cord up to the placenta, the edge of the placenta is sought. The uterus is steadied by the operator's other hand, which is holding the uterus through the anterior abdominal wall. The placenta is lifted off the uterine wall, not clawed off in pieces. The uterine cavity is then re-explored to remove any fragments left behind. Ergometrine 0.25 mg is given intravenously at the end of the procedure.

Manual removal of the placenta should only be undertaken by an experienced obstetrician, with the strictest aseptic precautions, with expert anaesthesia and with blood available.

Should a patient deliver away from a major unit and the placenta be retained, then the obstetric flying squad or emergency ambulance should be called.

The first *Report on Confidential Enquiries into Maternal Deaths in England and Wales 1952–54* (see Chapter 10) showed that transfer of a patient with the placenta *in situ* was a major cause of death, the patient not infrequently bleeding during transfer and arriving dead or moribund at the major unit. Obstetric flying squads were developed in consequence. More recently, emergency ambulances have largely replaced flying squads. The ambulance crews are trained to resuscitate patients and institute intravenous therapy. They also have basic obstetric training and have the major advantage of arriving at the scene much more quickly than the flying squad.

Examination under anaesthesia

If bleeding continues after delivery in spite of a well-contracted uterus, the genital tract must be inspected under anaesthetic. This should be carried out with the patient in the lithotomy position with operating theatre facilities.

The episiotomy or tear may not be adequately sutured at the top end. It may have extended into the posterior fornix.

A vaginal haematoma may be accumulating from an undetected vaginal wall laceration.

The cervix may be torn, especially at 3 and 9 o'clock. The apex of any tear must be defined to ensure that the tear does not extend into the uterus.

The uterine cavity must be gently explored to confirm its integrity. If more conservative measures fail to stop the haemorrhage, the abdomen should be opened without delay. Quite commonly an undetected uterine rupture will be revealed. Internal iliac artery ligation or hysterectomy may be necessary.

Clotting defects

These are usually suspected either following a history of abruption or when it is noticed that the blood taken for cross-matching does not clot, the patient is oozing from the site of venepuncture and the blood from the genital tract fails to clot.

The common defect is hypofibrinogenaemia, and the fibrinogen level and fibrinogen degradation products may be measured to confirm the diagnosis. Fibrinogen or fresh frozen plasma may be given, but treatment is most effective when absolutely fresh blood is transfused.

Sequelae of primary PPH

Five per cent of maternal deaths are due to PPH and over half of these are avoidable. Following hypovolaemic shock there is renal shutdown, anuria and possibly irreparable renal damage. Chronic anaemia in the puerperium, which is responsible for many minor ills, irritability, tiredness, depression, apathy, insomnia and so on, often goes unrecognized and frequently follows the less dramatic PPH.

Prolonged hypotension may cause damage to the blood supply to the pituitary, resulting in panhypopituitarism (Sheehan's syndrome). The features are not usually apparent until several weeks or months after delivery, but it should be suspected if lactation fails to become established.

Secondary PPH

This is discussed in Chapter 9.

MATERNAL TRAUMA
The vulva

A vulval haematoma is readily diagnosed. The very painful tense collection of blood is due to rupture of a subcutaneous blood vessel or ineffective repair of episiotomy or vaginal tear. The haematoma must be incised, the clot evacuated and the bleeding vessel ligated if it can be found.

The perineum

A first-degree tear involves the skin only at the fourchette, a second-degree tear involves the perineal body and posterior vaginal wall and a third-degree tear involves the external anal sphincter and often the anal mucosa as well as the posterior vaginal wall.

All tears need careful repair. Dyspareunia is commonly seen following inadequate or overenthusiastic repair, and in later life prolapse may occur if the perineal body is not reconstituted correctly. An unrecognized or ill-repaired third-degree tear leaves the patient incontinent of faeces and flatus.

Repair should be undertaken immediately after delivery since oedema will obscure the field if repair is delayed. The greater the tear, the greater the skill required for adequate suture.

Adequate analgesia, exposure, lighting and experience are necessary for satisfactory repair of a tear or episiotomy. The distress caused by improper repair is not seen until much later after discharge, and then rarely by the person responsible for the suturing. Vulval and perineal oedema can be very distressing, as can prolapsed haemorrhoids. Ice packs and sitting on a rubber ring or sheepskin will ease the condition locally. Oral analgesics are required.

The vagina

Lacerations must be defined and repaired. General anaesthesia may be required and certainly adequate exposure, lighting, experience and an assistant are necessary. A vaginal haematoma may occur during delivery, either from spontaneous rupture of a subcutaneous blood vessel or from an undetected laceration. There may be no visible blood loss. The patient usually complains of perineal pain or of a continuing desire to bear down after delivery of the fetus and placenta. Blood transfusion may be needed and the patient should be resuscitated before the haematoma is evacuated.

It is rarely possible to see a bleeding point. Sometimes the cavity can be obliterated by mattress sutures, but at other times firm packing is required to obtain haemostasis. The whole vaginal wall must be inspected for tears after rotational forceps. Fistulae are rare in the UK, but in some remote areas abroad prolonged obstructed labour not infrequently produces vesicovaginal or rectovaginal fistulae through pressure necrosis.

The cervix

Small tears are common and of little importance but larger tears, which often occur at 3 and 9 o'clock, may extend into the lower uterine segment or into the broad ligament. A broad-ligament haematoma may be palpable abdominally and will displace the uterus laterally. Transfusion is usually required but the haematoma will resolve spontaneously. This may take several weeks. Rarely it becomes infected and then has to be drained.

The uterus

Inversion of the uterus

Inversion usually occurs when cord traction has been applied before placental separation and in the absence of uterine contractions. It is rare but should be recognized at once since immediate replacement forestalls shock, which may be fatal. The fundus may appear at the introitus or be felt in the vagina, and the uterus will be impalpable on abdominal examination.

Shock occurs both because of traction on the tubes and ovaries, which are drawn down into the inverted fundus, and because of blood loss. Shock may be avoided if immediate replacement is carried out, before the uterus has contracted. If there is delay the inverted fundus becomes fixed in position by the uterus contracting. Bleeding may be profuse. After initial resuscitation, replacement by saline (O'Sullivan's hydrostatic method) is favoured in the UK. The hydrostatic method entails filling the vagina with warm saline while closing the vulva manually to prevent escape. Gradually, as the pressure of saline increases, the inversion reduces.

Rupture of the uterus

A complete rupture with tearing of the peritoneal covering may result in extrusion of part or all of the fetus and placenta accompanied by severe haemorrhage. This catastrophic event for both the mother and fetus is very rare in the UK today. A rupture occurring in the lower segment may produce a broad-ligament haematoma. The rupture may occur at the site of a previous operative scar or in a previously intact uterus.

Scar rupture

The classical caesarean section scar ruptures in 3% of cases. Half of these ruptures occur before the onset of labour. Rupture is usually sudden and complete, with death of the fetus and often death of the mother. The lower-segment caesarean section scar ruptures in 0.5% of cases and very rarely occurs before the onset of labour. Rupture is usually gradual and usually diagnosed before the fetus or mother is in serious trouble. Hysterotomy scars carry risks similar to classical Caesarean section scars. Myomectomy scars carry a very small risk of rupture.

Rupture of the previously intact uterus is extremely rare in this country and usually results from some form of obstetric mismanagement, such as neglected obstructed labour, particularly in parous women, overdosage of oxytocic drugs, traumatic deliveries or ill-advised intrauterine manoeuvres, such as destructive operations on the fetus other than in very experienced hands. Spontaneous rupture of the previously intact uterus does occur and when it does so it is usually in a grand multipara in labour.

Diagnosis of uterine rupture

In pregnancy

The patient may feel the scar 'give way', and this sensation may be associated with pain. If the contents are completely extruded and the uterus contracts, there may be little bleeding, shock and pain, but there may be sudden collapse with severe bleeding. The degree of shock and abdominal pain due to intraperitoneal bleeding depends on the amount of intraperitoneal bleeding.

In labour

Rupture of a lower-segment scar may be silent, and it is not uncommon to find a partial dehiscence at the time of repeat caesarean section.

Rupture in obstructed labour is usually associated with pain and quite profound shock, since intraperitoneal bleeding is a feature of rupture and the exhausted uterus fails to contract. Infection is usually present too.

In the immediate puerperium

If a patient collapses with or without bleeding, the possibility of uterine rupture must not be overlooked. The uterus should be explored under general anaesthesia.

Treatment
Resuscitation is the first concern and this includes blood transfusion. If there is doubt about the diagnosis, an examination under anaesthesia is done. Having made the diagnosis, laparotomy is performed. If the rupture is due to scar dehiscence, then simple suture is often all that is required. Hysterectomy is indicated if the uterus is too damaged.

Causes of shock in obstetrics

These may be summarized as follows:

1 Haemorrhage.

2 Amniotic fluid embolism.
3 Bacteraemia.
4 Anoxia and inhalation under anaesthesia.
5 Pulmonary embolism.
6 Cardiac failure.
7 Trauma.

FURTHER READING

O'Driscoll, K. and Meagher, D. (1980) *Active Management of Labour*. W. B. Saunders, Eastbourne.

9
Postnatal care

The 6-week period following the birth of a baby is called the puerperium and is defined as the phase during which the reproductive organs return to a non-pregnant state. It is the time during which the mother recovers from the effects of child-bearing but is not synonymous with returning to her prepregnant state since that is impossible for some structures, e.g. the perineum, skin pigmentation and striae (stretch marks), although the last two fade considerably. Also, sadly, childbirth can result in psychological scars which may never heal. Happily most women feel fit within 2 weeks, although tired, but some systems, e.g. the renal tracts, take up to 3 months to return to normal.

PHYSIOLOGICAL CHANGES

It is important to have an understanding of the physiological changes that occur in the puerperium since these dictate the pattern of care for the mother and baby and also explain potential problems.

Immediately after delivery the mother is tired, though usually elated. After time alone with her partner and baby, rest is important. The importance of rest is often neglected and adequate sleep should be ensured throughout the puerperium. Her temperature after delivery often falls and shivering is a frequent symptom. In the first 24 hours the temperature rises slightly above normal, perhaps as a catabolic reaction, but then should be normal. After 24 hours a rise of more than 0.5°C (1°F) is abnormal and a cause should be sought.

The uterus continues to contract regularly in the puerperium and the contractions may be so strong as to give rise to pain. These 'after-pains' are especially noted during suckling, because of the reflex release of oxytocin.

Lochia

Until the uterine cavity is healed there is a serosanguineous discharge, which lasts for 2–6 weeks and is known as the lochia (from the Greek *lochos*, meaning childbirth). The passage of lochia is often marked during suckling due to the induced uterine contractions. For the first few days the discharge is mainly blood, then for the next 7–10 days it is a paler serosanguineous loss and becomes yellowish for up to 6 weeks. The lochia consists of red blood cells, leukocytes, decidual cells and fibrinous products. Lochia from the uterus is alkaline. It becomes acid in the vagina and its constituents decompose due to the action of bacterial saprophytes. If lochia is retained in the uterus it becomes offensive-smelling.

The bacterial flora normally found in the vagina return within 72 hours and may include anaerobic streptococci, *Escherichia coli*, staphylococci and *Clostridium welchii*. A mixed growth of such organisms is *not* necessarily evidence of infection of the genital tract. However, slow or delayed involution of the uterus (see below) together with heavy lochia suggests retained products of conception (fragments of placenta or membrane, or clots) and if the uterus is tender, the lochia offensive and the woman pyrexial, then infection is present.

Prevention of ascending genital tract infection

The mother should be in a clean environment with, ideally, access to a shower or bath and bidet. She can care for the vulva herself but should be advised to pay special attention after defecation, and avoid drawing anal organisms forward to the vulva. Strict aseptic techniques should be observed if ever a vaginal examination is done.

Statutorily in England and Wales a mother is seen by a midwife daily for the first 10 days. The midwife takes her temperature, observes the lochia and measures the height of the fundus, looking to detect early evidence of infection or retained products.

The perineum

Lacerations or an episiotomy should be inspected daily to note healing and non-absorbable sutures are removed on day 5 or 6, by which time skin healing should have occurred. Complete deep tissue healing occurs in 3 weeks. The pain from a bruised or swollen perineum may be relieved by ice packs (a bag of frozen peas conforms readily to perineal anatomy), local analgesic sprays (but beware allergic reactions) and mild oral analgesics. Mega-pulsed ultrasound may also be helpful to reduce oedema and bruising, as it does in sports injuries.

Involution of the genital tract

The dramatic shrinkage of the uterus after delivery is called involution. It is brought about by the disappearance of the placental hormones oestrogen and progesterone. The uterus atrophies, the excess uterine tissue of pregnancy is autolysed, i.e. enzymatically resorbed, and leads to increased nitrogen excretion. Blood flow ceases in the hypertrophied spiral arteries and veins and they become thrombosed and hyalinized. Figure 9.1 shows the normal progress of involution of the uterus.

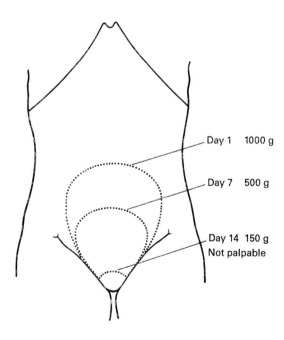

Day 1   1000 g

Day 7   500 g

Day 14 150 g
Not palpable

Fig. 9.1   Involution of the uterus following delivery.

The cervical os admits one to two fingers for 7–10 days after delivery. The external os never regains its nulliparous appearance, being stretched or lacerated to some extent in labour (Fig. 9.2). The pouting endocervical mucosa so commonly seen on the ectocervix during pregnancy (and often misnamed erosion of pregnancy)

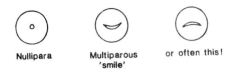

Nullipara   Multiparous   or often this!
             'smile'

Fig. 9.2   Appearance of the cervical os.

gradually disappears during the puerperium and has usually gone by 6 weeks. The vagina slowly shrinks and rugae reappear in the third week.

Ovarian function

If the mother is breast-feeding, prolactin is released at each feed and the high pregnancy levels of prolactin are maintained, so ovarian function remains suppressed, ovulation does not occur, the endometrium remains thin even when healed and the mother is amenorrhoeic and hypo-oestrogenic. The vaginal epithelium becomes atrophic and sexual intercourse can be uncomfortable, even after lacerations have been completely healed.

However ovarian suppression cannot be guaranteed and breast-feeding is not a reliable contraceptive for the individual, though by generally delaying the next pregnancy, it is demographically important in many developing countries. Basal prolactin levels gradually fall, high levels later occur only during suckling, so the suppressive effect on the ovarian axis is reduced, particularly when breast-feeding is spaced out, as is typical in western countries. Obviously, ovarian function will return earlier in women who introduce complementary bottle-feeding and reduce breast-feeding.

If the mother does not breast-feed, ovarian function returns with little delay and ovulation can occur as early as 4 weeks and thus pregnancy is possible too. The first menstrual period often occurs about 6 weeks after delivery.

Contraception should have a high priority, ideally before 4 weeks, whether the mother is breast-feeding or not, but she often gives no thought to it, being totally absorbed with her new baby and inevitably tired from interrupted nights and busy days. It is an important duty of the carer to offer contraceptive advice to the family soon after the baby is born, though the matter should have been considered even earlier, during pregnancy.

Urinary tract

After delivery micturition may be delayed due to dehydration in labour and reflex inhibition caused by perineal and vulval pain, but should occur at the latest within 12 hours. By day 2 a diuresis occurs and most of the fluid retained during pregnancy is excreted. The changes in glomerular filtration rapidly revert to normal, but the dilatation of the ureters seen in pregnancy does not disappear until 12 or more weeks after delivery.

Urinary tract infection is very common within a day or two of birth, especially if the patient has been catheterized in labour.

Acute retention, often with overflow, may occur, particularly following operative vaginal delivery especially if epidural anaesthesia is used, due to reflex inhibition caused by perineal pain. The bladder is flaccid and causes no complaint, and with intermittent urinary loss due to overflow the condition can easily be overlooked. If overlooked, permanent damage to the kidneys (due to pyelonephritis) and bladder function may occur. Catheterization is required and may need to be repeated. If the patient is still unable to micturate then bladder drainage with an indwelling catheter is required. If the patient is catheterized, bacteriological examination of the urine is necessary and prompt treatment with antibiotics is needed if infection develops.

Continuous urinary incontinence suggests a fistula. This is extremely rare in this country, being more common after prolonged obstructed labour, difficult intravaginal manoeuvres or inexpertly executed caesarean section.

Blood

The increased plasma volume of pregnancy disappears with the early postpartum diuresis. The haemoglobin level rises and is stable by day 5. The leukocytosis of pregnancy (which may reach 30 000 cells per mm^3 in labour) falls to 10 000 cells per mm^3 by day 4. The platelet count increases by day 4 and rises to a maximum by day 10. There is an increase in platelet stickiness and immature platelet forms appear in the blood. These changes, together with increased fibrinogen, tissue trauma and bed rest, explain the liability to puerperal thromboembolism. The changes in the clotting factors during pregnancy gradually revert to normal.

Gastrointestinal tract

The mild gastrointestinal disturbances of pregnancy should disappear soon after birth. There is however a tendency to constipation, which is enhanced by the lack of exercise, fluid loss, restriction of food intake during labour and fear of pain if the perineum is sore, but defecation should occur by the third day. Constipation is often a source of concern to the patient. Fruit, fluids and bran are to be encouraged, but a mild laxative may be needed. Analgesic suppositories and cream will ease discomfort from congestion of any haemorrhoids, which should improve during the puerperium. The mother should eat whatever she wishes but if she is lactating, at least 2 litres of fluid each day is necessary to include provision for the milk.

Metabolism

There is an increase in urinary nitrogen due to intense myometrial breakdown, and peptones are present for the first 10 days. It is not unusual to find lactose and traces of albumin during this time. The basal metabolic rate and glucose tolerance return to normal within 48 hours.

Psychology

Minor emotional disturbances are very common, the elation of the first 48 hours classically giving way to a reactive depression called 'fourth-day blues', which may be related to the rapid fall in oestrogens during this time. These changes gradually settle over the next few days. However, chronic tiredness can lead to depression. All new mothers get tired through disturbed sleep at night during the puerperium. It is sound advice to sleep when the baby sleeps but that can be difficult to follow if there are other children or commitments at home. New mothers need advice to organize help and unbroken periods of rest. Low-dose oestrogen replacement therapy may be valuable prophylactic therapy to prevent depression in susceptible individuals, as mentioned later.

OBJECTIVES OF CARE IN THE PUERPERIUM

Briefly the objectives of maternal care in the puerperium may be summarized as:

1 To establish bonding with the baby.
2 To establish breast- or bottle-feeding and suppress lactation as necessary.
3 To prevent or promptly treat mental and physical complications: depression, urinary retention, bleeding, sepsis and thromboembolism.

Bonding

An intimate psychological unity between mother and infant is normally achieved in the first hours and days after delivery. Such a relationship has profound beneficial effects on the child, especially during its formative years, and for the mother. Bonding can of course be achieved later as seen in the case of very premature babies who cannot be handled much, but the mother's involvement at this time should be encouraged in every possible way.

The mother and baby should be together as much as possible. She should hold the baby at the time of delivery and continue to hold the baby, under supervision if necessary, for as long as she wishes. The baby should be put to the breast as soon as convenient if the woman has decided to breast-feed. If the father is present he should be encouraged to handle the baby and other children should be introduced to their new sibling at the earliest appropriate time. Bonding of the whole family is of major importance but should not interfere with that of the mother and her new baby.

Ideally the mother and baby should only be separated at the wishes of the mother but if, for medical reasons, the infant is taken into a special care unit then free and frequent access is to be encouraged. If the mother is ill the baby should be brought to her as often as their condition permits, or if visiting is not possible a Polaroid photograph should be given to the mother. Any separation should be bridged by the father and other children as appropriate. The young primipara may need encouragement and guidance to establish her confidence but ideally she and the father will have been prepared during antenatal parentcraft classes.

Feeding

Breast-feeding should be encouraged. Breast milk is instantly available, of the right consistency and content, at the ideal temperature and is free. It also contains important antibodies and these are also present in the initial colostrum. Recent studies have demonstrated that breast-feeding reduces lifetime risks of breast cancer by a third, thus preventing three times more deaths than the cervical smear programme.

Bottle-feeding is perhaps slightly faster because the teat is bigger. It is, however, expensive, requires lengthy preparation, and carries the hazards of protein allergy, excessive salt ingestion and infection. This last is due to poor sterilization and the lack of antibodies. Also it can interfere with bonding.

The decision about how to feed the baby is the mother's, but the decision should be made during the antenatal period after full discussion and explanation of the facts about breast- and bottle-feeding. The arguments against breast-feeding – 'I'll be slower to get my figure back', 'It ties me down as only I can do it' and 'It takes too long to learn' – are really excuses. However, the mother who decides she does not wish to breast-feed or finds she does not lactate should not be made to feel guilty. She will need as much assistance and supervision during the early days while bottle-feeding as the mother who breast-feeds.

Feeding technique

When she feeds her baby the mother should be relaxed with no other concern. She should be settled wherever she is most comfortable; this is usually in or on the bed, or in a low chair which gives good support. She may find a footstool comfortable. Some breast-feeding mothers enjoy the closer contact obtained by baring the top half of the body and the baby undressed except for a nappy and shawl.

The mother should support the baby's head. If breast-feeding, she should ensure that the baby's nose is clear of her body and she may need to depress the baby's tongue to help it to take in the nipple. The whole nipple and most of the areola are taken into the baby's mouth; this is called 'fixing' on the breast, as shown in Figure 9.3. If bottle-feeding then the entire end of the teat is taken into the mouth over the depressed tongue.

Feeding is not all instinctive: it has to be learned by both mother and child, and it is essential that guidance and help are readily available during that time. Fashions change about how often and how long babies should feed. However, the baby should not be allowed to remain on the breast for more than a few minutes at first, to avoid soreness and cracking of the nipples before they have hardened. A

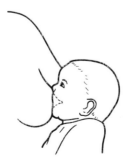

Fig. 9.3 A baby 'fixed' on the breast.

nursing bra needs to give good support for comfort and a little lanolin cream applied to the nipples will prevent excessive drying and cracking.

Poor lactation is often due to poor motivation, but occasionally is due to general ill health. Poor milk production can sometimes be improved by giving the mother metoclopramide, an antiemetic which stimulates prolactin secretion by its action as a dopamine antagonist. If the breast is not emptied at feeding and the remaining milk not expressed then lactation will subside. Inverted nipples and sore cracked nipples can interfere with suckling and lead to poor lactation. The same can happen if the baby has difficulty starting to suckle because of a tense, engorged breast; initial manual expression of some of the milk to soften the breast can help the baby take in the nipple and areola properly.

When bottle-feeding is chosen, suppression of lactation is most satisfactorily achieved by avoiding stimulation of the nipples and binding the breasts firmly. Mild analgesics may be required about the third day because as the milk comes in the breasts become engorged and tender. Should it be necessary to suppress already established lactation then the dopamine agonist bromocriptine may be given to suppress prolactin. The dosage is 2.5 mg initially, then 2.5 mg b.d. for 14 days.

GOING HOME

Most mothers and babies delivered in hospital go home within 2–3 days and some mothers elect to leave within 6 hours if the birth was normal. If normally delivered, mothers and babies can be discharged from hospital by midwives. Hospital medical staff have little to do with normal puerperal care. The community midwife visits at home for the first 10 days, as a statutory duty, and after that the health visitor and primary health care team, including the general practitioner (GP), help the family as necessary.

Before leaving hospital it is important to check and arrange if necessary:

1 Rubella immunity: vaccinate if not immune
2 Rhesus state: give anti-D gammaglobulin if appropriate.
3 Contraception: plan
4 Home conditions: is extra help necessary?
5 Six-week postnatal check: make an appointment with the GP/hospital.

These matters should be communicated clearly to the mother, the community midwife and the GP. Most mothers will see their own GP for their 6-week check but those who have had operative deliveries or complications will be offered an appointment to see the hospital obstetric team so that explanation can be made and plans for the future agreed.

THE MAJOR PUERPERAL COMPLICATIONS

The major puerperal complications are bleeding, uncorrected urinary retention, sepsis, thromboembolism and pathological depression. Observations should be particularly directed at the likelihood of bleeding and urinary retention during the first 24 hours, infection after 2–7 days, thromboembolism until fully mobilized, and depression at any time for several weeks and sometimes later.

Bleeding

Primary postpartum haemorrhage

The first hour following delivery and primary postpartum haemorrhage are discussed in Chapter 8. Careful observation of the uterus, vaginal loss and mother's pulse and blood pressure should be made regularly during the first 4 hours to detect evidence of excessive bleeding. If the other signs occur without obvious bleeding, it is often due to clots hidden in the uterus or vagina, but very occasionally there may be bleeding into the abdomen from a ruptured uterus. Massage of the uterus and expression of the clots, together with an injection of ergometrine and further observation, are indicated. If further bleeding or signs of bleeding occur the vagina and uterus should be explored under general anaesthesia.

Secondary postpartum haemorrhage

This is defined as excessive blood loss from the genital tract after the first 24 hours following delivery. No precise volume is specified.

If bleeding occurs in the first few days after delivery, it is likely to be due to retained fragments of placenta, retained membranes or blood clot. Bleeding occurring later may be due to infection of retained products or the endometrium.

On examination the uterus is usually larger than expected and tender, and the cervical os may be open. The blood may be offensive and the mother pyrexial. A high vaginal swab should always be taken, and if there is any clinical suspicion of infection systemic antibiotics started before the culture result is available. If there is no evidence of infection and the bleeding is slight the patient may be kept under observation. Ergometrine is of dubious value here, but if bleeding is heavier or continuous the uterus must be explored and parenteral ergometrine (0.5 mg ergometrine intramuscularly) may be given. Evacuation of the uterus should be done in all such cases under general anaesthesia. It is easy to damage the uterus and such operations should be done by an experienced operator.

Sepsis

In past centuries childbed fever carried millions of women to their graves and it still does in developing countries, but it is now an uncommon cause of maternal death in the UK. Before the discovery of microbes by Pasteur, 'childbed fever' or 'milk fever' was thought to be due to 'cosmic telluric influences hovering in the upper miasmata'. However, in Vienna Semmelweis noted the connection with medical students sent straight from the postmortem rooms in the morning to the bedside and delivery suite. There were no gloves or hand-washing. Semmelweis made all attendants wash their hands in soda of lime between patients and pushed the crowded beds apart. These simple measures dramatically reduced the deaths from puerperal sepsis and Semmelweis is acknowledged as the father of aseptic techniques.

Puerperal pyrexia

This is specifically defined by the Department of Health in England and Wales as 'any febrile condition occurring in a woman in whom a temperature of 38°C or more has occurred within 14 days after confinement'.

Causes

1 Ascending genital tract infection – most important: it can lead to sterility and death. Signs are tender bulky uterus, offensive lochia.
2 Urinary tract infection – most common. There are often no specific symptoms or signs.
3 Deep venous thrombosis – very important – can lead to pulmonary embolism and death. Signs include fever only if pelvic veins are involved. Classic leg signs may be absent.
4 Mastitis – important whether breast-feeding or not. Signs include tender red area, often segmental (i.e lobar).
5 Respiratory infection – especially after general anaesthesia.

6 Wound infection – episiotomy, lacerations or caesarean section scar.
7 Unrelated causes – e.g. appendicitis.

Diagnosis and treatment

1 Detailed history of relevant systems, but specific symptoms of genital and urinary infection are often absent.
2 General physical examination, to include throat, chest, breasts, abdomen, uterus, perineum, wounds and legs.
3 Microbiology: high vaginal swab; clean specimen of urine; throat swab; (wound swab); (blood culture); milk if the breast is infected.
4 Antibiotic therapy: There should be *prompt* urgent prescription of broad-spectrum antibiotics after taking swabs but without waiting for laboratory reports. Antibiotics must be effective against anaerobic as well as aerobic organisms and a frequently used combination is cefuroxime and metronidazole. (Consider using intravenous preparations if the mother is severely ill.)
5 Isolation: Consider the need to isolate the mother and baby if significant uterine infection is present to prevent cross-infection to others.

Genital tract infection

The patient is particularly vulnerable to ascending genital tract infections during the early puerperium, and every effort must be made as described earlier in this chapter to prevent infection. The site of placental separation is an extensive raw wound and the perineum and/or vagina may have been damaged by laceration or episiotomy. The natural defence mechanisms of the vagina and cervix have been compromised by pregnancy and delivery. The uterus contains a great deal of cellular debris and small pieces of necrotic tissue in a relatively anaerobic atmosphere – an ideal environment for the growth of organisms. Infection is particularly common after prolonged labour and prolonged rupture of the membranes. The effects are aggravated by debility due to exhaustion, dehydration, anaemia and ill health. Figure 9.4 shows the pathways of spread of infection.

The organisms usually responsible are the common commensals from the patient's rectum, but can come from attendants. They are mostly coliforms and anaerobic streptococci. Staphylococci and *Clostridium* are now rare. β-Haemolytic streptococci can cause little local signs but present with septicaemia and associated toxaemia.

Clinically the patient may feel unwell, complain of pain and tenderness in the lower abdomen and of offensive lochia which may

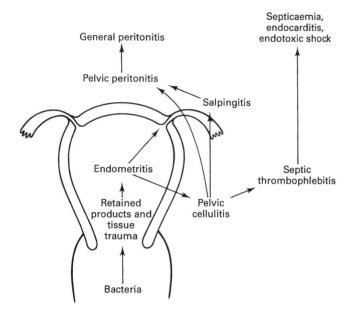

Fig. 9.4   Spread of genital tract infection following delivery.

become a deeper red and heavier. On examination she may be found to be pyrexial with a tender uterus.

The management priorities are definitive microbiology, appropriate antibiotic therapy, adequate analgesia, rest and adequate hydration, and measures to avoid spread of infection to others. The risks of death, chronic ill health or sterility should be avoidable by early detection and prompt treatment.

Urinary tract infection

Urinary tract infection is common in the puerperium. It may present with the standard symptoms of frequency and dysuria but will sometimes produce no symptoms or signs apart from pyrexia. Culture of urine from all women with puerperal pyrexia but no clear cause must therefore be routine.

Thromboembolism

This continues to be one of the most frequent causes of maternal death and half occur postnatally.

Prevention

Early ambulation is to be encouraged, particularly after caesarean section or operative vaginal delivery when the risks of thromboembolism are greatest. Deep venous thrombosis occurs in leg and pelvic veins. The mother should start postnatal exercises on the day of delivery to help reduce the risks, including leg exercises and deep breathing. Prophylactic anticoagulants (in the form of subcutaneous heparin 5000 units b.d.) should be used in selected cases: the obese, poor movers, those who were bed-rested antenatally. Graduated compression stockings may be worn.

It is important to establish a diagnosis of pulmonary embolism or deep venous thrombosis properly since the diagnosis has implications for the woman's future pregnancies, operations and contraception. A venogram or ventilation/perfusion scan should be arranged forthwith but treatment should be started at once with full anticoagulant doses of heparin. If the investigations confirm the diagnosis then oral anticoagulant therapy should be commenced and continued for at least 6 weeks.

Depression

The minor emotional lability and 'fourth day blues' so common in the early puerperium can progress unrecognized to serious, debilitating and sometimes fatal depression. Doctors, midwives and health visitors need to be alert to the possibility and appreciate the insidious effects of sleeplessness and tiredness.

Although true insomnia, excessive mood change and depression may be premonitory signs of puerperal psychosis in the immediate puerperium, the manifestations may not be apparent until some weeks after delivery. Poor bonding with and inadequate care of the child and loss of interest may also be early signs. Depression is the main feature and, if not detected early and treated promptly, can lead to major disability, family breakdown, infanticide and suicide. Most psychiatric hospitals have special mother-and-baby units for patients with puerperal psychosis so that the mother is not separated from her baby but is supervised with it.

Postnatal depression should be anticipated if there is a history of depression or if it has occurred before, and it must be remembered that it may last for many months after the puerperium. The help of the psychiatric team may be invaluable. Low-dose oestrogen therapy combined with progestogen to replace the acutely deficient hormones in the puerperium seems to be effective in reducing the risk of depression. A low dose of a natural oestrogen, as used for hormone replacement therapy in postmenopausal women, is safer than a synthetic oestrogen, to minimize the risk of thromboembolism.

FURTHER READING

Department of Health (1994) *Report on Confidential Enquiries into Maternal Deaths in the United Kingdom 1988–1990*. HMSO, London.

Kakkar, V.V. (1984) Venous thromboembolism. In: Brudenell, M. and Wilds, P. (eds) *Medical and Surgical Problems in Obstetrics*. Wright, Bristol, pp. 175–192.

Kumar, R. (1984) Psychological disorders. In: Brudenell, M. and Wilds, P. (eds) *Medical and Surgical Problems in Obstetrics*. Wright, Bristol, pp. 50–59.

10

Maternal and perinatal mortality

OBSTETRIC PRACTICE – HISTORICAL PERSPECTIVE

The first hospitals were to provide destitute women with a place where they could be delivered of their babies. Unfortunately, they proved relatively unsafe because of cross-infection. Puerperal sepsis ('childbed fever') killed one in four mothers little more than 100 years ago, and the babies lost were not even counted. Then, Albert Semmelweis in Vienna and Budapest reduced the death rate dramatically by antiseptic methods to stop cross-infection, long before Pasteur's identification of the bacterial cause.

The next major advance was anaesthesia, which enabled the more liberal use of caesarean section and in turn the development of the more refined lower-segment rather than upper-segment operation. Nevertheless, 50 years ago three mothers and 60 babies in every 1000 still died from childbirth (Figures 10.1 and 10.2) and many of today's grandparents remember their fear at the time.

Caesarean section remained an operation of last resort because of bleeding and sepsis. Antibiotics and the development of efficient blood transfusion services nearly 60 years ago altered the outcome dramatically, although it then took another generation of experience to appreciate that caesarean section was an inherently safe operation if done when mother and baby were still in good condition.

Prolonged labour was the real threat. The development of oxytocin therapy 35 years ago helped overcome that problem. The present philosophy of management of labour is directed at avoidance of prolonged labour, by early recognition and early treatment with oxytocin or caesarean section if unsuccessful. As a consequence, puerperal sepsis is rarely a problem, mothers return very quickly to normal fitness, and the well-being of the baby during labour and soon after birth is protected. Care is now directed as much to the baby as the mother; as much to morbidity as mortality; and as much to emotional needs as safety.

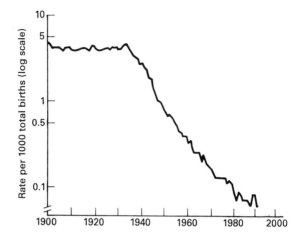

Fig. 10.1   Maternal mortality in England and Wales since 1900. Note the logarithmic scale for rate.

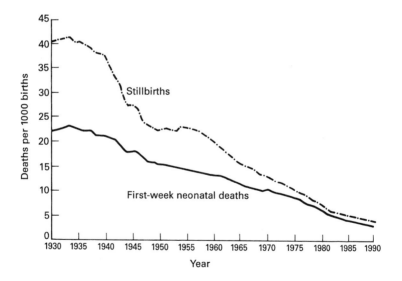

Fig. 10.2   Stillbirth and first-week neonatal death trends, together representing perinatal mortality, in England and Wales since 1930.

The use of epidural anaesthesia has been a great influence on obstetric practice in the last 30 years. It has freed many women from the fear of pain of labour and especially of surgical vaginal delivery. However, by reducing the mother's urge to push to help normal vaginal delivery of her baby, it leads to increased use of instrumental delivery and has therefore received unwarranted criticism. Spinal or epidural anaesthesia for caesarean section not only allows the mother to be awake to experience the baby's birth but also facilitates her partner's presence, involvement and emotional support.

Advances in neonatal paediatrics have transformed obstetric practice in the last 20 years. They largely account for the continuing reduction in perinatal mortality from rates which would have been considered impossible to achieve even a decade ago. Survival of babies born from 30 weeks' gestation onwards is now virtually 100%, and at 26–28 weeks 85% (see Chapter 6, Fig. 6.9, which includes deaths from all causes). Babies as early as 23 weeks' gestation can now sometimes be saved. Yet barely 15 years ago there was virtually no hope when complications of pregnancy arose as late as 30–32 weeks, so many babies were left to be stillborn. The present improved survival depends on the baby being delivered before suffering the effects of severe malnourishment or hypoxia, and without injury. Therefore obstetricians now tend readily to deliver babies however prematurely, and often by caesarean section, when serious complications arise.

Apart from these medical advances, it must be recognized that improvement in the general health of the population through rising socioeconomic conditions and reducing family size has also been an important contributor to the steady and continuing fall in maternal and perinatal mortality rates (Figs 10.1 and 10.2). Partly for this reason, and because pregnancy and childbirth now seem so safe, there is increasing questioning of medical intervention and criticism of delivery in hospital. Also, inexperienced medical staff easily lose sight of the need for vigilant care. The lessons of history should not be lost.

MATERNAL MORTALITY

Maternal death is defined as occurring during pregnancy or within 6 weeks of delivery or abortion, and attributable to complications of pregnancy, childbirth or the puerperium. The definition in the UK has recently changed – deaths occurring within 12 months used to be the criterion.

There is about one maternal death from every 17 000 pregnancies – less than the mortality risk in non-pregnant women of reproductive age. About half the deaths are due to pregnancy ('true maternal deaths') and the others are due to associated causes such as heart disease. Complete and detailed information is available from a series of *Confidential Enquiries into Maternal Deaths* which are published every 3 years. The most recent report, based on the years 1991–93, is the third to include data for the whole of the UK, rather than for England and Wales alone with separate reports for Scotland and Northern Ireland. By providing audited data since 1952, the reports have highlighted and focused attention on specific situations where the mother is at increased risk and made recommendations for improvements in clinical practice and risk reduction. The main causes of true maternal deaths in the latest report are shown in Table 10.1 in diminishing order:

Table 10.1   Causes of true maternal deaths in the UK

Cause of death	Per cent
Pulmonary embolism	27
Hypertensive disease	16
Haemorrhage	12
Amniotic fluid embolism	8
Sepsis	7
Ectopic pregnancy	6
Abortion	6
Anaesthesia	6
Ruptured uterus	3

Factors associated with maternal deaths are given in Table 10.2.

Table 10.2   Factors associated with maternal deaths in the UK

Associated factor	Per cent
Caesarean section	39
Cardiac disease	18
Anaesthetic complications	9

The prevention of pulmonary embolism, one of the leading causes of maternal death, remains elusive. Predisposing factors often cannot be avoided but they need to be recognized: obesity, bed rest for any reason, caesarean section and increasing age and parity. Oestrogens should never be used to suppress lactation.

One unfortunate factor reported is that in about 40% of cases maternal deaths were considered to be associated with substandard care. This was not necessarily a failure of clinical care; it also included situations where the action of the mother or her relatives was contributory or where the infrastructure of resources and facilities available to the mother was below the standard which should have been offered.

Controversy continues about whether to concentrate deliveries in large specialist units where clinical expertise and technological resources are always available, or whether to provide greater facilities for community maternity care and delivery. The latter requires careful and accurate selection of women at low risk for delivery in the community, either in general practitioner units or at home. However, selection and prediction of risk are unreliable. As many as 15% of women considered at low risk will require transfer to a consultant unit in labour. It remains to be seen whether the psychological and emotional advantages of delivery in the community will be more than outweighed by an increased risk to mother and baby.

PERINATAL MORTALITY

Perinatal deaths are defined as stillbirths after 24 weeks' gestation and neonatal deaths within the first week after birth. The rate is defined as per 1000 total births, and at present is about 8.

This definition is now unfortunately too inaccurate to serve its purpose. Perinatal mortality is intended to reflect the effectiveness of obstetric practice. It was therefore defined to include only first-week deaths rather than all neonatal deaths, which are those occurring up to 4 weeks after birth. However, now that obstetricians more readily deliver babies prematurely there is likely to be a reduction in stillbirths, but consequent neonatal problems are more likely to be prolonged. Therefore deaths up to 4 weeks should be included. On the other hand, babies born before 24 weeks – which previously have been classed as abortions – now sometimes receive neonatal care, and those that die are added to the perinatal mortality rate.

Other major determinants of perinatal mortality are developmental abnormality and the mother's parity and socioeconomic class, which are beyond obstetric control (see below). For all these reasons, therefore, there is a growing international movement towards standardizing reporting of perinatal mortality to babies weighing at least 1000 g and without lethal developmental abnormalities, and separating first-born from the others.

Causes

The main causes, of both stillbirths and neonatal deaths, are shown in Table 10.3.

All these complications are more likely with multiple pregnancy, and other causes include maternal diabetes mellitus and rhesus isoimmunization.

Lethal developmental abnormality varies greatly in incidence

Table 10.3 Main causes of stillbirths and neonatal deaths (figures are approximate)

Cause of death	Per cent
Developmental abnormality	33
Prematurity	33
Chronic starvation and hypoxia	20
Acute intrapartum hypoxia	5
Birth injury	3

around the world. It is particularly high in the UK, and varies significantly even within the country, increasing westwards in England and in Wales and Ireland, and northwards in Scotland. The commonest malformations affect the central nervous system – anencephaly, hydrocephaly, spina bifida and meningomyelocele – and next come cardiac and renal abnormalities.

The importance of low birth weight (<2500 g), whether due to prematurity or chronic starvation and hypoxia, is clear from the fact that these babies constitute fewer than 7% of total births in England and Wales, but account for approximately 60% of stillbirths and nearly 50% of infant deaths in the first year of life.

Prematurity is mostly due to spontaneous premature labour, which remains one of the outstanding unresolved problems in obstetrics today, rather than due to obstetric intervention.

Chronic starvation and hypoxia result from placental insufficiency, which is commonly due to hypertensive diseases and partial placental abruption. However, it often occurs without any evident cause and is expressed only by fetal growth retardation, which is therefore so important to look for in the course of antenatal care.

Acute hypoxia is caused by major placental abruption but usually occurs during labour, either due to relative placental insufficiency or to abnormal uterine activity, including iatrogenic overstimulation. Early recognition of the signs of fetal hypoxia is therefore a major aim of monitoring in labour, because hypoxia causes not only death but in survivors it can cause permanent cerebral damage.

Birth injury, usually to the brain from intracranial haemorrhage, also needs to be carefully avoided because it can cause not only death but also permanent disability. There is therefore no longer a place for difficult vaginal delivery as the risks can usually be overcome or significantly reduced by caesarean section.

Contributory factors

Risk of perinatal loss is significantly increased by the following background factors in the mother, which need to be taken into account when considering the type and place of antenatal care and delivery:

1 Age: under 20 and over 35 years.
2 Parity: 0 and 4 or more.
3 Social class: reducing from V to I.
4 Ethnic origin: women from developing countries.
5 Social habits: smoking, alcohol, drugs.

MANAGEMENT OF STILLBIRTH AND NEONATAL DEATH

Tending to the bereaved is always difficult, but it is an essential role that doctors must not shirk. Grief is essential to overcome bereavement, and in helping parents to grieve for their dead baby the first priority is contact with the baby, even if it is deformed. The parents' imagination may be worse than the reality and cannot be put out of mind. Some parents may choose not to hold or even see their baby, but later they often desperately regret that and photographs should always be taken so as to be available when needed.

The second essential is explanation. Parents must be fully informed. Indeed, if a baby's death, before or after birth, can be anticipated the parents must be closely involved in discussion about management. Postmortem and other investigations may not be complete for several weeks and a subsequent opportunity must be given to parents for further explanation, not only of the possible cause of death but also to give advice for the future.

It is essential to keep the family doctor and community midwife well-informed as they will be closely involved with the parents during their grieving time. Others whose help may also be required include, for instance, social workers, and the parents may find useful support from the local branch of the Stillbirth and Neonatal Death Society (SANDS).

Investigations

The first essential is postmortem examination of the baby. Sensitive explanation is necessary to gain permission from the parents. The following basic investigations should be made:

Baby

1 Cord or cardiac blood for haemoglobin and group.
2 Deep ear swab for culture.
3 Skin biopsy for chromosome analysis.
4 X-ray whole body.
5 Autopsy.

Maternal blood

1 Cytomegalovirus antibody assay.
2 Toxoplasma antibody assay.
3 Rubella antibody assay.
4 Rhesus antibody assay.
5 Kleihauer test (for fetal red cells).
6 Wassermann reaction (WR) and Venereal Disease Research Laboratory (VDRL) test.
7 Free thyroxine index or thyroid-stimulating hormone (TSH).
8 Glycosylated haemoglobin and/or glucose tolerance test (within 24 hours).

FURTHER READING

Chamberlain, G.V.P. (1981) The epidemiology of perinatal loss. In: Studd, J. (ed.) *Progress in Obstetrics and Gynaecology*, vol. 1. Churchill Livingstone, Edinburgh, pp. 1–17.

Department of Health (1996) *Report on Confidential Enquiries into Maternal Deaths in the United Kingdom 1991-1993*. HMSO, London.

Macfarlane, A. and Mugford, M. (1984) *Birth Counts. Statistics of Pregnancy and Childbirth*. HMSO, London.

Macvicar, J. (1981) The effect of race on perinatal mortality. In: Studd, J. (ed.) *Progress in Obstetrics and Gynaecology*, vol. 1. Churchill Livingstone, Edinburgh, pp. 92–104.

Thompson, M. (1951) *The Cry and the Covenant (the Semmelweis Story)*. Heinemann, London.

11

Contraception, sterilization and therapeutic abortion

The demand for medical provision of contraception, sterilization and therapeutic abortion has increased dramatically in recent years, and each of these related topics will form a substantial part of the workload of most gynaecologists and general practitioners. Although sterilization operations will generally be performed in specialist units, they really form part of the range of contraceptive methods, and all doctors should be able to provide information to patients about sterilization as well as contraception. For the foreseeable future, contraceptive methods as well as patients are likely to remain fallible, and there will be a place for abortion as the long stop of family planning methods.

CONTRACEPTION

Four groups of contraceptive methods will be considered:

1 Hormonal.
2 Intrauterine devices.
3 Barrier methods.
4 Other methods.

In the past barrier and other methods were predominant, but the 1960s and 1970s saw a swing to the more reliable methods of the first two groups. The spread of acquired immunodeficiency syndrome (AIDS) has more recently re-emphasized the importance of barrier methods.

Hormonal contraception

Oestrogen–progestogen combinations

Actions

The principal action is suppression of ovulation. Three secondary actions assist contraception:

1 Inhibition of cervical mucus changes that normally allow sperm migration at the time of ovulation.
2 Interference with ovum transport by altering smooth-muscle activity in the fallopian tubes and uterus.
3 Prevention of the physiological cycle in the endometrium. It is not prepared for implantation.

Effectiveness

Typical accidental pregnancy rates for combined oral contraceptives would be 0.4 per 100 women-years.

Formulation

Since the Scowen Committee Report in 1969 linking thrombo-embolic side-effects with higher doses of synthetic oestrogens, all combinations used include no more than 50 µg of either ethinyl-oestradiol or mestranol and most now contain only 20–35 µg. Mestranol has a lesser oestrogenic effect than ethinyloestradiol (approximately 60%).

The progestogens are synthetic compounds varying widely in molecular structure and potency. Their action is similar to proges-terone in that they induce progestational changes in the oestroge-nized endometrium, but if used continuously they tend to inhibit endometrial growth altogether. The most commonly used progesto-gens are levonorgestrel and norethisterone.

Most preparations contain the same amount of oestrogen and progestogen in each of the 21 pills taken in a cycle, but phased formulations are also available. In these the amount of progestogen is low in the early part of the cycle, increasing in two or three phases for the rest of the cycle. Overall these phased formulations provide slightly more oestrogen and less progestogen than the uniphasic preparations of similar dosage. A number of combined pills are marketed in ED forms where the addition of seven placebo pills allow the preparation to be taken every day without a break.

Method of use

The pills are taken one daily for 21 days with a gap between each pack of 7 days. Protection against conception is continuous after the first seven pills of the first pack if they are started on day 5 of the cycle, or immediately if started on day 1. Combined oral contraceptives may be started immediately after a termination or miscarriage, or 3 weeks after delivery. Protection continues if one pill is forgotten, provided it is taken within 12 hours with the next day's pill being taken at the usual time. If more than 12 hours late, extra precautions should be taken for 7 days after resuming normal pill-taking. During the interval between packs there is usually, but not always, some uterine bleeding. It is possible to delay menstruation to a more convenient time by taking further pills at the end of the course.

With ED preparations the pills are taken continuously. The first pill is taken on day 1 of the period and alternative precautions should be taken for the first 14 days.

Hazards

Oestrogen–progestogen combinations can only be obtained on medical prescription as there are various hazards associated with their use. Some are mild, some very serious, but their prevalence is fortunately slight and certainly far less than most non-medical people believe. They are certainly small compared with the risk of an unwanted pregnancy. The major hazards are as follows.

THROMBOEMBOLISM

There is an increased incidence of deep vein thrombosis, pulmonary embolus and cerebral thrombosis related to the synthetic oestrogen component of the pill. With the lower-oestrogen-dose pills the mortality risk from these conditions is of the order of 2–3 per million women per year – less than a tenth of the risk associated with a pregnancy and minute compared with the risk of smoking even a few cigarettes per day. Total deaths for venous thromboembolic disease in the 11 million women in England and Wales aged 15–44 were 18 in the year 1989. For comparison, there were 260 deaths for myocardial infarction and stroke in the same group. In 1995 information was released by the Committee on Safety of Medicines indicating that oral contraceptives containing desogestrel or gestodene are associated with risks of venous thromboembolism roughly twice those of the older norgestrel-based formulations.

METABOLIC EFFECTS

Changes in virtually every aspect of metabolism have been recorded in pill-users. These changes tend to alter the normal female metabolic pattern marginally towards either the male pattern or that found in early pregnancy. Probably the most important of these changes are those affecting cholesterol and high-density lipoprotein (HDL), which almost certainly accounts for the observed slightly increased incidence of ischaemic heart disease in the older (over 35 years) long-term oral contraceptive user. Progestogens and androgens increase cholesterol concentrations and decrease HDL, whereas oestrogens do the reverse, so that the hormonal balance of the preparation is of importance, and a low progestogen content may be more important than a low oestrogen content. Desogestrel and gestodene are said to have a lesser adverse effect on lipid metabolism than levonorgestrel at the same dose level, and there is the distinct possibility that formulations based on these progestogens may have mortality savings in relation to heart disease and stroke which comfortably outweigh their increased venous thromboembolic risks. Glucose tolerance is also reduced (as in pregnancy), very occasionally producing overt diabetes in a latent diabetic.

HYPERTENSION

In the occasional patient blood pressure is significantly elevated while taking oral contraceptives.

DEPRESSION

A few patients will get quite severe depression while taking the pill. This has been shown to be related to disturbances in tryptophan metabolism, and is partly treatable by pyridoxine (vitamin B_6).

NEOPLASIA

There has naturally been considerable concern about the possibility of pill usage increasing the risk of cancer of the genital tract or breast. A number of studies have shown clear evidence of a reduced incidence of ovarian and endometrial cancer in pill-users. The evidence in relation to breast cancer is more equivocal with some studies showing an increased risk and some a decreased risk. There is no evidence to link the pill with cervical cancer (although barrier methods have a modest protective effect).

Medical care

Before prescribing oestrogen–progestogen pills, the doctor should ensure as far as possible that there is no predisposition to thromboembolism which the pill might potentiate. Also, the medical history should identify disturbances of liver function, which might interfere with steroid metabolism, and the pre-existence of conditions such as migraine, the later occurrence of which might be ascribed to the pill. Family history of thromboembolism or of heart disease may also be relevant.

An assessment must be made of any intercurrent illness or condition which might be affected by taking the pill. If necessary, specialist advice should be sought. Examples are diabetes mellitus, essential hypertension, renal disease and psychiatric illnesses. It is important in making this assessment not to forget the possible harm resulting from further pregnancy.

The physical examination should include measurement of body weight and blood pressure, and also exclude a carcinoma of the breast that might be adversely affected by administered sex steroids.

Women over 35 years should be discouraged from long-term pill usage if an acceptable alternative exists. Smoking significantly increases the risk of thromboembolic disease and ischaemic heart disease and one should discourage long-term pill usage in smokers (or better still, discourage smoking!).

Pill-taking should be stopped immediately in case of pregnancy, thromboembolism, jaundice, migraine or severe headache (as a new symptom) or visual disturbances. It should be discontinued 6 weeks prior to major elective surgery.

Contraindications

The following conditions should be considered contraindications to combined oral contraception:

1 Any history of thromboembolism.
2 A known predisposition to thromboembolism.
3 Significant liver disease.
4 An oestrogen-dependent tumour (i.e. breast or endometrium).

Choice of preparation

The higher-dose preparations give better cycle control and virtually always control dysmenorrhoea, but the associated metabolic disturbances and hazards are greater.

The available preparations are shown in Table 11.1.

Table 11.1   Available preparations of combined oral contraceptives

Preparation	Oestrogen (mg)	Progestogen (mg)
Combined (ethinyloestradiol and progestogen)		
Loestrin 20	20	1 Norethisterone acetate
Loestrin 30	30	1.5 Norethisterone acetate
Conova 30	30	2 Ethynodiol diacetate
Brevinor	35	0.5 Norethisterone
Ovysmen	35	0.5 Norethisterone
Neocon 1/35	35	1 Norethisterone
Norimin	35	1 Norethisterone
Microgynon 30	30	0.15 Levonorgestrel
Ovranette	30	0.15 Levonorgestrel
Eugynon 30	30	0.25 Levonorgestrel

Table 11.1 *cont.*

Ovran 30	30	0.25 Levonorgestrel
Ovran	50	0.25 Levonorgestrel
Mercilon	20	0.15 Desogestrel
Marvelon	30	0.15 Desogestrel
Femodene	30	0.075 Gestodene
Minulet	30	0.075 Gestodene
Cilest	35	0.25 Norgestimate

Combined (mestranol and progestogen)

Norinyl-1	50	1 Norethisterone
OrthoNovin-1	50	1 Norethisterone

Biphasic/triphasic (ethinyloestradiol and progestogen)

Binovum	35/35	0.5/1 Norethisterone
Synphase	35/35/35	0.5/1/0.5 Norethisterone
Trinovum	35/35/35	0.5/0.75/1 Norethisterone
Logynon	30/40/30	0.05/0.075/0.125 Levonorgestrel
Trinordiol	30/40/30	0.05/0/075/0.125 Levonorgestrel
Triadene	30/40/30	0.05/0.7/0.1 Gestodene
Triminulet	30/40/30	0.05/0.7/0.1 Gestodene

Progestogen-only pills

Actions

These are similar to those of oestrogen–progestogen combined pills, except that ovulation is not reliably suppressed. They rely on:

1 Changes in the maturation of endometrium which inhibit implantation.
2 Constant hostility of cervical mucus to penetration by sperm that lasts throughout the cycle.
3 Interference with the tubal transport of ova.

Formulation

The dose of progestogen is generally less than that in the combined pills, and oestrogen is entirely absent. The preparations available are:

1 Micronor (norethisterone) 0.35 mg.
2 Noriday (norethisterone) 0.35 mg.
3 Femulen (ethynodiol diacetate) 0.5 mg.
4 Microval (levonorgestrel) 0.03 mg.
5 Norgeston (levonorgestrel) 0.03 mg.
6 Neogest (norgestrel) 0.075 mg.

Method of use
The pills are supplied in packs of 28 or 35 and one is taken every day at the same time of the day. Note that there is no interval: the tablets are taken continuously. The first packet is started on day 1 of the period and becomes effective immediately.

The timing of pill-taking is more critical than with the combined pill, and a progestogen-only pill should be considered 'missed' if taken 3 hours or more late. Extra precautions should be taken for 48 hours if only one pill is late. The pill should be stopped immediately in the case of pregnancy, jaundice or thromboembolism. There is no need to stop progestogen-only contraception before elective surgery.

Hazards and medical care
Adverse effects are very uncommon, except for irregular uterine bleeding. This may be severe enough to prevent patients continuing. It usually settles to a more or less regular cycle after 9 months. Other problems are rare but include skin reactions, breast discomfort and occasional symptoms of premenstrual tension.

ACCIDENTAL PREGNANCY
This is the most serious drawback to the use of progestogen-only pills. Rates reported vary considerably from 2 to 6 per 100 women-years, and a disproportionate number of these pregnancies are ectopic.

INDICATIONS
Progestogen-only pills are suitable for patients who suffer adverse effects from pills containing oestrogen. They are also useful in lactation as milk supply is not affected.

DEPOT CONTRACEPTION
Progestogens have been used in depot form, given as an intramuscular injection (usually medroxyprogesterone acetate 150 or 300 mg in oil) to last 3–6 months. Irregular bleeding or amenorrhoea with anovulation are common side-effects. Recently studies have shown increasing loss of bone density in women using depot progestogen contraception, similar to that of the postmenopausal woman. The only real advantage (shared with intrauterine contraceptive devices (IUCDs)) is the total lack of dependence on patient co-operation once administered.

Postcoital contraception

The aim is to inhibit implantation of the fertilized ovum by giving an oral dose of hormone. This form of contraception is not really suitable for long-term use, but can be useful as a 'first-aid' measure.

An abnormally high dose of an oestrogenic combined pill (tabs ii stat and repeated after 12 hours) is given. Schering PC4 is the only preparation currently licensed in the UK for postcoital contraception. It has the same formulation as the combined contraceptive pills Ovran and Eugynon 50, which may be available in other countries.

Patients should ideally begin the treatment within 72 hours of unprotected intercourse.

History-taking should aim to exclude those in whom high oestrogens would be particularly hazardous (e.g. any predisposition to thromboembolism, any liver dysfunction). The exposure is brief and the risk of thromboembolism is not yet known. The effect on the fetus, if pregnancy occurs, is not known. In many cases termination of pregnancy would be advisable. Pregnancy rates are 1–1.5%

Alternatively an IUCD may be fitted within 3 days with a high degree of effectiveness.

Intrauterine contraceptive devices

There are stories dating back to biblical times of pebbles being inserted into camels' uterine cavities as contraceptive devices, but practical intrauterine contraception started with the Graefenberg ring in the 1930s and more especially with the Lippes loop in the 1960s. A very wide variety of devices have been designed since, but litigation, particularly in the USA, has led to the withdrawal of many of them, notably the Dalkon Shield, which was associated with a high risk of septic mid-trimester abortion.

Inactive devices

These are small objects made of polyethylene or nylon (previously gold or silver).

They are designed to fit into the uterine cavity and have various configurations. Usually the shape has led to the commonly used name, e.g. shield, ring, coil, loop (which is not a loop but a zig-zag shape), together often with the name of the inventor.

Many of the IUCDs have one or two nylon threads fixed to the lower end which normally protrude from the cervical canal. These assist simple removal and also demonstrate the presence of the IUCD in the uterus.

Mode of action
IUCDs are considered to inhibit the implantation of the blastocyst in the endometrium, possibly by altering the pH of the uterine

secretion and thus inhibiting the essential enzymes. There is a small round-cell infiltration in the endometrium when an IUCD is present but normally this does not proceed to full-scale inflammation. The mildness of the reaction is possibly due to the short length of time that the endometrium is in contact with the IUCD before being shed in menstruation. Changes in tubal motility, possibly affecting egg transport, have also been demonstrated.

Effectiveness
The devices vary in their effectiveness against conception (from 1 pregnancy or less per 100 women-years for copper devices to 3 per 100 or worse for the small inert devices). The important facts are that they are generally not as effective against pregnancy as combined oestrogen–progestogen pills, but there is much less chance of 'user-failure', e.g. by forgetting to take pills regularly or running out of supplies.

Complications and side-effects
IUCDs may be a nearly perfect method of contraception for many patients, but over a period of 2 years of use, about 30% of Lippes loops will have to be abandoned for reasons other than planned pregnancy.
Removals are most common on account of:

1 *Bleeding*: Periods may be unduly heavy or prolonged. Less commonly, there is constant intermenstrual bleeding. Iron-deficiency anaemia can occur in women with IUCDs, even without subjectively excessive losses.
2 *Pain*: In some patients uterine pains occur after insertion and gradually subside. In a small number the pains continue and are not tolerable.
3 *Expulsion*: If unnoticed, expulsion may lead to unplanned pregnancy.
4 *Pregnancy*: With the device in the uterus (accidental pregnancy).
5 *Infection*: Occasionally tubal or intrauterine infection occurs. Most cases can be treated with the device in. If there is not a good response immediately or the infection is initially severe, the IUCD should be removed. The overall risk of pelvic infection with an IUCD is small, and several studies have shown that the risk is least with copper-containing devices. The nulliparous woman appears to be at greater risk of infection compared with parous women, and the consequences are of course more serious. It is difficult to put a figure on the risk of infection associated with an IUCD when pelvic infection is so common anyway. It has almost certainly been exaggerated in the past and may well be no more than 1 per 1000 users.

Insertion

In most parous women, insertion of an intrauterine device is an easy outpatient procedure. If there is any substantial difficulty the operator should not continue the attempt. It can always be carried out at another time under theatre conditions, if necessary with a general anaesthetic, or a local intracervical block.

In nulliparous women, insertion is more difficult and painful and the side-effects in use more severe.

After insertion, hypotension and bradycardia may occur, even if insertion has been very easy. All patients should not leave for 10 minutes and should be able to lie down if necessary.

IUCDs should never be inserted in the presence of pelvic inflammatory disease.

Perforation of the uterus is a rare complication following insertion.

At present there is no evidence to suggest that inactive IUCDs need to be replaced routinely unless they cause symptoms.

Active intrauterine devices

Background

Owing to poor long-term continuity rates with inactive devices, attempts have been made to incorporate active antifertility agents in smaller IUCDs.

Active agents used so far are metals and hormones. Virgin copper wire has been used very successfully in the Endouterine T (Copper-T) and Graviguard (Copper-7) and Multiload devices.

Progesterone was tried in a T-device (Progestasert). This had the advantage of a low pregnancy rate and a lower incidence of bleeding problems, but it was relatively large and difficult to insert, needed to be changed annually, was very expensive and had a high ectopic pregnancy rate. More recently, encouraging results have been reported with a modified Nova T releasing levonorgestrel, known as the Mirena, lasting 6 years and associated with a good pregnancy rate (0.5 per 100 women-years) and a reduced ectopic pregnancy rate. It has the additional advantage of substantially reducing menstrual blood loss and may have a role in the management of menorrhagia.

Insertion

Insertion of the small devices is much easier for the patient. The Copper-7 introducer is only 3 mm in external diameter. This allows it to be a feasible method for women who have never been pregnant, in contrast to the inactive devices. Results of its use in nulliparous women are good. Care is required in inserting the Copper-7, to ensure that the transverse limb reaches the fundus of the uterus in a full open position.

Perforation is rare, but there is a marked omental reaction to a copper device in the peritoneal cavity, and misplaced devices should be removed within a few days. This is usually possible through a laparoscope.

Mode of action
The small plastic shape alone has very little contraceptive effect. The action of copper and similar metals is not known for certain, but traces of copper ions are known to inhibit enzymes, such as alkaline phosphatase which may be required for implantation. Cupric ions are toxic to sperm in lower mammals and, incidentally, to many bacteria.

Effectiveness
The copper devices are highly effective against pregnancy, giving accidental pregnancy rates of around 1 per 100 women-years. The initial trials of the Mirena show pregnancy rates of 0.5 per 100-women years, which compares well with those of combined oral contraception.

Complications and side-effects
These are of the same kind as those of other IUCDs, but removals for bleeding and pain are greatly reduced with the copper devices because of their smaller size. Infection with a copper-containing IUCD *in situ* may be caused by actinomycosis-type organisms and specific culture for this type of organism should be undertaken if a coil is removed for suspected infection.

The copper is not significantly absorbed systemically, and in the case of accidental pregnancy the evidence suggests that there is no danger from teratogenicity. All active agents are slowly lost by elution, and active devices require replacement at intervals. Replacement of the copper devices is recommended every 5 years.

Pregnancy with an IUCD
A relatively high proportion of pregnancies occurring with an IUCD *in situ* will be ectopic pregnancies (although the absolute rate of ectopic pregnancy probably does not exceed that in the general population). Dalkon Shields (*in situ*) were shown to be associated with a high rate of middle-trimester septic abortion, and have been withdrawn from the market. All coils (*in situ* in pregnancy) are associated with a high spontaneous miscarriage rate, and probably a higher late pregnancy complication rate, and should, if possible, be removed in early pregnancy, whether or not the woman wants to continue with the pregnancy.

Barrier methods

Barrier appliances are designed to prevent the direct insemination of the cervical mucus with spermatozoa. They are used with spermicidal substances which are placed so as to be in direct contact with the seminal fluid in the vagina. They have the advantage of offering some protection against venereal infection, and particularly human immunodeficiency virus (HIV).

The condom, sheath or 'French letter'

This is rolled on to the erect penis before coitus and retains the ejaculated semen. Spermicides are not always used with condoms, but if they are effectiveness is increased, the risk of them bursting is reduced and they are lubricated. It is important that the sheath is put on before there is any penile contact with the vagina as initial secretions may contain spermatozoa. Quoted failure rates for long-term use are 4–7 pregnancies per 100 women-years.

The diaphragm or 'Dutch cap'

This is the most commonly used and probably the safest (against pregnancy) female barrier method. It fits like a ring pessary between the posterior fornix and the anterior vaginal wall just above the symphysis pubis. It is not as heavily constructed as a ring pessary and is surprisingly unobtrusive during coitus if correctly fitted. The woman places it in the vagina herself before coitus and it must remain in position for at least 8 hours afterwards. The correct size is estimated by a doctor or specially trained nurse, and the patient is carefully instructed in the correct manner of use. In fitting a diaphragm it is important to ensure:

1 That the cervix is covered.
2 That the lower edge fits snugly into the sulcus above the symphysis.
3 That the width of the vagina is filled at the cervical level without causing undue lateral stretch, leading to ridging of the posterior vaginal wall.

Most women take a 70–75-mm cap. Routine checks of fit should be made, initially after a week and then every 6 months. Variation is caused by age, pregnancy, change in pelvic muscle tone and change in intrapelvic fat tissue related to changes in body weight.

Other caps

Other forms of cap to cover the cervix have been employed in the past (cervical, vault and vimule caps) but their use now is very limited. A female condom (Femshield) is available but has not gained wide acceptance.

Effectiveness
It has been said that the use of a barrier and spermicide by a well-motivated couple gives results at least as good against pregnancy as an inert intrauterine device, and without the problematical side-effects. The crucial factor is motivation, with perseverance in correct use, and it is often in this that the method breaks down. Many people find caps and condoms 'messy' and inconvenient by comparison with their expectations from more up-to-date methods, and will fail to use them on every occasion. This means that the general figures obtained from studying their use often give high rates of failure. Overall pregnancy rates for caps of around 4% per year can be expected.

Other methods

All other methods are relatively inefficient, with pregnancy rates probably in excess of 10 per 100 women-years in general use.

Coitus interruptus (withdrawal)

Here the male aims to withdraw his penis from the vagina just before ejaculation occurs. The method frequently fails because he may not possess the necessary degree of control, because some sperm may leak before the main ejaculation occurs, and because semen deposited on the vulva may still allow a pregnancy to occur.

The safe period (rhythm method or natural family planning)

Pregnancy is only likely to occur in the few days leading up to ovulation. The safe-period method relies on estimating when this is likely to be, and avoiding coitus during that time. The reliability of the method can be increased by recording the basal temperature or assessing cervical mucus, to give a closer estimate of ovulation timing. However, it has been reliably shown that sperm can survive for 8 days in preovulatory mucus and precise prediction of the ovulation date is, in practice, difficult.

Chemicals

A number of pessaries, sponges, creams, foams and other chemical preparations have been produced for use as sole contraceptive agents. The results are so poor that they cannot be recommended, except as adjuncts to the barrier methods.

STERILIZATION

The use of male and female sterilization for social rather than medical indications has only been widespread since the late 1960s, but it now forms a major part of the world's contraceptive efforts. It is estimated that in the USA 1 million sterilization operations are carried out annually, and 20% of all married couples have had one partner sterilized.

Female sterilization

This may be performed laparoscopically, or through a small suprapubic incision, or through an incision in the posterior vaginal fornix. Laparoscopically the tubes may be occluded by diathermy or by applying clips or plastic rings. Diathermy carries some risk of bowel damage and is now rarely used. The umbilical incision leaves no significant scar, and hospital stay is brief, most surgeons discharging the patient on the same day.

At open operation a wide variety of techniques for tubal ligation may be employed. With the Pomeroy method a knuckle of tube is tied and excised on each side, while the Oxford technique separates the cut ends of the tubes by the round ligament in order to minimize the possibility of recanalization. Hospital stay is longer and tubal ligation is now rarely performed except at the time of caesarean section.

Through the posterior fornix the tubes can be diathermized or a simple ligation technique used. The complication rate and hospital stay are comparable to that of laparoscopic sterilization.

Failure rate

About 3 or 4 per 1000 women can be expected to become pregnant after a Pomeroy tubal ligation. Failure rates for laparoscopic or culdoscopic (posterior fornix) sterilization are possibly slightly better (i.e. 1–2 per 1000), depending on the experience of the operator. The more sophisticated tubal ligation methods such as the Oxford technique have failure rates of 1 per 1000 or less.

Reversibility

Female sterilization may be reversed with 50% or better success, as long as minimal amounts of tube were destroyed by the original operation. Simple ligation without removal of a segment of tube or laparoscopic clip sterilization are the most reversible techniques. Success rates are considerably reduced if more than 3 years have elapsed since the sterilization and if the woman is over 40.

Side-effects

Apart from operation complications, side-effects are rare. There is no evidence for the common belief that female sterilization causes menstrual problems.

Male sterilization – vasectomy

This is a simple procedure that can be done under local anaesthesia. The vas is divided and tied off through small scrotal incisions. Sperm are still produced in the ejaculate for several months afterwards, and continued contraception with semen examination starting at 3 and 4 months after operation and continuing until the ejaculate is spermfree is essential.

Failure rate

As long as adequate follow-up procedures are employed, failures should be less than 1 per 1000, but about 5 per 1000 do not become sperm-negative after the initial operation – which makes follow-up checks vital.

Complications

Haematoma formation or local infection occurs in about 3% of cases.

Reversibility

Vasectomy can be successfully reversed in approximately 50% of cases. Removal of more than 2 cm vas or removal of the convoluted part of the vas limits success.

Counselling for sterilization

Both partners should be seen together. The choice of which partner to sterilize will usually be determined by the attitudes of the couple,

234 Undergraduate Obstetrics and Gynaecology

and it is rarely profitable to persuade them otherwise. A simple explanation of the procedure and any follow-up routine should be given. Some enquiry into their sexual stability should be made. Sterilization should have no effect on a normal sex life, but is no cure for sexual problems and may in fact aggravate them. The procedure should be presented as basically irreversible, and the possible circumstances that could lead them to regret their decision should be fully discussed.

ABORTION

The 1967 Abortion Act made abortion legal in the UK. Amendments were introduced in 1991 to limit termination to gestations of no more than 24 weeks except in the most serious circumstances. The conditions under which terminations may now be carried out are if:

1 The continuance of the pregnancy would involve risk to the life of the pregnant woman greater than if the pregnancy were terminated.
2 The termination is necessary to prevent grave permanent injury to the physical or mental health of the pregnant woman.
3 The pregnancy has *not* exceeded its 24th week and the continuance of the pregnancy would involve risk, greater than if the pregnancy were terminated, of injury to the physical or mental health of the pregnant woman.
4 The pregnancy has *not* exceeded its 24th week and the continuance of the pregnancy would involve risk, greater than if the pregnancy were terminated, of injury to the physical or mental health of any existing child(ren) of the family of the pregnant woman.
5 There is a substantial risk that if the child were born it would suffer from such physical or mental abnormalities as to be seriously handicapped.

Two doctors are required to certify that they have seen and examined the woman and that one of these clauses applies to her. Over 150 000 legal abortions are performed in this country annually.

METHODS OF TERMINATION
Early medical termination

Abortion may be produced with fair reliability up to 8 weeks with a combination of an antiprogesterone drug Mifepristone (taken orally) and a prostaglandin pessary. The process has to take place in hospital and a proportion will need surgical evacuation. There are cost advantages compared with surgical termination but some would feel that the discomfort of aborting while awake does not outweigh the advantage of avoiding an anaesthetic.

Aspiration termination

The cervix is dilated in proportion to the size of the uterus. The uterus is then evacuated with a suction curette. This technique is relatively safe and simple until 12 weeks. Up to 8 weeks aspiration termination can be done with a local anaesthetic, and this is the safest of all methods of termination. The mortality risk for aspiration termination is about 1 in 100 000 and this, it may be noted, is significantly less than the maternal mortality rate.

Late termination

After 12 weeks aspiration termination is more hazardous. Abortion may be induced with prostaglandins vaginally with pessaries, extra-amniotically (introduced through a cervical catheter) or intra-amniotically (introduced by amniocentesis). Intra-amniotic hypertonic saline and hysterotomy are more hazardous and now rarely used.

Complications

Serious complications are rare and termination before 12 weeks carries less risk than a term pregnancy, but the following may occur:

1 Incomplete abortion with subsequent sepsis or haemorrhage.
2 Sensitization of rhesus-negative women (give anti-D – see Chapter 6).
3 Cervical damage leading to subsequent middle-trimester abortion (mainly if the cervix is dilated more than 10 Hegar).
4 Uterine perforation.

FURTHER READING

Burkman, R.T. (1989) *Handbook of Contraception and Abortion.* Little, Brown, Boston.
Szarewski, A. and Guillebaud, J. (1992) Contraception. Current state of the art. *British Medical Journal* 302:1224–1226.

12

Fertility and infertility

Infertility presents a problem with many interesting but subtle facets which need clear understanding: the statistical facts, the emotional pain, profound ethical issues, and social priorities for national funding of services.

Most people have a deep and instinctive desire to have children. Infertility causes a form of grief like that of bereavement. Unlike bereavement, however, the infertile grieve for children that never were and the grief is usually never-ending. They often feel unfulfilled and worthless, and therefore suffer in secret while putting on a brave face or denying their problem as defence. The fertile majority rarely appreciate the pain and sadness.

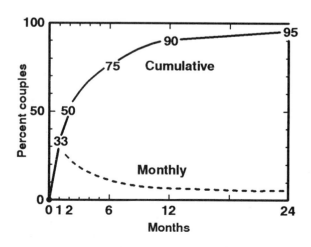

Fig. 12.1 Normal conception rates in couples of proven fertility.

NORMAL FERTILITY

Figure 12.1 illustrates conception rates in couples of proven fertility, during their first 2 years of trying; ultimately they all conceived, by definition. The peak rate is 33%, in the first month of trying, and it then falls quickly, settling to about 5% each month. That represents the lower limit of the normal range, which accounts for 95% of the fertile population. Ten per cent of normal couples take more than a year to conceive, and 5% more than 2 years.

The average normal monthly chance of a young fertile couple conceiving is 20–25%. That is therefore the best that can reasonably be expected of fertility treatments, though repeated treatments – if tolerable – should lead to a high cumulative chance of success.

It is essential to appreciate the chance nature of fertility, and of fertility treatment. As with trying to throw a 6 with dice, success can never be guaranteed. On the other hand, infertile couples usually still have some chance of conceiving naturally, though low, and the true success of any treatment must be evaluated against that chance of natural conception by prospective comparative study.

The woman's age is a major factor. Fertility declines slowly from age 30, more quickly after about 37, and sharply after 40, reaching almost zero by 45. Also the risks of miscarriage and genetic abnormality rise exponentially, all due mainly to declining oocyte quality. Ideally women should not delay their first attempts to conceive beyond 30, and fertility treatment if needed should not be delayed beyond 35.

DEFINITIONS: FERTILITY, INFERTILITY, SUBFERTILITY

There are several terms used often inconsistently or loosely. **Fertility** is a state of being fertile, which requires demonstration of having achieved pregnancy. **Infertility** is thus a state of not having achieved a pregnancy, though the individual may later become fertile. **Sterility** means permanently infertile.

What matters is the chance of conception each monthly ovulation cycle or within a defined time interval, called **fecundity** or **fecundability**. That is expressed as cycle-specific or time-specific fertility rates.

Thus any definition of infertility must be time-specific. For practical clinical purposes infertility is usually required to have lasted at least 1 or 2 years, as by then 90–95% of fertile couples would have conceived. In some cases, however, investigation and treatment are needed sooner given an obvious indication of a cause of infertility or when the woman is over 35 years old.

Infertility is seldom absolute, however, with a zero chance of conception. That occurs only if, for example, the woman's Fallopian tubes are both completely blocked or she has a premature menopause, or the man has complete lack of sperm (azoospermia). Infertility is mostly some degree of **subfertility**, which is therefore the preferred term, there being a chance of conceiving naturally, although it may be small.

In practice diagnosis is aimed not only at defining a possible cause but also at accurately assessing the degree of subfertility, to decide whether treatment is needed at all; and if so, the choice between different treatments depending on their relative effectiveness, complexity and cost.

Primary infertility or subfertility means that a pregnancy has never been achieved before. **Secondary** implies a previous pregnancy, though it may have ended in miscarriage or ectopic loss. The terms primary and secondary can apply separately to a couple and to the individuals. Two individuals who achieved a pregnancy with a previous partner and therefore have secondary infertility may as a couple have primary infertility.

CAUSES OF SUBFERTILITY

Any of the key requirements for conception can fail:

1 Ovulation.
2 Oocyte transport along the fallopian tube.
3 Timed coital delivery of sperm.
4 Cervical mucus secretion and receptivity.
5 Sperm motility to penetrate cervical mucus and reach the fallopian tubes.
6 Fertilization.
7 Uterine/endometrial receptivity for implantation.

Main causes and approximate frequencies

1 Sperm defects or dysfunction: 30%
   (including primary spermatogenic failure: 1–2%, seminal anti-sperm antibodies: 5%, varicocele: 1–2%).
2 Ovulation failure (amenorrhoea or oligomenorrhoea): 25%
   (including primary ovarian failure: 1–2%).
3 Tubal infective damage: 20%.
4 Unexplained infertility: 25%.

Other causes

1 Endometriosis (if causing damage): 5%.
2 Coital failure or infrequency: 5%.
3 Cervical mucus defects or dysfunction: 3%.
4 Uterine abnormalities (e.g. fibroids): rare (? true cause).
5 Genital tuberculosis: rare in developed countries.
6 General debilitating illnesses: rare.

The causes add up to more than 100% because some couples have more than one cause. In primary infertility endometriosis and sperm disorders are relatively more frequent (because they are usually present from the start), whereas in secondary infertility tubal infective damage is more frequent (because that is acquired, sometimes due to complications of childbirth, miscarriage or termination of pregnancy).

Other 'causes' are often cited which are **spurious**, i.e. apparent abnormalities which however controlled studies have shown do not reduce fertility, or corrective treatment improve it. These include:

Intermittent 'luteal deficiency'.
'Hyperprolactinaemia' in ovulating women.
Endometrial polyps.
Minor endometrial adhesions (common after normal pregnancy).
Endotubal (cornual) polyps.
Fibroids (at least in most cases).

INVESTIGATIONS OF SUBFERTILITY

Bearing in mind the main causes of subfertility, it is necessary to investigate all the key functional requirements for conception. A history and examination of both partners can give clear indications of a likely diagnosis needing early specialized investigation. Some couples will seek help from their family doctor at a very early stage and need only simple screening checks and basic advice initially.

Preliminary ethical and safety considerations

Even before investigating a couple, and certainly before offering treatment, consideration should be given to the welfare of any offspring. That takes priority over the needs of the immediate patients facing a doctor: an unusual and sometimes conflicting position in medical practice.

Obvious examples that would usually exclude couples from

treatment are a history of child abuse, hard drug abuse or HIV infection. Other considerations may include the possible importance of a stable and heterosexual partnership. There is a specific legal requirement in the UK (when offering licensed treatments like *in vitro* fertilization (IVF)) to consider the child's need for a father. And what about terminal illness or old age? A man may want his semen freeze-stored before cancer treatment. Women long past their menopause may want eggs from a young donor.

Couples with a medical or social history suggesting increased risk of infections which could pass to the fetus should be tested accordingly by serology for hepatitis, human immunodeficiency virus (HIV) and syphilis.

As in any woman planning pregnancy, routine steps should be taken to minimize dangers to the fetus by, for example, ensuring prior immunization against rubella and dietary supplementation with folate (see section on basic advice to couples, below, and Chapter 7.

History and examination

General illness is unlikely to be a cause of infertility in either partner but a basic medical history and haematological screening are appropriate.

Oligomenorrhoea or amenorrhoea is clear indication of ovulatory disorder or failure and needs specific endocrine investigations as discussed in Chapter 15: serum follicle-stimulating hormone (FSH), luteinizing hormone (LH), prolactin, thyroid-stimulating hormone and progestogen challenge test (to assess oestrogen state) and clomiphene stimulation test.

Tubal infective damage is suggested by a history of:

1 Sexually transmitted infection.
2 Abdominal inflammatory conditions and/or surgery such as appendicitis.
3 Complications of miscarriage or childbirth.
4 Complications of an intrauterine contraceptive device.
5 Deep dyspareunia.
6 Pelvic tenderness or tumour on examination.

Serum *Chlamydia* antibodies in high titre (see section on investigations, below), even without any suggestive history, also suggest tubal infective damage.

Male genital defects of significance seldom come to light in the history – mainly surgery for cryptorchidism, congenital hernia or testicular trauma or torsion – but important abnormalities to be found unexpectedly on examination include:

1 Undescended testes.
2 Small testes, indicating spermatogenic failure, usually primary. Failure secondary to gonadotrophin deficiency would present with impotence and other signs of diminished virilization.
3 Epididymal cysts, suggesting obstructions.
4 Varicocele, i.e. varicosities of the spermatic veins, usually the left (see below). Appears like a 'bag of worms', enhanced by the Valsalva manoeuvre.

Coital failure or inadequacy is defined by the history. The details are too important to be avoided due to embarrassment, but can be approached easily with sensitivity and personal confidence. Vaginal penetration and ejaculation must be questioned but the commonest issue is frequency and timing. Less than twice a week reduces the chance of conceiving substantially. Attention to accurate preovulatory timing is then valuable, though all couples, including those having more frequent intercourse, feel helped by being given practical advice about timing (see below).

Investigations

Semen microscopy

Sperm production is assessed by measuring the seminal volume (normally ≥ 2 ml), sperm concentration (≥ 20 million/ml) and the proportions with forward-progressive motility ($\geq 50\%$) and normal morphology ($\geq 50\%$). Thus the normal ejaculate usually contains at least 10 million normal motile spermatozoa (in total), though usually a lot more.

Unfortunately such simple sperm counts in semen are a poor predictor of a man's fertility, except in the case of azoospermia or severe oligospermia (overall concentration < 5 million/ml). There are men with normal seminal sperm counts with severe sperm dysfunction, and vice versa. Testing function is of overriding importance.

Azoospermia and severe oligospermia

Severe oligospermia may be due, like azoospermia, to spermatogenic failure or occlusion though incomplete. The differential diagnosis is:

1 Gonadotrophin deficiency (and secondary spermatogenic failure; rare): impotence, small testes, low testosterone, low/normal FSH.
2 Primary spermatogenic failure: virilized, small testes, raised FSH.
3 Occlusion: virilized, normal testes, normal FSH.

The final diagnosis may require surgical exploration within the scrotum of the epididymis and vas deferens (which may both be congenitally absent), including vasography using radio-opaque dye, and testicular biopsy for histology.

Sperm function

Seminal plasma acts only as a brief transport and buffering medium but is otherwise unfavourable to sperm, which begin to lose fertilizing ability within half an hour. Motility and long-term survival must be tested by and after migration into a physiologically favourable medium, either natural cervical mucus or an artificial medium. Other more complex tests are also available if indicated.

Seminal antisperm antibodies

These can be tested by various agglutination reactions, either non-specifically employing red blood cells (the mixed antiglobulin reaction or MAR test) or specifically for immunoglobulin A (IgA) and IgG. Such antibodies are only relevant if they can be demonstrated to block sperm penetration of cervical mucus, due to attachment to the mucoprotein mesh-like matrix.

Cervical mucus

The quality of mucus secretion needs to be checked during the preovulatory mucus 'surge', which usually lasts only about 2 days. It should be copious, clear and ductile, like the raw white of a hen's egg.

Receptivity to sperm is also checked at that time. Timing is critical. Sperm penetration from a semen sample can be tested *in vitro*. Alternatively, sperm penetration and survival can be tested *in vivo* by examining the mucus around 12 hours (6–24 hours) after intercourse for the presence of progressively motile sperm – the so-called postcoital test (PCT). The PCT has the added advantages of testing not only sperm survival in the mucus but coital competence, ejaculation and any adverse effect of the acidic vaginal environment. It is therefore directly relevant to the chance of conceiving naturally.

Negative PCTs, if properly timed, are in fact mostly due to defective sperm. Deficient mucus secretion occurring despite adequate oestrogenic stimulation in ovulatory cycles is uncommon and usually due to surgical damage to the cervix, such as cone biopsy for intraepithelial neoplasia.

Ovulation

Follicular growth and rupture can be observed by serial ultrasonography. Of greater importance, however, is the functional maturity of the follicle, which is best indicated by production of oestradiol and progesterone. The peak mid luteal serum progesterone concentration is the simplest reliable index of normal ovulation. Although, strictly, it is an index only of the functional capacity of the corpus luteum, that is directly determined by the degree of preovulatory follicular maturation (granulosa cell proliferation) and of course an adequate LH surge. Corpus luteum development follows preovulatory follicular maturation as night follows day.

Because variation between cycles is normal – about 20% are subnormal – it is necessary to check several cycles to be representative. In fact, persistent ovulatory failure is rare in women with normal menstrual cycles. It is usually reassuring, however, to measure the mid luteal progesterone level in two or three cycles.

Indirect indication of progesterone production is given by biological responses: secretory changes of the endometrium and a rise in body temperature. However, such responses are too sensitive to progesterone (occurring at quite low levels) and quantitative measurement of the hormone level is required if it is to be assessed at all. The basal (early morning) body temperature (BBT) chart can sometimes be useful, in oligomenorrhoeic women responding unpredictably to clomiphene treatment, to check retrospectively whether and when ovulation *might* have occurred. In general, however, keeping a BBT chart is an unhelpful nuisance.

The decline in oocyte quality which leads to progresssive reduction in implantation after 40 years of age, despite normal ovulatory cycles, is linked to critical reduction in ovarian follicle numbers and is thus reflected by rising serum FSH levels long before reaching the menopause. However, the decline may occur prematurely. Basal serum FSH measurement, i.e. early in the folllicular phase (menstrual phase), is therefore a generally useful prognostic index for potential fertility, and for urgency of any required treatment.

Tubal/pelvic state

The simplest method of checking tubal patency is by hysterosalpingography (HSG), injecting radio-opaque dye through the cervical canal as an outpatient procedure. HSG cannot, however, reveal pelvic adhesions surrounding the tubes and ovaries, or endometriosis.

Laparoscopy is therefore the definitive investigation, coloured dye being passed through the cervix to check tubal patency also. The degree of tubal damage, particularly affecting the fimbria, and the severity of adhesions – whether filmy or dense – are critical determinants of the chance of successful surgery.

Fertilization

Testing fertilization is beyond the scope of routine practice. It is only usually done as a step in chosen treatment with a view to transferring embryos to the uterus. In fact, fertilization failure is rarely a problem except due to otherwise evident sperm dysfunction.

Implantation

Nor can implantation be tested in practice. The main factor reducing implantation is the quality of the oocyte (despite normal ovulation and fertilization occurring), which diminishes greatly after the age of 40 years. The uterus and endometrium are not affected (as indicated by the success of oocytes from young donors), unless grossly distorted or damaged (see below).

Uterine state

HSG provides an outline of the uterine cavity (as well as the tubal lumen) and can show enlargement and distortion by encroaching fibroids, or ragged defects due to severe adhesions (Asherman syndrome). These are directly visualized, however, by hysteroscopy (via the cervical canal), which can conveniently be done along with laparoscopy. Transvaginal ultrasonography can also be used to assess the shape of the endometrial lining and its changing thickness through the ovarian cycle.

Nothing of practical value is known about how to assess endometrial receptivity for implantation, and it is not worth attempting. Fortunately, the endometrium appears to be a reliable slave to the hormone signals it receives. Endometrial biopsy is only required for histology and culture when tuberculosis is suspected.

Summary of history and basic investigations

Female history

1 General health.
2 Smoking.
3 Excess alcohol.
4 Menstrual cycle.
5 Menstrual loss.

6 Pain (menstrual, coital, other).
7 Sexually transmitted disease.
8 Surgery (abdominal, pelvic).
9 Pregnancy complications.

Coital history

1 Penetration.
2 Ejaculation.
3 Frequency.

Female examination

1 Pelvic tenderness.
2 Tumours.

Female investigations

1 Rubella serology.
2 *Chlamydia* serology.
3 Basal (i.e. menstrual-phase) serum FSH.
4 Optional: mid luteal serum progesterone ×2–3 cycles.

Male investigations

1 Semen microscopy (counts of sperm concentration, percentage motile, percentage normal forms (morphology)).
2 Semen antisperm antibody test or assay.

BASIC ADVICE TO COUPLES

Couples are helped and encouraged by clearly understanding their diagnosis and prognosis. Most are intelligent enough to understand the statistical graphs shown in this chapter, and their intelligent cooperation is essential to successful management. Many at an early stage will not need active treatment, only advice.

All feel helped by knowing how to optimize coital timing, to ensure that no ovulatory opportunity is missed. Self-recognition of the preovulatory cervical mucus surge is simple for most women, with a view to having intercourse daily during that (usually) short time. Some women like to use a self-test kit to check their urinary LH surge. That is usually sufficient in just one cycle to show that their recognition of the mucus surge does coincide with the LH surge.

A serious – contraceptive – mistake that some couples make through misunderstanding is to keep a BBT chart to 'save up' intercourse until the temperature has risen. That is too late. Progesterone causing the temperature rise has already opposed the action of oestrogen on the cervical mucus and effectively 'closed the door' to the sperm. Second, abstinence for more than 7–10 days leads to sperm senescence. Ejaculation every couple of days seems best. More frequent intercourse is, however, no disadvantage. Though sperm numbers in frequent ejaculates are reduced, the sum total delivered is at least the same and may be more favourable.

Incidental fertility factors

Smoking tobacco damages reproduction in several ways. Not only does it increase the risks in pregnancy of miscarriage and fetal growth retardation (Chapter 7), it reduces fecundity – the monthly chance of conception – by one-third. Although in general most smokers catch up eventually with non-smokers, those who are already subfertile and perhaps needing treatment are putting themselves at a substantial disadvantage by smoking. Furthermore, even if they conceive, their chance of a successful outcome is considerably reduced, which seems particularly tragic.

Smoking products reach both seminal plasma and follicular fluid. Smoking seems to reduce the fertilizing ability of sperm although that has not been well defined. However, it clearly reduces the fertilizing ability of the oocyte, and this is probably achieved by passive as well as active smoking. Even light smokers are affected. Both partners should be advised to stop smoking.

High alcohol intake (particularly in men, and they are more commonly the heavy drinking partner) and high caffeine (tea and cola drinks as well as coffee) appear to be associated with reduced fertility although the effects are not so clearly defined as for smoking. Couples should be advised to moderate their intake of alcohol and caffeine or switch to decaffeinated products.

Incidental preparation for pregnancy

In trying to help an infertile couple to conceive it should be remembered to give them the usual advice about healthy preparation for pregnancy (Chapter 7). This includes a balanced diet supplemented with folic acid, as well as to stop smoking and to moderate alcohol intake. Certain disorders such as diabetes mellitus may need optimization of control even before conception. The tragic risk of rubella infection in pregnancy should be prevented by preliminary immunization if susceptible, and immunity should be checked.

TREATMENTS AND OUTCOME

Choice of treatment

In couples with subfertility – as opposed to absolute infertility – the choice of treatment depends on a balance of factors:

1 Knowing the chance of pregnancy:
   a. Without treatment.
   b. With simple but only modestly effective treatment.
   c. With more complex but more successful treatment.
2 Duration of infertility
3 The woman's age

The outcomes of standard treatments aiming at natural conception in the three main causes of subfertility – sperm disorders, ovulation failure and tubal infective damage - are shown in Figure 12.2. The results of assisted conception treatments are shown later.

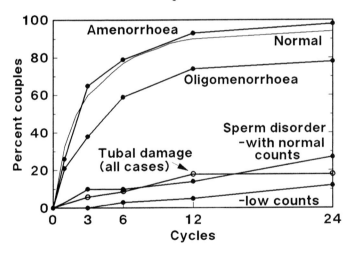

Fig. 12.2 Overall cumulative conception rates resulting from treatment of the main causes of subfertility, compared with normal, excluding the use of donor insemination, *in vitro* fertilization or surgery for reversal of sterilization. Data drawn with permission from Hull *et al.* (1985) *British Medical Journal* **291**:1693.

Sperm disorders

The results shown in Figure 12.2 demonstrate a poor prognosis. The chance of conceiving each month is about 1% or less. There is no treatment of proven benefit for natural conception, though many are tried, including hormone stimulation with clomiphene, vitamin E and artificial insemination. None works because the sperm have diminished fertilizing ability as well as usually reduced numbers. Standard IVF treatment concentrating about 100 000 sperm with each of numerous oocytes offers only a moderate chance of conception (about 10–15% per cycle of treatment), but not in severe cases. It is usually possible, however, even in severe cases to achieve fertilization and a good chance of conception (20% or greater) by injecting a single spermatozoon directly into each oocyte (intracytoplasmic sperm injection, or ICSI). That is of course more difficult and expensive than standard IVF treatment, but even just a few live spermatozoa collected surgically from behind an epididymal block or from biopsied testicular tissue are sufficient. The resulting children appear healthy but there is a possibility of specific genetic defects affecting the fertility of the males, which will not become apparent for many years.

Seminal antisperm antibodies

Antibody levels can be partly suppressed using high-dose glucocorticoid therapy, but the chance of pregnancy is only slightly improved and there are potentially severe risks of the treatment, which is therefore a difficult choice. Fertilizing ability is reduced by standard IVF methods due to the attached antibodies, but ICSI is effective.

Varicocele

Varicosity of the spermatic vein within the scrotum (varicocele) damages sperm development and consequent function by overheating the testes. About 10% of normal men have at least a small varicocele and the true relation to sperm disorder remains unclear. Surgical occlusion of the spermatic vein remains of unproven benefit for fertility, but is commonly done if there is severe sperm dysfunction and the prognosis for fertility is poor to try to avoid turning to the complexity and cost of IVF or ICSI.

Azoospermia or severe oligospermia

Spermatogenic failure secondary to gonadotrophin deficiency is rare and usually presents with impotence because of associated testosterone deficiency, but infertility can be successfully treated by gonadotrophin therapy, which requires several months to be effective.

Occlusive conditions are usually difficult to correct surgically. Tapping of sperm from behind the blockage, even in the epididymis, can be done for IVF treatment by ICSI as described above. However, occlusion due to congenital bilateral absence of the vas deferens can be associated with the genetic risk of cystic fibrosis, which must be considered.

Primary spermatogenic failure cannot be successfully treated. However, if the condition is not quite complete there may be a few spermatozoa recoverable from biopsied testicular tissue sufficient for ICSI treatment.

Donor insemination

Because sperm disorders are associated with severe subfertility and therapeutic options are complex and costly, anonymous donor insemination is often chosen as offering the most realistic hope of achieving a pregnancy. Such treatment however involves profound ethical and emotional issues, and requires special counselling of both the recipient couple and donors. It is also subject to specific legal regulation.

Semen collected from usually anonymous normal donors is carefully checked for health and infection risks and freeze-stored to enable quarantine for later HIV serology on the donor. Physical characteristics of a donor are matched to those of the infertile husband. The semen is simply injected into the cervical canal, just before the time of ovulation. The chance of conception is not normal, however – about 5–10% each cycle – because of the damaging effect of cryopreservation on many of the sperm, but the chance of success builds up with repeated treatment and it is simple.

Ovulation failure

The results shown in Figure 12.2 demonstrate that with accurate diagnosis and appropriate selection of treatment women with ovulation failure can expect a virtually normal chance of conceiving. Only primary ovarian failure cannot be treated to induce ovulation, and in such cases the only hope of pregnancy is by IVF using donated oocytes.

Paradoxical though it may seem, the results in women with oligomenorrhoea are not quite so good as in those with complete amenorrhoea. That is due to the greater subtleties of disorder associated with polycystic ovaries (PCO). PCO account for 90% of cases of oligomenorrhoea and about a third of amenorrhoea, often without obesity and hirsutism, the other features of the classical PCO syndrome (see Chapter 15).

A few patients can be treated by specific methods to correct the underlying cause (see below) but most will depend on hormonal stimulation of ovulation.

Specific treatments

These include:

1 Dietary and psychological measures to overcome weight loss-related amenorrhoea.
2 Thyroxine replacement to overcome primary hypothyroidism.
3 Glucocorticoid therapy to suppress adrenal hypersecretion of androgen (adult congenital adrenal hyperplasia).
4 Ablation of a pituitary or suprasellar tumour by surgery or irradition. Most tumours are however prolactinomas and their size and activity can be suppressed using bromocriptine.

Bromocriptine is a synthetic ergot alkaloid which acts as a dopamine agonist to suppress pituitary prolactin secretion. In hyperprolactinaemic amenorrhoea reduction of prolactin levels to normal removes the inhibition of hypothalamic gonadotrophin-releasing hormone (GnRH) secretion and leads to normal ovulatory cycles. Bromocriptine is taken orally every day until conception, when it is no longer needed except to keep a large tumour under control. Initial intolerance (nausea and dizziness) can usually be avoided by starting with a low dose, taken with the evening meal. New longer-acting alternatives include cabergoline and quinagolide.

Hormonal stimulants of ovulation

Bromocriptine and related agents do not stimulate ovulation but merely remove the inhibitory influence of hyperprolactinaemia. In most other cases, however, empirical therapy is needed to stimulate ovulation, often resulting in mulitple ovulation.

Clomiphene is an oral synthetic non-steroidal weak oestrogen. In oestrogenized women with active hypothalamus, pituitary and ovaries – typically with PCO – clomiphene acts by competition as an antioestrogen, to reduce negative feedback on the pituitary and consequently enhance FSH (and LH) secretion. Clomiphene is taken for only 5 days at the start of induced or natural menstruation, to stimulate follicular recruitment. Subsequent follicular maturation, the LH surge and ovulation evolve due to independent activation of the normal feedback-control mechanisms. Clomiphene is thus generally a mild and safe stimulant which is easily administered and should therefore always be tried first to induce ovulation. Its effect is not improved by increasing the dose above the standard 50–100 mg daily, but can adversely affect cervical mucus receptivity due to its antioestrogenic action.

GnRH is a synthetic decapeptide like the natural form, used to stimulate pituitary gonadotrophin secretion in women with hypo-thalamic failure or disorder. It is given in pulsatile manner to mimic the physiological pattern, though at fixed intervals of 90 minutes, subcutaneously via an indwelling needle and tubing from a portable battery-driven syringe pump. A normal pituitary–ovarian cycle usually with uniovulation evolves in 2–3 weeks. Though such treatment is very effective in women with chronic anorexia nervosa, the risks of pregnancy in underweight women would be better avoided by specific dietary and psychological measures to restore natural fertility if possible.

Gonadotrophins are needed to stimulate the ovarian follicles directly in women with pituitary failure due to ablation, but much more often empirically because of failure to respond to appropriate therapy with clomiphene, bromocriptine or pulsed GnRH. Increased FSH is the key requirement to stimulate follicular maturation but LH may need to be added in women with profound deficiency. Treatment is administered by daily injection, and the ovarian response must be monitored closely by serial – eventually daily – ultrasonography and oestradiol measurements to prevent hyperstimulation and the risk of high-order multiple pregnancy. Ovulation is finally induced with an injection of human chorionic gonadotrophin (hCG) to mimic the LH surge. Even with careful control, however, about 25% of pregnancies are twin and higher-order pregnancies cannot be entirely avoided. If uncontrolled, numerous large luteinized cysts which are highly permeable can develop in the ovaries in response to the hCG, leading to massive ascites, haemoconcentration and hypercoagulability, which are life-threatening. If too many follicles develop, ovulation and the hyperstimulation syndrome can be prevented by withholding the hCG.

Tubal/pelvic infective damage

The results shown in Figure 12.2 demonstrate a generally poor prognosis, even after surgery. However, the type and degree of damage vary widely and surgery needs to be offered selectively. Only a minority of cases are favourable for surgical correction. They are those due either to flimsy avascular adhesions (which can be easily divided without reforming) or limited occlusion close to the uterine horn (allowing that section of the tube to be excised and accurate reanastomosis performed), offering a 50% chance of conception within 2–3 years. The essential favourable feature required is that the fimbria and tubal mucosa are otherwise healthy. That is why reversal of simple clip sterilization is particularly successful. The common simple procedure of distal salpingostomy – to open up a baggy hydrosalpinx – is particularly unsuccessful because of the irreversible functional damage to the tubal mucosa caused by previous salpingitis. That also leads to increased risk of ectopic pregnancy. In most cases IVF offers a better chance of success in just one cycle of treatment, and it can be repeated.

Endometriosis

Figure 12.3 shows that endometriosis causes severe subfertility when there are damaging adhesions or blood-filled chocolate cysts. Surgical correction of the structural problems is the definitive treatment, though preoperative hormonal suppression of the endometriotic activity may be surgically helpful. The chance of conception depends on surgical feasibility but at best amounts to about 50% after 2–3 years. IVF, and gamete intrafallopian transfer (GIFT) if there is a healthy accessible tube, are favourable alternatives.

Even when the disease is only superficial, however, there is fairly marked subfertility (Fig. 12.3), although the endometriosis does not appear to be the underlying cause. Subtle disorders of follicular and oocyte function are present, and probably others. Hormonal suppression of the endometriotic activity – like the endometrium,

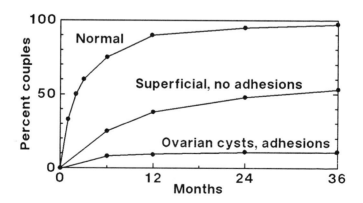

Fig. 12.3   Cumulative conception rates without treatment in women with endometriosis related to the severity of disease. Data drawn with permission from Hull (1992) *Human Reproduction* **7**, 785.

leading to amenorrhoea – does not improve the subsequent chance of conception and only delays the opportunity during the course of treatment. If natural conception has not occurred after 2–3 years, IVF or GIFT offers a favourable choice.

Unexplained infertility

Infertility is classified as unexplained when all the main critical factors appear favourable: ovulatory cycles, normal pelvic organs, normal semen, normal sperm–cervical mucus interaction and normal coital frequency. Not all those investigations are done in some centres and the diagnosis given of unexplained infertility can be unsatisfactory.

Accurate diagnosis of unexplained infertility is important because many such couples are really normal and have a good chance of conceiving naturally, having simply been unlucky so far. That applies to most couples with unexplained infertility of less than 3 years' duration, as shown in Figure 12.4. They need only advice and encouragement.

After more than 3 years' duration, however, the chance of natural conception falls and offers unrealistic hope. That seems to be due to the compounded effect of both partners functioning at the lower

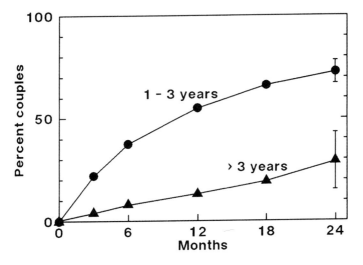

Fig. 12.4 Cumulative conception rates without treatment in unexplained infertility related to duration of infertility when investigated. Data drawn with permission from Hull *et al.* (1985) *British Medical Journal* **291**:1693.

limit of the normal range for fertility. There is no effective treatment to boost the chance of natural conception. However, if sperm function has been properly defined as normal, IVF and GIFT offer favourable options, with a chance of success each cycle that is as good as normal (see below). A less effective option is a combination of superovulation with intrauterine insemination (see below). Clomiphene is often used empirically to try to boost ovulation but is of only marginal benefit to the chance of conception.

Assisted conception methods of treatment

These are considered together because they are the common solution to a variety of infertility problems, though with varying degrees of success depending on the underlying disorder and age of the woman. The term assisted conception refers to methods involving:

1 Stimulation of multiple ovulation.
2 Delivery of specially prepared motile sperm to the oocytes.

There are three main distinct types – IVF, GIFT and intrauterine insemination (IUI):

1 *IVF*: Oocytes are collected and mixed with the sperm to fertilize *in vitro* (literally in glass), and the resulting embryos – maximum of three – are transferred to the uterus after 2–3 days. It is the only appropriate method when there is tubal damage. ICSI is a form of assisted fertilization *in vitro* by injecting a single spermatozoon directly into each oocyte, essential in severe cases of sperm dysfunction or depletion of sperm numbers.
2 *GIFT*: The collected oocytes – maximum of three – and sperm are placed immediately into the Fallopian tubes to fertilize there. GIFT is appropriate if the tubes are healthy as in endometriosis or unexplained infertility, and if sperm function is favourable. If there is sperm dysfunction and few of the oocytes would fertilize, IVF is better, or preferably ICSI, to enable transfer of the oocytes which actually fertilized.
3 *IUI*: Sperm prepared as for IVF or GIFT are injected high into the uterus to help them reach the tubes, which must be healthy. IUI is less precise and less effective than IVF or GIFT, without taking too great a risk of high-order multiple pregnancy by over-stimulation of the ovaries, as the oocytes are not collected but released in the natural way. Superovulation/IUI may seem to offer a reasonable initial compromise compared with GIFT.

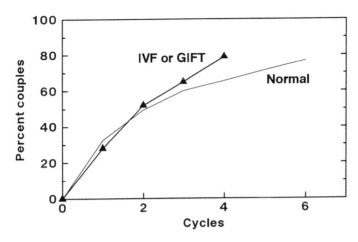

Fig. 12.5 Cumulative conception rates by *in vitro* fertilization (IVF) or gamete intrafallopian transfer (GIFT) treatment for tubal damage (only IVF in those cases), endometriosis or prolonged unexplained infertility (limited to women under 40 years and men with normal sperm). Data drawn with permission from Hull *et al.* (1994) *Fertility and Sterility* **62**:997.

Results of IVF and GIFT treatment are illustrated in Figure 12.5. Such treatments, along with ovulation induction for the ovulatory failures (Fig. 12.2), are the only methods that can offer a normal chance of conception (provided, of course, the woman is under 40 years and the man has normal sperm). However, IVF and GIFT are so complex and costly that couples usually manage only two or three cycles. IUI with multiple ovulation is about half as successful, but simpler and half the cost and can often be managed for more cycles.

OUTCOME OF PREGNANCY AFTER TREATMENT OF INFERTILITY

Prolonged delay to conception is associated with increased risk of early miscarriage (about 20%). That suggests subtle impairment of reproductive ability in several respects, probably principally of gamete quality. After ovulation induction when required because of gonadotrophin deficiency states, which lead simply to inactivity of otherwise normal ovaries, miscarriage rates are low (about 10%), but high (40%) in association with PCO and raised LH and androgen levels. The risk of miscarriage associated with PCO can be minimized by prior pituitary desensitization (using a superactive GnRH analogue) to suppress LH and consequently androgen levels.

PCO also involves increased risk of gestational diabetes and hypertension due to the effects of associated hyperinsulinaemia on lipid and fatty acid metabolism (see Chapter 15).

The woman's age is a major factor, particularly after about 37 years. Not only does the chance of conception fall but the risks of miscarriage and genetic abnormality rise exponentially (miscarriage 30% at 40 years, 50% and more after 42 years), all due to defective oocyte quality.

The main risk directly referable to treatment is multiple pregnancy, particularly triplet and greater, associated with gonadotrophin usage, either to induce ovulation in cases of ovulation failure or purposefully to stimulate multiple ovulation for assisted conception methods. The most important risks to the offspring are fetal growth retardation and prematurity which can lead to permanent cerebral damage. Minimizing the chance of multiple pregnancy is an important aim in specialist fertility practice, but the price for that is a reduced chance of any pregnancy, which presents a dilemma.

FURTHER READING

Insler, V. and Lunenfeld, B. (eds) (1993) *Infertility: Male and Female*, 2nd edn. Churchill Livingstone, Edinburgh.

Speroff, L., Glass, RH and Kase, N.G. (eds) (1994) *Clinical Gynecologic Endocrinology and Infertility*, 5th edn. Williams & Wilkins, Baltimore.

Templeton, A.A. and Drife, J.O. (eds) (1992) *Infertility*. Springer-Verlag, London.

13

Miscarriage, ectopic pregnancy and hydatidiform mole

Miscarriage is a common event. One in seven of known pregnancies miscarries in the first 3 months, and probably twice as many miscarry before the woman knows she is pregnant, when development of the embryo stops and the woman has a 'silent abortion' indistinguishable from a period. Around 1% will miscarry in mid-trimester and a similar proportion have ectopic pregnancies. Hydatidiform moles are rare (about 1 in 2000 pregnancies in the UK) but have the added importance of possibly leading on to chorio-carcinoma. Miscarriage in any form can cause major distress to the patient, and sometimes real risk to her life. The management of miscarriage forms an important part of both general practice and gynaecology. Most forms of miscarriage have traditionally been referred to as spontaneous abortion, but this term has strong emotional overtones for most women and is better avoided.

FIRST-TRIMESTER MISCARRIAGE (ABORTION)

About one in seven of all pregnancies abort at this stage of pregnancy and the vast majority of those that do so are abnormal. In most cases there is no recurrent aetiological factor and the outlook for the subsequent pregnancy is not appreciably worse than average after one, two or even three spontaneous miscarriages. Very occasionally there is a recurrent factor, and it is usual to investigate women who have had three spontaneous miscarriages.

Threatened miscarriage (abortion)

A threatened miscarriage is diagnosed when there is any bleeding from the genital tract before the 24th week of pregnancy and as long as no products of conception have been passed and the cervix remains undilated. Three out of four threatened miscarriages settle down, and when this happens there is no increased risk of fetal abnormality. The remainder abort and the abortion rate is not materially affected by any treatment. It is traditional to confine patients with threatened miscarriage to bed until a few days after the bleeding has stopped, and to rest and to avoid intercourse for at least 2 weeks. There is no evidence that any of these measures has any effect other than a psychological one. There is also no evidence that hormones are of any help in the treatment of threatened miscarriage (or recurrent abortion) and as there are a number of known adverse effects of steroid hormones given in early pregnancy, they should not be used even for their psychotherapeutic effects. Human placental lactogen and progesterone estimations may give some indication of prognosis, but misleading results are common, and skilled ultrasound examination of the uterus provides a much better prognostic indicator. Once a fetal heart has been visualized (which is usually possible at 7 weeks) only 2% of women will miscarry.

Inevitable miscarriage

A miscarriage becomes inevitable when the cervic dilates significantly or products of conception are passed. Most inevitable miscarriages are accompanied by a considerable amount of vaginal bleeding and low abdominal pain. Before 14 weeks it is usual for the placenta to be expelled incompletely and the risk of continued bleeding or uterine infection means that such cases are best admitted to hospital for evacuation of the uterus. The bleeding in incomplete miscarriages can occasionally be severe and necessitate a resuscitation of the patient before admission to hospital. Blood loss is usually controlled at least in part by ergometrine 0.5 mg intramuscularly or intravenously. When the patient is seen a day or two after a miscarriage, signs that suggest it is incomplete are continued vaginal blood loss, a patulous cervix and a slightly bulky and tender uterus.

Complete miscarriage

Following complete miscarriage there should be no appreciable vaginal blood loss, only a slight reddish discharge. The uterus is not tender and fairly rapidly returns to normal size. The cervix should be closed. Complete miscarriage needs no further treatment, but if there is any doubt at all it is better to perform an evacuation.

Missed abortion

This is the term used when the fetus has died or failed to develop but miscarriage has not occurred. The placenta will continue to produce hormones and maintain the pregnancy, sometimes for several weeks after death of the fetus. Pregnancy symptoms persist, pregnancy tests may remain positive and the uterus may grow, although usually at a reduced rate. The diagnosis is readily made by ultrasound.

Septic miscarriage

An incomplete miscarriage may occasionally become infected with organisms from the vagina or bowel and this is particularly likely if abortion has been procured illegally. The infection may spread from the uterine cavity to the parametrium and to the tubes and thence to the pelvic peritoneum. Death from generalized peritonitis, septicaemia or renal failure may result. Cases of septic abortion must be admitted urgently to hospital and treated with high-dose antibiotics, blood transfusion and general supportive measures and early evacuation of the septic products. There is a danger of long-term tubal blockage and sterility.

Recurrent miscarriage

Recurrent miscarriage may be caused by the following:

1 Chromosome abnormalities in either parent (such as translocations).
2 Uterine abnormalities.
3 Serious chronic illness, such as renal disease, systemic lupus erythematosus or syphilis.
4 Incompetent cervix (although this usually produces middle-trimester miscarriage).
5 Mistaken diagnosis, where the woman wants to be pregnant and is having delayed periods
6 Polycystic ovarian disease.

In practice these factors only account for a few per cent of recurrent miscarriage when the woman has had three previous miscarriages. Nevertheless, in such cases it is usual to perform chromosomal investigations of the couple with renal function tests, blood sugar and lupus anticoagulant checks for the woman, and to have a hysterosalpingogram to exclude congenital uterine abnormalities and intrauterine fibroids. When recurrent causes have been excluded, the mainstay of treatment for recurrent first-trimester miscarriage is tender loving care. However, such patients are often advised prolonged rest, although it is doubtful whether this is necessary or effective.

Recently some evidence has accumulated to suggest that recurrent miscarriage may be related to failure of the mother to recognize that the conceptus is immunologically different. Some success has been claimed for infusing the husband's lymphocytes into the wife before attempting further pregnancy, but convincing evidence of efficacy is lacking.

SECOND-TRIMESTER MISCARRIAGE

The causes of middle-trimester miscarriage are as follows:

1 Uterine abnormalities.
2 Cervical incompetence.
3 Fetal abnormality.
4 Intrauterine death of the fetus.
5 High multiple pregnancy.
6 Maternal ill health, particularly undiagnosed diabetes.
7 Genital tract infection with TORCH (Toxoplasma, Rubella, Cytomegalovirus and Herpes) viruses or *Listeria*.

There is a strong tendency for middle-trimester miscarriage to be recurrent and all cases should be investigated after the first loss. If at all possible the fetus and placenta should be examined by a pathologist at the time of miscarriage, and if these are normal a hysterosalpingogram is advisable. Abnormalities such as a bicornuate uterus may sometimes be corrected surgically with subsequent pregnancies going to term. An incompetent cervix is treated by the insertion of a cervical suture (see Chapter 7).

HYDATIDIFORM MOLE

Hydatidiform mole is a tumour of placental tissue, consisting of vesicles formed by distended chorionic villi, with the appearances of small seedless grapes. Most moles are benign, but some are invasive and some give rise to the highly malignant choriocarcinoma. The term trophoblastic disease is used to cover this spectrum of abnormality. The management of trophoblastic disease is dealt with fully in Chapter 24 with other genital neoplasia, but the clinical features of hydatidiform mole are discussed here because it forms an important part of the differential diagnosis of miscarriage.
    Presenting features of hydatidiform mole include:

1 Recurrent vaginal bleeding.
2 Hyperemesis.

3 Large-for-dates uterus (but sometimes small).
4 Early-onset pre-eclampsia.
5 Passage of vesicles vaginally.
6 Presence of vesicles in evacuated products.

The diagnosis of hydatidiform mole is very easily made (before abortion) by ultrasound scan. The vesicles produce strong echoes, giving a snowstorm appearance to the scan. The diagnosis can also be made by finding excessively high levels of human chorionic gonadrotrophin (hCG) in blood or urine, but scans are usually more readily available. If any vesicles are seen in products aborted or evacuated it is essential that they are sent for histological examination, so that appropriate follow-up may be instituted for those with trophoblastic disease. Sometimes innocent vesicular degeneration of the placenta will mimic the appearances of a partial mole. Appropriate follow-up of all hydatidiform moles allows the virtual elimination of mortality for the previously invariably fatal condition of choriocarcinoma.

ECTOPIC PREGNANCY

In about 1 in 100 pregnancies (in this country) an embryo may develop in a site other than the uterus, most commonly in the fallopian tube but occasionally in the ovary or the pelvic peritoneum. The incidence has increased in this country and varies around the world, principally in relation to the occurrence of pelvic inflammatory disease, although there is also an increased risk of ectopic pregnancy after tubal surgery, and with the use of intrauterine contraceptive devices or progestogen-only pills.

Clinical features of tubal ectopic pregnancies

The clinical picture depends on whether the embryo has implanted in the narrow part of the fallopian tube (the isthmus) or in the wider outer portion (the ampulla). The lumen of the isthmus is 1 mm or less and the developing conceptus rapidly erodes its way through the tubal wall, presenting the features of a ruptured ectopic pregnancy:

1 Onset of symptoms around the time of the first missed period.
2 Severe pain in the pelvis and lower abdomen, and sometimes shoulder tips (diaphragmatic irritation).
3 Collapse – due to intraperitoneal haemorrhage, sometimes progressing rapidly to the death of the patient.

4 Slight, dark red vaginal loss.
5 Marked tenderness on vaginal examination, particularly on moving the cervix. Vaginal examination may provoke further bleeding and should probably be delayed until the patient is in hospital if the other features suggest the possibility of a ruptured ectopic.

If implantation occurs in the ampulla there is more room for the pregnancy to expand, and the features are usually those of a leaking ectopic pregnancy:

1 Onset of symptoms usually 6 weeks or more from the last menstrual period.
2 Moderate pain in the pelvic region, usually unilateral, often intermittent.
3 Collapse and serious intraperitoneal blood loss is uncommon.
4 Moderate tenderness and palpable adnexal mass may be present.
5 Diagnosis may be difficult and is often only made after considerable delay.

Management

With a ruptured ectopic, the diagnosis of intraperitoneal haemorrhage is usually readily made. The patient should be admitted to hospital, using the obstetric flying squad or emergency ambulance service in most cases, and laparotomy should be performed without delay. It is then a simple matter to remove the bleeding tube. Attempts at resuscitation should not be allowed to delay laparotomy as the patient is likely to bleed more rapidly than blood can be replaced.

With a leaking ectopic the diagnosis is more difficult and treatment not so urgent. β-hCG tests will be positive. Ultrasound scan will fail to demonstrate an intrauterine pregnancy (normally visible from 5 weeks onwards). Scanning with a vaginal probe may show an intrauterine or a tubal pregnancy somewhat earlier, and either form of scan may show a collection of blood or blood clot in the pelvis. Quite often one is left with a patient with pelvic pain, a positive β-hCG and no intrauterine pregnancy visible on scan. In this situation, and in any other case of doubt, a laparoscopy should be performed. Failure to visualize a tubal pregnancy by scan certainly does not exclude an ectopic.

The standard treatment for a tubal ectopic pregnancy is to remove that tube. It is possible to treat the ectopic by injecting methotrexate into it or by removing the pregnancy while leaving part, or all, of the tube. The chance of repeated ectopic pregnancy in the same tube is considerable. If the tube is removed, subsequent pregnancies involve at least a 10% risk of ectopic pregnancy in the other tube. Ectopic pregnancies in sites other than the tube are so rare that they are of concern only in specialist practice. Very rarely an ectopic pregnancy implanted in the abdomen may progress and survive to term.

PSYCHOLOGICAL ASPECTS OF EARLY PREGNANCY LOSS

It is important to realize that a miscarriage even very early in pregnancy can have a devastating emotional impact on a woman, her partner and her family. The sense of loss, of personal failure and of the unfairness of it can be as strong as with losing a member of the family, and the problems are accentuated if the pregnancy has occurred after prolonged infertility. In a gynaecological ward where many incomplete miscarriages may be admitted in a single day, it may be all too easy to treat the matter as a minor problem of no great consequence, and so to add considerably to the woman's misery. A sympathetic and sensitive approach by the medical and nursing staff is essential. The woman will go through a bereavement process which may last many weeks or months and she should not be hurried through this. She should be given the opportunity to talk about possible causes and the outlook for the future, and she may well find it helpful to be put in touch with a local miscarriage support group.

14

Gynaecological problems of childhood and puberty

CHILDHOOD

Genital problems are uncommon in childhood. Abnormal sexual differentiation is rare but profoundly important and easily overlooked. Tumours are extremely rare (see Chapter 24). Most genital disorders presenting in children seem trivial, but there is growing awareness that some cases are due to sexual abuse.

In the newborn girl vaginal bleeding or breast engorgement and secretion ('witch's milk') may occur due to the previous stimulation by placental hormones now withdrawn, but it is transient.

Vaginal discharge in young girls is usually bacterial, unlike the usual protozoal and yeast infections in young adults (see Chapter 18), and sometimes due to the presence of a small foreign body in the vagina, often long forgotten. Speculum examination may, therefore, be necessary and can only be successfully done under general anaesthesia. Often the cause is bad hygiene, not only due to neglect but also sometimes misplaced fastidiousness, which is easily corrected.

Vaginal bleeding may be due to trauma, perhaps self-inflicted by a sharp object out of curiosity. Since the vaginal vault might have been penetrated it is important to examine the abdomen in case of peritoneal bleeding or peritonitis. Rarely, bleeding in young girls may be due to urethral prolapse or sarcoma botryoides of the cervix.

Abnormal sexual differentiation (intersex)

In practice this is defined as indeterminate external (phenotypic) gender. Gender can be defined in chromosomal, gonadal, phenotypic or psychological terms, but in children it is abnormality of the external genitalia that presents itself. The abnormality may not be recognized and so the gender may be interpreted wrongly with respect to the chromosomal and gonadal gender, i.e. pseudohermaphroditism. The mistake will only become apparent at puberty, with potentially disastrous consequences for the individual because of the need for plastic operations and, worse, the psychological upheaval necessary to change the accustomed gender. If these tragedies are to be avoided it is extremely important to examine the external genitalia at birth routinely with care (see below), and deal with any abnormality early.

Every degree of abnormality is possible, but for illustration only the most typical, i.e. extreme, examples will be described.

Female pseudohermaphroditism

Female pseudohermaphroditism means female chromosomal and gonadal gender associated with apparently male external genitalia. The commonest cause is congenital adrenal hyperplasia in which there is excessive androgen production by the female fetus's adrenal cortex due to any of a variety of enzymic defects which block the synthetic pathway for cortisol. The precursors and androgen side-products are secreted in excess because the cortisol deficiency, by lack of negative feedback on the pituitary, leads to excessive secretion of adrenocorticotrophic hormone (ACTH). The fetus may be partly protected, however, by maternal cortisol which crosses the placenta, and masculinization may only occur later. At birth there is likely to be clitoral enlargement and labial fusion, resembling a boy with hypospadias and undescended testes (see Chapter 3, Fig. 3.9b,c). In some cases the baby's life is endangered by a salt-losing syndrome due to associated aldosterone deficiency. Virilization of a female fetus can also be caused by administration of androgens, including some progestogens, to the mother during pregnancy.

Male pseudohermaphroditism

Male pseudohermaphroditism means male chromosomal and gonadal gender but with apparently female external genitalia. The testes are undescended, often intra-abdominal, and the vulva may be typically female, but the vagina is absent or short, and the uterus is missing. The abnormality may be recognized at birth only by separating the labia and looking for the (absent) shadowy depth of the normal vaginal canal. Congenital inguinal hernias are often also present.

The condition may occur due to deficiency of fetal testosterone at the critical stage of development of the external genitalia (see Chapter 3), but it can also be caused by antiandrogen treatment of the mother for hirsutism. Internal genital development occurs appropriately in response to anti-Müllerian hormone secreted by the testes. If the external and internal genital anomaly is overlooked at birth the problem will present at puberty with irreversible clitoral enlargement and deepening voice due to testosterone, and severe emotional distress.

By contrast, **testicular feminization** is due to insensitivity to androgens (on the part of all normally responsive target tissues), whether the androgens are of testicular or adrenal origin, so masculinization does not occur, nor does axillary and pubic hair grow (see the section on puberty, below). The testes secrete normal amounts of hormones. In the fetus, anti-Müllerian hormone prevents development of the uterus and upper vagina. At puberty there is enough oestradiol to induce otherwise normal secondary female development (of breasts, external genitalia and body fat) and skeletal growth. Thus the individual usually presents first as an apparently normal pubescent girl but lacking sexual hair and with delayed menarche. Simple genital examination at birth (as described above) might have provided the warning.

True hermaphroditism

True hermaphroditism, in which there is a testis and ovary, or ovotestes, with mixed development of the internal and external genitalia, is extremely rare.

Management of intersex

Management of intersex depends on the age at which it is recognized. Once the child is accustomed to its gender it is usually better not changed, but a female pseudohermaphrodite with very inadequate external male differentiation may well be better converted from the accustomed male gender. Psychological factors are most important. Whatever the age at discovery, it is essential to define the exact genital configuration by examination under anaesthesia and laparoscopy and/or laparotomy. Abdominal testes should be excised because of the risk of developing dysgerminoma in later life, and oestrogen therapy will be required at the age of puberty. Cosmetic surgery on the external genitalia may be necessary, and later the young adult 'woman' will usually require a functional vagina constructed, or developed non-surgically by a gradual process of mechanical invagination from the existing vaginal entrance.

PUBERTY AND ADOLESCENCE

Puberty

The proper meaning of puberty is procreative capability but the word is usually applied to the events leading up to this state. Thus in this book puberty is taken to be the time of development of the genitalia and secondary sexual characters leading up to the menarche (first menstruation). The time of further maturation to adulthood is adolescence.

The endocrine events of puberty

The neuroendocrine changes that initiate all the other recognizable events of puberty are imperfectly understood, but are clearly the result of maturation of the hypothalamus rather than of any primary change in the gonads. Puberty can be induced prematurely in monkeys by administering pulsed gonadotrophin-releasing hormone (GnRH) in the usual adult dosage, and patients with delayed puberty can be treated successfully in the same way. However, pubertal development also involves independent maturation and contribution of the adrenal cortex, and normal ability to secrete growth hormone (GH).

1 The first endocrine change is increased adrenocortical secretion of androgens (dehydroepiandrosterone (DHA) and DHA sulphate) from about 7 years of age. Levels rise steadily until about 14 years. Increased secretion is associated with an increase in specific enzymic androgenic capacity, although the regulatory mechanism is not understood. An unidentified specific adrenal androgen-stimulating hormone of either pituitary or adrenal origin is postulated. The increased adrenal androgens, although only weak androgens, stimulate growth of ambisexual hair (see Chapter 15, section on hirsutism), notably in the axillae and pubic regions – so-called adrenarche (see below). All other features of pubertal development occur independently of, and can occur in the absence of, adrenal androgen secretion.

2 Pulsatile secretion of GnRH by the hypothalamus is released from the suppression which has been applied throughout childhood (see Chapter 5, section on gonadotrophin and sex steroid cycles through life and Fig. 5.7), due it is believed to non-steroidal inhibition of central nervous origin via the posterior hypothalamus. (Thus lesions in that region can cause precocious puberty.) Gonadotrophin and consequently gonadal steroid levels rise steadily from around 9 years of age until ovulatory cycles are established. Oestradiol in girls and testosterone in boys induce the characteristic secondary sexual features. Oestrogen also stimulates skeletal growth, by direct action on cartilage and bone to stimulate local production of insulin-like growth factor-1 (IGF-1). In addition, oestrogen and testosterone stimulate GH secretion.

3 Increased GH secretion stimulated by the rise in gonadal steroids also has an important role in stimulating the skeletal growth spurt associated with pubertal development. The effect is mediated by stimulation of IGF-1 production (in the liver and various target tissues) and IGF-1 levels in blood rise during pubertal development. The GH effect on skeletal growth is additional to the effect of oestrogen. Hypopituitary patients deficient in both GH and gonadotrophins have an impaired growth spurt if only GH, or only oestrogen or testosterone, is replaced.

The physical events of puberty

There are two separate sequences of events, each closely coordinated, but the two may vary in their relative timing, being determined separately in girls by rising gonadal oestrogen levels on the one hand and adrenal androgens on the other.

Oestrogen effects
1 Breast development (thelarche, i.e. the first appearance of breast development) is the first externally noticeable change, starting at 11 years on average (normal range 9–13 years), and takes longest (up to 5 years) to complete.
2 Growth and maturation of the genital organs.
3 Body growth accelerates, reaching peak velocity about 11 months before menarche, with remarkable constancy in the relative timing of these two events. The point of peak velocity is, however, not distinguishable at the time.
4 Menarche occurs at 13 years on average (normal range 11–15 years).

Adrenal androgen effects
1 Pubic hair (adrenarche) usually begins to appear around the time of first breast development.
2 Axillary hair (the second feature of adrenarche) may begin to grow before or after menarche.

The relative timing of all those pubertal events is illustrated in Figure 14.1. The age of pubertal development is determined not only genetically but by nutritional and health factors associated with socioeconomic conditions. The average age of menarche in industrialized countries has fallen steadily by 4 years during the last 150 years. Fatness is a factor. The average body weight at menarche is 47 kg, but short fat girls tend to reach menarche earlier than tall thin girls.

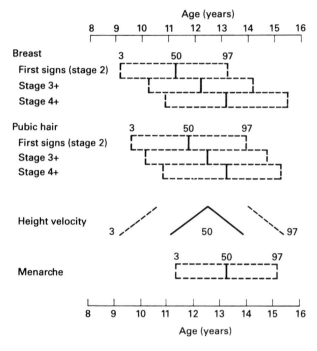

Fig. 14.1 Relative timing of pubertal changes in girls, showing the third, 50th and 97th centiles.

Adolescence

This is the time from menarche to adulthood when physical, mental and reproductive maturation occurs. The physical and reproductive events that occur in girls are:

1 Further slow growth in body height for 3–4 years until closure of epiphyses due to oestrogens.
2 Further maturation of breasts and labia.
3 Extension of pubic hair growth to inner thighs and sometimes lower abdomen.
4 Main growth of axillary hair.
5 Regularization of menstrual cycle and gradually increased frequency of ovulation up to about 20 years. This is not to say that the fertility of adolescent girls is negligible!

Once the various features of secondary sexual development have begun it can be difficult to tell when maturation is complete, or

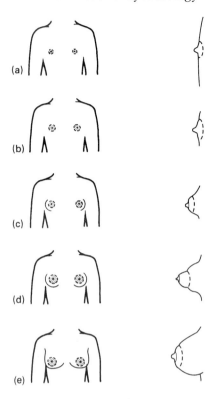

Fig. 14.2 Stages of breast development (as classified by Professor J.M. Tanner). Note that the nipple consists of both the papilla (often alone called the nipple) and the surrounding pink areola, shown here demarcated by a dotted line. (a) Stage 1: prepubertal; elevated papilla only. (b) Stage 2: breast bud; small mound of breast with areolar enlargement. (c) Stage 3: enlargement and elevation of breast, the areola remaining within the same contour. (d) Stage 4: projection of areola and papilla above the contour of the enlarging breast. (e) Stage 5: mature breast; areolar recession into the enlarged breast contour; projection of papilla only.

whether progress might have been arrested. The several distinct stages of breast and female external genital development are illustrated for reference in Figures 14.2 and 14.3.

Problems of puberty and adolescence

The most common problems are due to inadequate sex education. The deficiency applies less to the physical aspects, more often to the

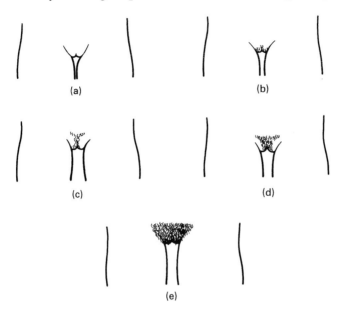

Fig. 14.3 Stages of external genital and pubic hair development (as classified by Professor J.M. Tanner). (a) Stage 1: prepubertal. (b) Stage 2: slight labial enlargement; sparse, slightly pigmented downy hair along labia. (c) Stage 3: darkening, coarsening and curling hair spreading sparsely over pubis; further labial enlargement. (d) Stage 4: dark, coarse, curly pubic hair, but not on full pubic area or on to medial thigh; labial enlargement complete. (e) Adult pubic hair with full female triangular distribution and involving medial thigh but not extending up linea alba.

development of interpersonal relationships, love and the value of sex. For these reasons venereal disease, contraceptive problems, pregnancy and the need for abortion are becoming rapidly more common at this age.

Reproductive disorders particularly associated with puberty and adolescence include the following, in order of frequency. The common problems of painful and heavy menstrual periods or secondary amenorrhoea and oligomenorrhoea are discussed in the relevant chapters dealing with such problems, which are similar in principle at any age.

1 Spasmodic dysmenorrhoea (see Chapter 19).
2 Dysfunctional (excessive) uterine bleeding (see Chapter 16).
3 Secondary amenorrhoea or oligomenorrhoea (see Chapter 15).

4 Delayed puberty.
5 Delayed menarche, i.e. primary amenorrhoea.
6 Abnormal sex differentiation (see above).
7 Precocious puberty – very rarely.

Delayed puberty and menarche

Delayed puberty means failure of development of all the secondary sexual characteristics including menarche. It can be recognized as early as 14 years by failure of breast development (more than 3 standard deviations above the normal mean). Menstruation will inevitably be delayed and in practice there is no need to wait to discover that.

The cause is nearly always *primary failure* of one of the components of the hypothalamic–pituitary–ovarian axis (primary here meaning inherent in the endocrine organ, not a chronological term):

1 Primary ovarian failure due to ovarian dysgenesis is the commonest cause of delayed puberty. The ovaries are typically mere streaks of tissue without any follicles, depleted as a result of excessive rate of atresia. That is classically associated with Turner syndrome (karyotype 45,XO). This condition demonstrates the importance of the second X chromosome to protect the ovarian complement of follicles from excessive loss by atresia. The initial differentiation of the gonad to an ovary is determined only by the absence of a Y chromosome (see Chapter 5, section on oogenesis). In many cases of ovarian dysgenesis, however, no karyotypic or phenotypic abnormality can be found except for the streak ovaries. In such cases it is assumed that there is a mosaic chromosomal abnormality affecting only the ovaries.
2 Primary hypothalamic failure may be temporary (true delayed puberty, which will resolve spontaneously) or permanent. One can be certain of permanent failure given a history of hyposmia, i.e. impaired sense of smell, indicating Kallmann syndrome. Kallmann syndrome is rare, particularly in girls, but of interest because it demonstrates the embryonic link between the olfactory tract and the GnRH-secreting neurones. The GnRH neurones reach the hypothalamus, remarkably, by migration along the olfactory nerves from their common origin in the olfactory placode. The nerves grow through the cribriform plate of the skull to synapse with the olfactory tracts of the brain, but if that fails to occur the Kallmann syndrome ensues. In the absence of a history of hyposmia or anosmia it is not possible to distinguish between temporary or permanent failure of pubertal development, and hormone replacement therapy must be started empirically.

3 Primary pituitary failure is rare, and then usually due to a large pituitary tumour or a craniopharyngioma compressing the pituitary or its stalk.

Other *functional disorders* (discussed in Chapter 15) which cause secondary amenorrhoea can at an earlier age delay puberty. Anorexia nervosa and hyperprolactinaemia causing suppression of hypothalamic secretion of GnRH and consequent secondary ovarian failure rarely occur early enough to interfere with puberty. A well-recognized although rare example of hypothalamic suppression is due to extreme exercise, as occurs in female gymnasts. They are often at their best in their early teenage years and the severe physical training of top-class competitors can delay their pubertal development and skeletal growth. Hypothyroidism can cause secondary hyperprolactinaemia and consequent hypothalamic suppression.

Treatment

In the absence of any specific treatment that might be appropriate, oestrogen replacement therapy is needed without delay because of the distress – often hidden by meekness – caused in a teenage girl by her continuing infantile condition. The main concern with oestrogen therapy is to avoid inducing premature epiphyseal closure by keeping to a low dose until growth to full height has occurred (e.g. ethinyloestradiol about 5 µg/day). That is one-quarter or less than in a contraceptive preparation. Bone is even more sensitive to oestrogen than the breast. A higher dose inhibits bone growth and can cause premature epiphyseal closure and thus permanent stunting of growth. In addition a higher dose of oestrogen can cause distorted and permanently disfiguring growth of the breasts due to ugly prominence of the areolar region. It is important to start treatment without delay, but equally important to be patient once started.

Delayed menarche means failure to menstruate by 16 years. It may or may not be associated with other delayed pubertal development (see above). When secondary sexual development otherwise appears normal the causes may be:

1 Atresia of the vagina or cervix, resulting in retention of the normal menses (cryptomenorrhoea). Most commonly the atresia is lower vaginal and very limited in extent, presenting as a thin transverse membrane, often mistakenly called imperforate hymen. It is very easily corrected. The key feature in all cases is a pelvic mass formed by the collected menses. Heavy retrograde flow of the trapped menses can cause severe pelvic endometriosis.

2 Polycystic ovarian (PCO) disorder. The condition is explained in Chapter 15. Essentially, there are very numerous small antral follicles (cysts) arrested in their maturation but actively secreting androgen (in excess) and oestrogen, and there is loss of normal cyclicity.

   The disorder is inherent in the ovaries and lifelong. Thus secretion of oestrogen induces normal and timely secondary sexual development, but lack of normal cyclicity may lead to delayed menarche and subsequently usually oligomenorrhoea or sometimes more prolonged episodes of amenorrhoea. The diagnosis can be made presumptively by inducing menstruation in response to a short course of progestogen, indicating oestrogenization (of the endometrium; see Chapter 15); or sometimes definitively by ultrasonography of the ovaries (done transabdominally in a girl of that age). Treatment at this stage simply requires cyclical progestogen to induce regular menstruation, partly for psychological reasons and partly to protect the endometrium in the long term from the carcinogenic effect of prolonged unopposed oestrogen.

3 Testicular feminization, rarely (see the section on male pseudohermaphroditism, above). The key features are normal female development of the breasts, external genitalia and body shape, but absent androgenic features (axillary and pubic hair), absent or short vagina, and absent uterus. The testes may be intra-abdominal or may be palpable in the inguinal or labial region. There is a 30% risk of malignant neoplasia (dysgerminoma) which requires orchidectomy after puberty and subsequent oestrogen replacement.

Precocious puberty

This is defined as breast development commencing (thelarche) before 8 years of age or menarche before 10 years (more than 3 standard deviations from the normal means). Pregnancy has been recorded in a 5-year-old (see *Guinness Book of Records*!). That demonstrates the occurrence of **true precocious puberty**, i.e. precocious pulsatile secretion of GnRH leading to normal pituitary–ovarian function. By contrast, a steroid-secreting ovarian or adrenal tumour leads to so-called **precocious pseudopuberty** because there is no hypothalamic–pituitary–ovarian (follicular) activity. True precocious puberty can be induced by a tumour or cyst in the posterior hypothalamic region, blocking the central nervous inhibitory pathway which normally suppresses GnRH secretion during childhood. Mostly, however, no cause is found and in such cases precocious puberty represents one extreme of normal.

In very young girls precocious puberty presents a desperate problem. Epiphyseal closure leads to gross limitation of height, and libido and aggression can cause major behavioural problems. A tumour must always be sought, by cerebral and abdominal imaging and sometimes by laparotomy. Steroidogenic tumours must be excised but cerebral tumours causing true precocious puberty may be too dangerous to remove. However, the effect of pulsatile GnRH secretion can be blocked by desensitizing the pituitary using a long-acting GnRH analogue, and pituitary–ovarian activity is thus effectively suppressed until the appropriate age.

FURTHER READING

Brook, C.G.D. (1982) *Growth Assessment in Childhood and Adolescence.* Blackwell, Oxford.

Hillier, S.G., Kitchener, H.C., Neilson, J.P. (eds) (1996) *Scientific Essentials of Reproductive Medicine.* W.B. Saunders, London.

Wilson, J.D. and Foster, D.W. (eds) (1992) *Williams' Textbook of Endocrinology*, 8th edn. Saunders, Philadelphia.

15

Amenorrhoea, oligomenorrhoea and other endocrine problems

Disorders affecting the hypothalamic–pituitary–ovarian endocrine axis usually lead to absent or infrequent menstruation and associated oestrogen deficiency or androgen excess and their consequent effects. Amenorrhoea and oligomenorrhoea have mostly the same endocrine causes, though different in frequency, but anatomical defects are a rare specific cause of amenorrhoea and for practical purposes are best included in this context. We will therefore deal first with amenorrhoea to cover the full range of possible causes, and later with oligomenorrhoea only to highlight the differences.

AMENORRHOEA

Amenorrhoea, the absence of menstruation, occurs as a physiological event during pregnancy and, of course, before normal menarche and after the menopause.

Pathological amenorrhoea is defined as the failure to menstruate for at least 6 months during the normal reproductive years in the absence of pregnancy, i.e. between 16 years (the limit for delayed menarche) and 40 years (the dividing line between normal and premature menopause). Some authors require 12 months' amenorrhoea for their definition, but any figure chosen is arbitrary and the diversity reflects the overlap between amenorrhoea and oligomenorrhoea (see below). It occurs in 1–2% of all women of reproductive age.

Amenorrhoea can be classified as *primary*, which is defined as for delayed menarche, i.e. failure to menstruate by the age of 16 years or later, or *secondary*, when menstruation has previously occurred. This distinction is of little practical value since the causes overlap. For instance, a partial form of ovarian dysgenesis can occur which, despite almost typical streak ovaries, can present with secondary amenorrhoea. The distinction can even be misleading because some girls describe having menstruated when that was clearly impossible, being the result of optimistic imagination or traumatic self-examination.

Amenorrhoea is only a symptom, not a diagnosis. It is the common presenting feature of a variety of distinct disorders. These are nearly always endocrine disorders (99%) and only occasionally due to anatomical defects (1%).

Anatomical causes

These can be summarized as follows:

1 Congenital:
   a. Intersex states (see Chapter 14).
   b. Vaginal atresia or uterine absence.
2 Acquired:
   a. Endometrial fibrosis.
   b. Cervical stenosis.

The congenital defects present of course with primary amenorrhoea, the acquired ones with secondary. Some intersex states are due, fundamentally, to endocrine disorder, e.g. congenital adrenal hyperplasia or testicular feminization (see Chapter 14).

Endometrial fibrosis (leading to occlusion of the cavity) may be due to tuberculosis, or to traumatic curettage, done usually after abortion or childbirth (Asherman syndrome). Amenorrhoea is of course the specific aim of endometrial destruction or resection done to relieve heavy menstrual bleeding (menorrhagia) in older women (see Chapter 16). Cervical stenosis may also result from surgery, particularly cervical cautery or conization.

Endocrine causes

Table 15.1 presents a nosological classification of the endocrine causes of amenorrhoea, according to their endocrine site of origin in the hypothalamic–pituitary–ovarian axis or other endocrine system. The table also shows how commonly each condition is seen in practice, its underlying causes and critical diagnostic features. It is worth also considering an alternative classification simplified from the ovarian standpoint:

1 Primary ovarian failure, whatever the cause. The critical endocrine features are raised follicle-stimulating hormone (FSH) levels as after the normal menopause and oestrogen deficiency.
2 Secondary ovarian failure due to gonadotrophin deficiency,

whether of hypothalamic or pituitary origin including hyperpro-lactinaemia (see below). The critical endocrine features are non-elevated FSH and luteinizing hormone (LH) levels, and oestrogen deficiency.

3 Polycystic ovarian disease. In most cases a genetically determined primary ovarian, hyperandrogenic condition, though its expression depends on associated hyperinsulinaemia (see below). The critical endocrine features are raised androgen levels and oestrogenization, in contrast to primary or secondary ovarian failure. The classically recognized presenting features of hirsutism and obesity affect only a minority of cases.

Primary hypothalamic or pituitary failure

Primary hypothalamic failure (see Chapter 14 on delayed puberty and menarche) is characterized by deficient pulsatile secretion of gonadotrophin-releasing hormone (GnRH), which results in deficient gonadotrophin secretion by the pituitary, but in practice those features cannot be reliably defined. Diagnosis is based on inference, due to the consequent ovarian failure (amenorrhoea and oestrogen deficiency), non-elevated FSH levels (unlike primary ovarian failure), and often specific historical features such as hyposmia (impaired sense of smell in Kallmann syndrome) or a known treated pituitary tumour (Table 15.1).

Kallmann syndrome, although rare in girls, is of basic interest because it illustrates the (disrupted) link between reproductive function and behaviour (due to pheromones) and the olfactory tract. The disorder arises due to failure of the GnRH-secreting neurones to migrate to the hypothalamus from their origin in the olfactory placode.

In hypothalamic failure ovulation can be induced by pulsed GnRH (given with a portable battery-driven syringe pump), and in pituitary failure by gonadotrophin therapy. Gonadotrophin therapy stimulates the ovaries directly, overriding normal feedback control, and therefore requires careful monitoring to avoid hyperstimula-tion, which can result in large ovarian cysts and massive peritoneal effusion, or high-multiple pregnancy.

If pregnancy is not desired, oestrogen replacement therapy is needed if there are symptoms due to deficiency, including lack of secondary sexual development, and to protect against osteoporosis, other connective tissue depletion and long-term cardiovascular risks. Oestrogen-deficient women aged in their 20s can suffer osteoporotic fractures, including crushed vertebrae leading to shortening and kyphosis, as usually seen only in old women (the so-called dowager's hump).

Table 15.1   Endocrine disorders causing amenorrhoea and their underlying conditions, relative incidence, diagnostic features and consequent oestrogen state

Cause	Percentage	Diagnostic feature	Oestrogen state
1 Primary failures of the hypothalamic–pituitary–ovarian axis			
(a) Primary hypothalamic failure:	2	Often specific history, and LH, FSH low (or not raised).	Deficient
Kallmann syndrome (permanent)			
Delayed puberty (temporary)			
Tumour			
(b) Primary pituitary failure:	1		
Tumour			
Ablation (tumour therapy)			
Necrosis (Sheehan syndrome)			
(c) Primary ovarian failure:	10	Serum FSH high	Deficient
Dysgenesis			
Damage (surgery, irradiation)			
Autoantibodies			
Premature menopause			
2 Functional disorders of the hypothalamic–pituitary–ovarian axis			
(a) Hypothalamic:	40	History and exclusion of other causes	Deficient
Psychological disorder			
Weight loss			
(b) Pituitary:			
Hyperprolactinaemia	15	Serum prolactin high	Deficient
Pituitary tumours (usually micro-prolactinoma)			
Primary hypothyroidism			
Drugs (dopamine antagonists)			
(c) Ovarian:			
Polycystic ovarian disease	30	Hirsutism if present	Normal or excessive
3 Other endocrine disorders	2		
(a) Thyroid disorders			
(b) Adrenal deficiency (Addison's)			
(c) Diabetes mellitus			

Primary ovarian failure

Whatever the cause, this is permanent and irreversible. It may present with primary or secondary amenorrhoea, depending on the cause. As in the postmenopausal woman, there is oestrogen deficiency and consequent high gonadotrophin levels, and some patients are troubled by hot flushes and atrophic vaginitis. High serum FSH (>40 iu/l) is the diagnostic feature, rather than LH which may be raised in other disorders, like the polycystic ovary (PCO) syndrome. There is no treatment, except oestrogen replacement for symptomatic deficiency and long-term protection as mentioned above (and see Chapter 23 on the menopause), but pregnancy can be achieved using donated eggs.

The resistant ovary syndrome is an uncommon variant which may correct spontaneously (although attempts to induce ovulation are fruitless). Recovery cannot be predicted, even by ovarian biopsy, and the diagnosis can only be made retrospectively. Rarely, recovery and failure can occur intermittently, as in some normal premenopausal women.

Hypothalamic disorders

The term implies disorder of the hypothalamic control of the hypothalamic–pituitary–ovarian axis, not due to primary failure but to extraneous influences, particularly psychological disorders and weight loss (see below). Their mode of action on the hypothalamus is unknown, but the fact that they disturb the hypothalamus is shown in research studies by deficient pulsatile secretion of GnRH and disorder of functions like body temperature control, and in practice by the normal pituitary–ovarian (ovulatory) response to pulsed GnRH therapy. Pulsed GnRH therapy can also overcome the negative feedback effect on the hypothalamus caused by pituitary hypersecretion of prolactin (see later).

The reproductive disturbance is severe. It is characterized by gonadotrophin deficiency and consequent oestrogen deficiency. There is also failure to ovulate in response to clomiphene due to lack of feedback control (on which to act) of gonadotrophin secretion by oestrogen. Induction of ovulation in these cases may be achieved by psychological and/or dietary treatment to correct the underlying disorder, but commonly it is necessary to use pulsed GnRH or to stimulate the ovaries directly with exogenous gonadotrophins.

Weight loss and psychological disorders

Psychological disorder or stress is the commonest cause of pathological amenorrhoea (Table 15.1) and accounts for its frequency in

young women leaving home for the first time and starting institu-
tional training. This is also commonly associated with loss of
appetite (true anorectic response to stress) and consequent weight
loss, which may be the main cause of the amenorrhoea. Another
common cause of weight loss leading to amenorrhoea, usually in
adolescence, is cosmetic dieting which gets out of control. A loss of
more than 10 kg seems to be the danger mark. Whatever the original
cause or motive for dieting, it is important to appreciate that for
some young women it becomes an obsession which can lead to
anorexia nervosa.

Anorexia nervosa is misnamed because there is no loss of
appetite. The girl (she is usually teenage) is obsessed with her size
and starves herself but cannot of course admit it. In its chronic form
anorexia nervosa is a lifelong disorder with distinct psychological
features still centred on obsession with weight control long after
most of the original weight loss has been restored. It accounts for
15% of all women complaining of amenorrhoea.

Altogether, a history of weight loss with or without the distinct
features of anorexia nervosa accounts for 25–30% of women with
amenorrhoea and is often referred to generally as weight-loss-
related amenorrhoea. It is important to appreciate that the major
weight loss usually occurred at the start of the amenorrhoea and
much of the original loss has usually been regained. These patients
are no longer extremely thin (although often well below average
weight: refer to Fig. 15.1 in practice). At first sight they appear

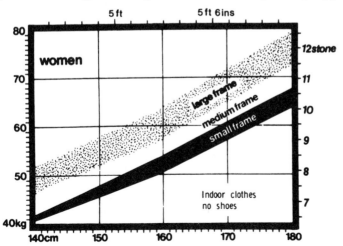

Fig. 15.1   Weight related to height and frame size in normal women.
(Reproduced from G.W. Thorpe (1974), *Medicine* Series 1, No. 28,
p.1658 with kind permission of the Editor).

unremarkable – perhaps modishly slim and a little reserved – and as a result their underlying condition is frequently missed. A careful history of weight fluctuation and psychological factors should always be taken in amenorrhoea. Much stress and unhappiness is likely to be uncovered. Also, regaining the lost weight is a sure means of restoring reproductive function, and preferable to hormone therapy because of the physical and psychological benefits, not only to the patient but also her offspring, during and after pregnancy. But the desire to stay thin is often too strong.

Exercise-related amenorrhoea

Heavy physical exercise is a well-known but uncommon cause of amenorrhoea which affects many competitive long-distance runners and ballet dancers. World-class gymnasts are usually at their best during the early teenage years and their pubertal development is often delayed. The effect depends on severe exercise involving endurance and extreme loss of fat, often compounded by intentional restriction of weight by ballet dancers. However, menstruation often returns soon after enforced rest due to injury, long before any increase in weight. The psychological aspects of competitive stress and ballet dancing were therefore thought to be important factors, but the key now seems to be that endurance athletes generally fail to provide adequately in their diet for their huge energy requirements. That leads to typical hypothalamic amenorrhoea as in cases due to weight loss. Oestrogen deficiency leads to reduction in bone mineral density even in such physically fit athletes and so-called stress fractures can occur.

Hyperprolactinaemia

Excess prolactin acts by negative feedback on the hypothalamus to reduce pulsatile secretion of GnRH, leading to reduced gonadotrophin secretion by the pituitary. Thus it causes secondary ovarian failure and consequent oestrogen deficiency.

Of all the trophic hormones of the anterior pituitary, only prolactin is controlled mainly by inhibition from the hypothalamus; the others are controlled mainly by releasing hormones. Thus tumours compressing the hypothalamus or pituitary stalk cause panhypopituitarism but hyperprolactinaemia. Since the prolactin-inhibiting factor from the hypothalamus is dopamine, many drugs with a dopamine-antagonistic action can cause hyperprolactinaemia and thus amenorrhoea. Such drugs have a wide range of therapeutic uses but most likely in young women are the phenothiazines for psychiatric disorders and metoclopramide for nausea. By contrast, and more commonly, since prolactin release can be stimulated by large amounts of thyrotrophin-releasing hormone, primary thyroid failure can present with secondary hyperprolactinaemia and amenorrhoea.

However, the commonest demonstrable cause of hyperprolactinaemia is a pituitary chromophobe adenoma secreting prolactin, called a prolactinoma. Prolactinomas are usually very small and evident only by computed tomographic or magnetic resonance image scanning, disturbing function because of hypersecretion of prolactin rather than damage to the normal pituitary tissue. Such damage associated with large tumours is usually due to surgery or radiotherapy. Prolactinomas are benign tumours which may grow very little in a whole lifetime, but may threaten sight and life by growing rapidly upwards to compress the optic tracts or laterally into the cavernous sinus to cause thrombosis or bleeding.

Since prolactin is the stimulus for normal lactation, galactorrhoea is a typical symptom of hyperprolactinaemia (see later). It occurs in less than half the cases, however, and is therefore an unreliable index. Serum prolactin must always be measured in women with amenorrhoea (but must be repeated if raised because that can occur misleadingly due to temporary stress).

Treatment

Except when there is a large tumour, prolactin secretion can be suppressed very easily, using a dopamine agonist such as bromocriptine, which is a synthetic ergot alkaloid. Similar newer agents include cabergoline and quinagolide. Prolactin levels fall quickly to normal, and the ovaries commence function almost immediately. The treatment is so effective and simple that it is easy to overlook the potential danger from a tumour if pregnancy ensues. The large amounts of placental oestrogens in pregnancy stimulate maternal prolactin secretion, causing the normal pituitary nearly to double in size, and a tumour may similarly undergo expansion with particular risk to the optic tracts. During pregnancy visual field perimetry should be done repeatedly to check the need for treatment. Bromocriptine, which is usually stopped when pregnancy occurs, although it is safe, can be reintroduced.

Surgery and/or radiotherapy are limited to exceptional tumours of dangerous size which do not respond to bromocriptine. Surgery even for easily removed small tumours (via a transnasal transsphenoidal approach) is often incomplete, leaving persistent hyperprolactinaemia (albeit at a lower level), and for larger tumours can damage the normal pituitary. Bromocriptine is now the first line of treatment because it usually suppresses tumour activity, leading to shrinkage, and that can sometimes be complete.

Polycystic ovarian disease and syndrome

This complex fascinating condition will be considered in relative detail because it is now recognized as the most frequent endocrine disorder of women of reproductive age and carries major long-term health risks apart from the familiar symptomatic problems of menstrual disorder, infertility and hirsutism. It presents with overt symptoms in at least 5% of young women and is hidden, though carrying related risks, in 10% of normally menstruating women. It accounts for about one-third of women with amenorrhoea and 90% with oligomenorrhoea, though often without the classically associated features of hirsutism and obesity.

The condition is characterized by excessive androgen production (androstenedione and testosterone) by the ovaries and/or adrenal cortex, which inhibits ovarian follicular ripening and may lead to peripheral features of virilization (hirsutism, male-pattern balding, clitoromegaly).

Numerous follicles – at least 15 in each ovary, often over 100 – develop abnormally, arrested at about 5 mm in diameter due to the atretic action of excess androgens. The numerous follicles account for the term polycystic, which is unfortunately misleading because the cysts are not large, distorting or neoplastic (*See* Plate 1). They are small, arrayed peripherally but within the ovarian cortex and enlarge the ovary evenly. When present in sufficient number they become closely crowded around the cortex and a sectional view on ultrasound scanning gives the typical necklace appearance, like a string of black pearls.

The ovary is further enlarged by hyperplasia and expansion of the stroma, which also contributes to the excessive production of androgen by the ovaries. The main source of the androgen hyper-secretion is the theca cells of the follicles, which are hypertrophied. The theca cells are of course related to the stroma by differentiation from it.

The follicles, being partly atretic, are deficient in their production of oestradiol. That applies to the individual follicle, but there are so many that together they secrete substantial amounts of oestradiol into the circulation and the patients are usually demonstrably oestrogenized.

The classical PCO syndrome is thus a combination of oligomenor-rhoea or amenorrhoea and hirsutism, also accompanied by obesity. The cause of the obesity is not clear but it is typically of the central type, particularly intra-abdominal – the so-called apple rather than pear shape. Obesity has an important effect, however, amplifying the PCO disorder by increasing insulin secretion, which is usually already excessive. Insulin resistance and hyperinsulinaemia are key

elements in the pathogenesis both of PCO and of important metabolic risks associated with PCO as described below.

First it needs to be emphasized, however, that many women with
PCO and oligo- or amenorrhoea do not have the classical features of
hirsutism or obesity. Nevertheless they nearly all have distinct –
though less marked – hyperandrogenaemia (raised serum androgen
levels) and insulin resistance with hyperinsulinaemia. The
differences in expression of hyperandrogen*aemia* as hyperandrogen*ism* depend on individual variation in the enzymic
conversion of testosterone to the more potent dihydrotestosterone
(by 5α-reductase) in the androgen-sensitive target tissues, and on
racial differences.

Pathogenesis and pathophysiology

The causes of PCO and the associated hyperandrogenic syndrome
include:

1 Primary ovarian androgen dysfunction (or primary PCO disease).
   This is by far the most common cause and is therefore discussed
   in more detail below. It is often associated with adrenal androgen
   dysfunction, and invariably linked with hyperinsulinaemia. The
   symptoms therefore usually begin around the onset of puberty
   and last throughout the reproductive age.
2 Secondary PCO disease (and dysfunction) due to other sources of
   excess androgen, such as:
   a. Androgenic forms of congenital adrenal hyperplasia, due
      to specific enzymic deficiencies on the pathway to cortisol
      (21-hydroxylase, 11-hydroxylase, 3β-hydroxysteroid δ5-4-
      isomerase). This condition can be difficult to distinguish from
      primary ovarian androgen dysfunction, necessitating specific
      ovarian suppression and adrenal suppression and stimulation
      testing.
   b. Androgenic tumours of the ovary or adrenal. The symptomatic
      history is usually short and testosterone levels in blood very
      high, sometimes with signs of marked virilization such as
      clitoromegaly.
   c. Exogenous administration of androgens – rare.

Primary PCO disease

This accounts for most cases of PCO syndrome. Knowledge and
theories of its pathogenesis have advanced rapidly. There appear to
be two primary functional defects which are interactive but each
apparently determined by separate genetic factors which both have
to be present for expression of the ovarian condition:

1 Increased enzymic capacity (of 17α-hydroxylase) for androgen production in the ovary and often the adrenal cortex. Full expression of the increased ovarian capacity for androgen hypersecretion depends on excessive stimulation by LH, which is one of the effects of hyperinsulinaemia.

2 Insulin resistance, probably due to a specific post-receptor defect, leading to hypersecretion of insulin by the pancreas as a compensatory mechanism to maintain glucose uptake and homeostasis. Hyperinsulinaemia has widespread metabolic effects of clinical importance (see below) associated with PCO, but the effects on ovarian androgen secretion are mediated via LH.

Both secretion of LH by the pituitary and its androgenic actions on the ovary (theca cells and stroma) are amplified. Those effects are probably due to excess availability of insulin-like growth factor-1 (IGF-1) caused by hyperinsulinaemia suppressing hepatic production of its main binding protein (IGF-1 BP-1).

LH secretion by the pituitary may be further amplified due to increased sensitivity to GnRH caused by prolonged exposure to acyclical oestrogen in circulation from the numerous though arrested ovarian follicles (see above).

Hyperinsulinaemia also suppresses hepatic production of sex hormone-binding globulin (SHBG), the main carrier protein for testosterone and oestradiol in the circulation, so increasing the free (unbound) proportion of testosterone and its consequent bioavailability.

Clinical endocrinology and diagnosis

The expected serum findings of raised testosterone, androstenedione and LH, reduced SHBG, and normal oestradiol are unreliable in clinical practice. The levels of total testosterone, which is largely bound to SHBG, are often normal and free testosterone is difficult to measure. Therefore calculation of the total testosterone : SHBG ratio is required in practice. LH levels in blood fluctuate greatly due to pulsatile secretion and are often normal unless measured several times, but a raised level is a reliable diagnostic index. Oestradiol is, like testosterone, largely bound to SHBG and the best index is a biological test of oestrogenization: progestogen-induced menstrual bleeding or endometrial thickening shown by ultrasonography.

Hirsutism is a common index of hyperandrogenaemia but is often absent. More marked signs of virilization are rare. Even when hirsutism is present it can be missed due to cosmetic measures on the face and embarrassment to admit to excessive hair elsewhere on the body, and must therefore always be enquired after. On the other hand it is essential to distinguish true hirsutism from the constitutional form (see later) found in women from naturally hairy and dark-complexioned races and families, which does not have an underlying endocrine disorder.

Vaginal ultrasonography of the ovaries can confirm the endocrinological diagnosis but requires refined technique and can therefore be misleading and unreliable.

Associated metabolic disorders and health risks

There are several important risks to general health associated with PCO mainly due directly or indirectly to the accompanying insulin resistance:

1 Inadequate compensatory hypersecretion of insulin leads to impaired glucose tolerance, mediated by increased (released suppression of) plasma free fatty acid concentrations, and eventual non-insulin-dependent diabetes mellitus (NIDDM).
2 Hyperinsulinaemia causes hypertension (indicated by animal experiments though the mechanism is unknown) and increased plasma concentrations of triglycerides and reduced high-density lipoprotein (HDL) cholesterol. Those are all factors along with impaired glucose tolerance/NIDDM which predispose to coronary artery disease.
3 Continuous exposure to oestrogen unopposed by cyclical progesterone in the absence of ovulation leads to increased risk of endometrial carcinoma and at a relatively young age – around 40 years.

Treatment of PCO disease

Specific treatment of *secondary* PCO disease is needed for congenital adrenal hyperplasia by lifelong glucocorticoid suppression/ replacement, or for an ovarian or adrenal androgenic tumour by surgery.

There is no specific treatment for *primary* PCO disease and the management is determined by symptomatic requirements and prophylaxis against incidental health risks as far as possible.

Ovarian activity including androgen production can be fully suppressed by pituitary desensitization using GnRH analogues, but this is not suitable for long-term use and requires added oestrogen replacement therapy. Regular though artificial menstrual cycles can be restored by cyclical oestrogen/progestogen therapy and additional advantages include reliable contraception and oestrogenic suppression of LH levels (at least partly) and raising of SHBG levels (so reducing free testosterone). Furthermore, choice of a progestogen with antiandrogenic activity like cyproterone acetate helps to reduce hirsutism (see later).

Ovulation failure causing infertility can be overcome by raising FSH levels to stimulate granulosa cell production of the aromatasing enzymes required to metabolize (to oestradiol) the excess thecal androgen causing granulosa cell inhibition and atresia. Endogenous FSH levels can often be raised sufficiently and simply by (oral) clomiphene, which blocks negative feedback of oestradiol on pituitary FSH secretion. Otherwise exogenous FSH must be administered by injection and the response monitored closely. Sometimes multiple deep electrocautery of the ovary can be temporarily effective, by partial damage to reduce ovarian androgen production. The operation is similar in principle to the outdated, much more damaging wedge resection of the ovaries.

Dietary reduction of obesity reduces insulin secretion and can as a result substantially reduce ovarian androgen production, sometimes greatly improving menstrual cyclicity and fertility. Exercise is the only known means of improving sensitivity to insulin. The combination of reducing obesity and increasing exercise also reduces the long-term risks of developing NIDDM, hypertension and coronary artery disease. They should be strongly advocated in women with PCO syndrome, but such profound changes in lifestyle are extremely difficult to achieve and sustain.

Protection against endometrial carcinoma could be achieved by cyclical progestogen therapy alone, but there are additional advantages of combination with oestrogen, as mentioned earlier.

Other specific endocrine disorders

Amenorrhoea is rarely found to be associated with thyroid disorders (1%), diabetes mellitus or Addison's disease (<1%), and their finding may be incidental. Primary hypothyroidism is a well-defined, if uncommon, cause of hyperprolactinaemia and consequent amenorrhoea. Hypothyroidism and Addison's disease can however be linked with primary ovarian failure due to a common autoimmune disease: so-called polyglandular autoimmune endocrine failure. Adrenal deficiency can be simply screened for by the typical clinical history and signs; thyroid disorders by the history and measurement of serum thyroid-stimulating hormone (TSH). Insulin-dependent diabetes mellitus is probably not a cause of amenorrhoea, but NIDDM can be linked via insulin resistance with PCO disease.

Other conditions incidentally linked with amenorrhoea

Obesity

In obese women there are minor changes in the differential release of FSH and LH, and there is increased adrenal cortisol and possibly androgen production. However, there is no clear association between amenorrhoea and obesity (unlike weight loss), except in the PCO syndrome due to amplification of hyperinsulinaemia. It is thus unpredictable (in contrast to weight restoration in the underweight) whether reduction of weight in obese patients will restore menstruation. It can however prove critical when ovulation induction therapy is otherwise ineffective, and it seems to be advisable anyway for wider reasons.

Oral contraception

There is often a slight delay in resumption of menstruation after stopping combined oestrogen–progestogen oral contraception. The average delay is only a week and it seldom lasts 6 months. The usual short delay is to be expected due to the relatively long life of the synthetic progestogens used, postponing the normal rise in gonadotrophin levels required to initiate follicular maturation.

In the case of prolonged delay the term post-pill amenorrhoea is commonly used to imply a causative association. However, evidence is against that. The endocrine disorders found are the same as in amenorrhoeic women who have not used oral contraception, suggesting that post-pill amenorrhoea is not an entity, and the need for investigation (see below) should not be disregarded. The coincidental nature of the association is explained by the artificially induced menstruation which masks the underlying condition for the duration of the oral contraception.

Amenorrhoea occurring during oral contraception is less easily explained – it is probably due to suppression of the endometrium by the progestogen given from the start of the cycle – but can be disregarded. It is mainly only a nuisance, causing concern about possible pregnancy.

Investigation of amenorrhoea

First, the possibility of pregnancy needs to be considered by a history of unprotected intercourse, specific symptoms (see Chapter 7) and urine testing for human chorionic gonodotrophin (hCG) if uterine enlargement is not already palpable abdominally.

The basic investigations needed for pathological amenorrhoea can be summarized as follows:

1 History:
   a. Weight fluctuation.
   b. Psychological factors.
   c. Thyroid symptoms.
   d. Drug usage (particularly prolactinergic drugs).
   e. Hirsutism.
   f. (Hot flushes: unreliable guide to primary ovarian failure but may need symptomatic relief).
   g. (Galactorrhoea: unreliable guide to hyperprolactinaemia but may need symptomatic relief).
2 Examination:
   a. Hirsutism (and other signs of virilization).
   b. Integrity of genital tract.
   c. Oestrogen state of the genital tract (cervical appearance, uterine size or endometrial thickness on ultrasonography).
3 Hormone measurements:
   a. FSH.
   b. LH.
   c. Prolactin.
   d. TSH.
   e. Testosterone (if there is hirsutism).
4 Dynamic tests:
   a. Progestogen challenge (menstrual response, to assess oestrogen state).
   b. Clomiphene test (ovulatory response, only when pregnancy is desired).

Treatment of amenorrhoea

Specific treatment of each cause (see Table 15.1) would be the ideal but is seldom possible. Patients with psychological causes or weight loss should be the most amenable to cure but are often very resistant to any change in their behaviour. Hypothyroidism can be overcome by thyroxine replacement, leading in turn to correction of the hyperprolactinaemia which caused the amenorrhoea. Pituitary prolactinomas might be excised but that can seldom be done with sufficient precision to be fully corrective.

When pregnancy is desired, in general ovulation induction is usually achieved not by fundamental correction of the underlying cause but by temporarily getting around the reproductive disorder using, most commonly, clomiphene, bromocriptine, pulsed GnRH or gonadotrophins as appropriate (see Chapter 12).

Alternatively, contraception may be needed. Since ovulation occurs sporadically in some disorders (e.g. PCO syndrome), and other common disorders may resolve spontaneously (e.g. due to psychological factors or weight loss), reliable methods should be used if contraception is needed. Since there is no evidence to implicate oral contraceptives as a cause of amenorrhoea or infertility they may be chosen as usual. Use of oestrogen preparations in hyperprolactinaemia should be checked by occasional prolactin measurements because of possible excessive stimulation of the growth of an existing pituitary tumour. An intrauterine device may be unsuitable for oestrogen-deficient women because of uterine atrophy.

Oestrogen deficiency may need replacement therapy to relieve acute symptoms such as vaginal dryness and dyspareunia, but other chronic effects like lack of libido and general energy are often not appreciated until – as, for example, occurs with chronic anaemia – the condition is corrected. Long-term prophylaxis is particularly important, however, to protect against progressive bone loss, which can reach an irreversible point when bone trabeculae break down. Bone loss is evident within 6 months of oestrogen-deficient amenorrhoea, and osteoporotic fractures including vertebral crush and shortening in height can occur in women aged in their 20s. Even if they escape such complications when young they are likely to suffer such effects long before other women after the normal menopause. Only a low dose of oestrogen is needed to stimulate bone growth, as used in postmenopausal women (see Chapter 23) but young amenorrhoeic women who are sexually active would be better receiving a standard contraceptive preparation.

Oestrogenized women, by contrast, need protection from endometrial carcinoma by cyclical progestogen therapy. Exposure of the endometrium to at least 12 days' progestogen each cycle is probably necessary as in the case of postmenopausal women undergoing oestrogen replacement therapy (see Chapter 23). Alternatively, a combined oestrogen–progestogen contraceptive preparation would provide endometrial protection, menstrual cycle control and contraception all in one.

OLIGOMENORRHOEA

Oligomenorrhoea is defined as menstrual cycles prolonged to between 6 weeks and 6 months. At one end of the spectrum it overlaps with normal, the cycles being ovulatory but infrequent. At the other, it overlaps with amenorrhoea and shares all the same causes (Table 15.1) except primary failure of the components of the hypothalamic–pituitary–ovarian axis, which causes permanent amenorrhoea.

Oligomenorrhoeic cycles may be ovulatory or anovulatory, depending on the cause. It is not important in practice to make this distinction, only to investigate possibly serious underlying causes which may need treatment, particularly a prolactinoma, androgenic tumour, thyroid disorder or psychological disturbance. If infertility is an associated problem and specifically treatable endocrine disorders can be excluded, it is easier to organize investigation of ovulation (which is difficult when cycles are long and irregular) in response to treatment with clomiphene. If effective, clomiphene shortens the cycle predictably and thereby also improves the chance of conception.

HIRSUTISM

Hirsutism is the occurrence of male sexual hair, namely:

1 Stout, pigmented (terminal) hair on the face, upper pubic triangle and chest, and spreading laterally from the lower pubic triangle, on the thighs and in the nose and ears.
2 Thin, unpigmented (vellus) hairs replacing terminal hairs in the temporal and vertical areas of the scalp (i.e. male-pattern balding).

In addition there is accentuation of ambisexual hair, i.e. terminal hair stimulated by low levels of androgens (from the adrenals and ovaries) in the axillae, pubic area, forearms and lower legs, as normally occurs in women as well as men.

Hirsutism is only one feature of virilism, which includes clitoromegaly, deepening of the voice and muscular prominence. However, hirsutism without baldness is usually the only presenting feature of virilism. In the absence of these other features it can often be difficult to distinguish between true and constitutional hirsutism. *True hirsutism* is due to excessive androgens, whereas *constitutional hirsutism* is a normal feature of certain races and tribes. There is much overlap in the hairiness of normal women and men, particularly evident when comparing southern European women with Mongoloid men. The majority of European women have terminal hair on the forearms and lower legs, and a quarter have it on the face, upper lip, upper pubic triangle or chest.

Associated menstrual disorder and ultrasonographic evidence of PCO support a diagnosis of true hirsutism, whereas constitutional hirsutism is more likely in swarthy women with normal menstrual cycles and hirsute male relatives. The hyperandrogenic basis for true hirsutism can be difficult to define in practice. Free (unbound) testosterone levels in serum are the best index but difficult to measure. Instead it is necessary to calculate the ratio of total testosterone to SHBG, as discussed in the section on PCO disease above. A very high level of total testosterone suggests an ovarian or adrenal androgenic tumour as the cause. The causes of true hirsutism and their investigation is as for the PCO syndrome (see section on amenorrhoea above).

Treatment

Although treatment is necessarily protracted and often unsuccessful, every effort should be made because hirsutism can be a distressing stigma. Success of treatment hinges on accurate diagnosis. An androgenic tumour should be excised, but it is rare. If hyperandrogenism originates in the adrenal cortex, glucocorticoid treatment is effective.

In hyperandrogenism due to primary PCO disease, oestrogen and cyproterone acetate therapy are both helpful, best given as a standard cyclical contraceptive regimen (Dianette). Oestrogen partly suppresses pituitary LH secretion and consequent ovarian androgen production, and increases serum SHBG levels, thus reducing free testosterone. Cyproterone acetate is a progestogen which also blocks androgen receptors by competition. It will therefore feminize a male fetus and should be combined with oestrogen as contraception. If pregnancy occurs, termination should be advised.

In all cases treatment must be continued for 12 months before the hirsutism can be expected to diminish because of the long growth cycle of the hair follicle (3 years). Androgen suppression or blockade does not interrupt hair growth, but only prevents initiation of new hair growth.

Dietary weight reduction and increased exercise should be encouraged because they reduce hyperinsulinaemia and increase sensitivity to insulin respectively, so reducing androgen production. Those measures are extremely difficult to achieve and maintain, however, due to the unhappiness often caused by hirsutism and the discouraging delay in evident response to any treatment. It is easier to encourage when hormonal therapy has shown some benefit.

When treatment is unsuccessful, or in cases of constitutional hirsutism, the only recourse is to cosmetic measures. When electrolysis of hair follicles is skilfully done it is remarkably good, but it needs repeating and is moderately expensive, and so is usually confined to the face. The alternatives are shaving, depilatory creams, bleaching and cosmetic make-up.

GALACTORRHOEA

Galactorrhoea is inappropriate, i.e. non-puerperal, lactation. In the majority of cases it amounts to only a few milky drops on firm manipulation of the breast and nipple, but can occur spontaneously and require constant wearing of absorbent pads. It is usually bilateral.

There are two main causes, which account about equally for most cases – hyperprolactinaemia and mechanical stimulation of the breasts. The few remaining cases have no recognizable cause, although in some galactorrhoea occurs only during oral contraception. Galactorrhoea itself is not harmful, although it might be a nuisance, but may be important as a symptom of hyperprolactinaemia, which is often due to a pituitary tumour (see section on amenorrhoea, above). Treatment should be aimed at the cause and bromocriptine should not be used indiscriminately. Since hyperprolactinaemia nearly always causes oligo- or amenorrhoea it is unlikely to be the cause of galactorrhoea when menstruation is normal.

Physical stimulation is the usual cause of galactorrhoea persisting after breast-feeding in a woman with normal menstrual cycles. It is even possible in this way to induce lactation long after breast-feeding (and even in nulliparous women), sufficient to feed another baby – hence the wet-nurses of old. The mechanism is by neuroendocrine reflex secretion of prolactin. The stimulation is often done out of curiosity 'to see if there is still any milk there', in which case avoidance is easy and effective. However, if the stimulation is sexual it may be hard to give up and there seems no need to insist on it, but temporary avoidance is worth trying because it may be permanently effective.

Galactorrhoea during combined oestrogen–progestogen contraception is also likely to be due to physical stimulation or hyperprolactinaemia. In the latter case, however, the expected clue of amenorrhoea will be masked by the artificially induced bleeds. Serum prolactin should be measured in all cases of galactorrhoea.

Galactorrhoea occurring only during oral contraception and not otherwise is difficult to explain. This is partly because the hormonal control of breast development and lactation (see Chapter 6) is remarkably complicated, involving not only oestrogens, progesterone and prolactin but also growth hormone, cortisol and thyroid hormones. The oestrogen–progestogen contraceptive pill certainly increases prolactin secretion, but not to abnormal levels. In addition to acting directly on the breast it also modifies the effect of other hormones by increasing the circulating amounts of their binding proteins. There seems no need to stop oral contraception just because of galactorrhoea.

FURTHER READING

Gilling-Smith, C., Franks, S. (1997) Hirsutism and virilization. In: *Gynaecology*, 2nd edn, edited by Shaw, R., Soutter, P. and Stanton, S. Churchill Livingstone, Edinburgh.

Hull, M.G.R. and Abuzeid, M.I.M. (1997). Amenorrhoea and oligomenorrhoea, and hypothalamic–pituitary dysfunction. In: *Gynaecology*, 2nd edn. edited by Shaw, R., Soutter, P. and Stanton, S. Churchill Livingstone, Edinburgh.

Speroff, L., Glass, R.H. and Kase, N.G. (eds) (1994) *Clinical Gynaecologic Endocrinology and Infertility*, 5th edn. Williams & Wilkins, Baltimore.

Tolis, G., Bringer, J. and Chrousos, G.P. (1993) Intraovarian regulators and polycystic ovarian syndrome. *Annals of the New York Academy of Science* **687** (whole volume).

16

Abnormal genital bleeding

This chapter is oriented to the clinical problems of abnormal vaginal bleeding, which is a very common symptom with a wide variety of causes, including carcinoma, and the differential diagnoses are of great practical importance. The individual causes and their management are described in other chapters.

Abnormal vaginal bleeding may be classified into:

1 Abnormal menstrual bleeding:
   a. Excessive.
   b. Reduced.
   c. Inappropriate (by age).
2 Non-menstrual bleeding.

A careful history can usually distinguish between menstrual and non-menstrual bleeding. The distinction is of great importance because, while menstrual disorders almost invariably have benign causes that originate beyond the endometrium, non-menstrual bleeding is often from a local lesion, commonly a carcinoma of endometrium or cervix, which must therefore be urgently sought. Menstrual bleeding is recognized by the typical loss (even when excessive it occurs in a typical pattern, uninterrupted for a few days with an early peak) and by its cyclicity (even when the cycle is irregular), whereas non-menstrual bleeding is non-cyclical and patternless. When in doubt one should assume the worse, i.e. non-menstrual bleeding.

ABNORMAL MENSTRUAL BLEEDING

Abnormal menstrual bleeding can easily be classified and defined in its various forms given the definition of normal menstruation (see Chapter 5).

Excessive menstrual bleeding

(Excessive menses but normal cycle, 'Menorrhagia')

Menorrhagia is derived from the Greek words *men* (month) and *rhegynai* (to rush out). Approximately 30% of women referred to a gynaecologist will complain of this symptom and it is the most frequent indication for hysterectomy.

With menorrhagia the blood lost in the menses is excessive enough to clot, and necessitates the use of towels rather than tampons and in excessive number. The duration of loss may or may not be prolonged. The actual blood lost at each menstruation, although of course not measured in practice, is regularly more than 80 ml. The causes to consider are:

Painless
1 Fibroids (see Chapter 24).
2 Ovarian endocrine disorder (dysfunctional bleeding).
3 Coagulation defects (rare).

Painful (i.e. congestive dysmenorrhoea and deep dyspareunia: see Chapter 19)
1 Pelvic inflammation or adhesions (see Chapter 18).
2 Endometriosis (see Chapter 17).
3 Sexual dysfunction (see Chapter 21).

Short cycle (≤21 days) but normal menses (epimenorrhoea or polymenorrhoea)

These cycles are always anovulatory and due to disorder of the hypothamic–pituitary–ovarian endocrine axis, often secondary to stress.

Short cycle and excessive menses (epimenorrhagia)

The causes are those responsible for menorrhagia or epimenorrhoea. Ovarian dysfunction is implied in all cases but is commonly secondary to vascular congestion due to extraovarian lesions.

Excessive menses at long intervals

The typical cause is anovulatory ovarian cycles in which there is prolonged oestrogen production. Oestrogen stimulates proliferation of the endometrium which, if unopposed by progesterone, results in cystic hyperplasia of the endometrium. This syndrome is called metropathia haemorrhagica. In many cases there will be occasional ovulatory cycles where typical endometrial hyperplasia is absent; indeed, secretory changes due to progesterone may be present. Thus the more appropriate term of ovarian endocrine dysfunction (or dysfunctional bleeding) is generally used.

Dysfunctional uterine bleeding

Dysfunctional uterine bleeding is essentially a diagnosis made by exclusion. It describes abnormal cyclical bleeding where any underlying organic cause has been ruled out by appropriate investigation. It usually results from endocrine dysfunction. Ovarian disorder (strictly disorder of the hypothalamic–pituitary–ovarian axis) results in menstrual abnormality, because the endometrium is generally merely a slave to the endocrine signals it receives. The disorder particularly affects the length of the menstrual cycle. The bleeding may appear to be totally disordered and patternless, but in those cases a local lesion must be carefully excluded first. The endocrine disorder can be proven by the absence or deficiency of progesterone. However, these conditions have been imperfectly studied, and in clinical practice there is no use in endocrine determinations unless infertility is an associated problem. Indeed, because these disorders commonly occur in the early and late menstrual years, contraception is the more frequent associated need.

Diagnosis and treatment of excessive menstrual bleeding

An accurate history is essential (see above). Pelvic tumours and tenderness must be sought and treated appropriately (see Chapters 17 and 24). Thyroid dysfunction – particularly hypothyroidism – commonly presents in women in their middle years, will be found in 1% of women with menorrhagia, and can be readily treated. If the pelvic organs feel normal the diagnosis is dysfunctional bleeding and is confirmed if there is a normal menstrual response to hormone therapy (see below). Outpatient endometrial biopsy, diagnostic curettage or hysteroscopy is unnecessary and unhelpful in most cases. It usually only needs to be done if hormone treatment is unsuccessful or contraindicated, to search for an endometrial lesion. Endometrial assessment should be considered more carefully in women over the age of 40 who are more likely to have local pathology. A preliminary transvaginal pelvic ultrasound scan may give useful guidance by demonstrating whether there is abnormal endometrial thickening or any distortion of the endometrial cavity. Coagulation disorders are rare causes of menorrhagia and need only be investigated if there is a specific lead given in the history, such as easy bruising or a familial association.

Treatment depends on the nature of any causative lesion and on the wishes of the patient, including her associated desire for contraception or pregnancy. She may be satisfied merely to know that the condition is harmless. Menstrual disorders resulting in anaemia always need treatment.

Dysfunctional bleeding is most reliably controlled with combined oestrogen and progestogen oral contraception preparations (see Chapter 11). When bleeding is heavy a preparation containing a relatively large progestogen dose is sometimes necessary (e.g. as in Ovran 30 or Loestrin 30). Many patients resume normal menstruation after the treatment is stopped, and treatment should, therefore, be limited initially to only two to three cycles unless, of course, it is also to be used to provide contraception.

If oestrogen therapy is contraindicated (see Chapter 11), then progestogen given alone in the second half of the cycle, days 15–25, is effective in about half the cases by direct action on the endometrium (e.g. norethisterone acetate 10–15 mg daily). Alternatively, progestogen can be given from days 5–25 to shorten the time of unopposed oestrogen stimulation and more fully suppress endometrial proliferation. Some progestogens (danazol, gestrinone) are additionally effective by relatively powerful negative feedback on the pituitary to reduce ovarian hormone secretion. They need to be given throughout the cycle without interruption in a dose, suited to each individual, not so large as to suppress ovarian function altogether, leading to amenorrhoea. However, danazol and gestrinone can cause unpleasant androgenic side-effects in some women (e.g. hirsutism, seborrhoea and voice change) and should be used with appropriate caution.

A number of non-hormonal medical treatments are available, the most effective being the non-steroidal anti-inflammatory drugs, particularly fenamates (e.g. mefenamic acid) which not only inhibit prostaglandin production but also block prostaglandin receptors. These reduce menstrual blood flow and are also effective treatment for any associated dysmenorrhoea. Alternatively drugs that modify capillary integrity (e.g. ethamsylate) or fibrinolysis (e.g. ε-aminocaproic acid) will be partially helpful in half the cases.

Medical treatment may be of limited use in women whose family is complete and who may have many years of menstrual disturbance to face before their natural menopause. Dysfunctional bleeding often recurs in time and repeated courses of medical treatment before a woman 'earns' definitive surgical treatment is only acceptable if it is at the woman's request. There has been recent interest and enthusiasm by patients and gynaecologists for hysteroscopic procedures which remove or destroy the endometrium rather than resorting to hysterectomy. Transcervical resection of the endometrium (TCRE) uses a diathermy loop to resect strips of endometrium down to a level beneath the basement membrane. These strips may then be assessed histologically, unlike after laser ablation where the endometrium is vaporized and destroyed. These operations have a number of potential hazards and have been incompletely evaluated in terms of long-term follow-up studies. The evidence which is currently available suggests there may be an unacceptably high risk of recurrent dysfunctional bleeding with time.

Hysterectomy is always available as a last resort, but the patient's sometimes fervent desire for the operation may hide psychological or sexual problems that need to be properly explored. Nevertheless, there should not be unnecessary delay in discussing the option of hysterectomy. For many women it offers a cure rather than temporary respite from a distressing problem which restricts their quality of life.

Reduced menstrual bleeding

Unlike excessive menstrual bleeding, reduced bleeding is often due to endocrine disorder of serious origin, and frequently occurs in the middle reproductive years when pregnancy is desired, so that proper endocrinological investigations are needed. They are mainly dealt with in Chapter 15. However, they are classified as follows:

Scanty menstrual bleeding (hypomenorrhoea)

The loss usually amounts to no more than a smear lasting not more than 2 days. It is occasionally a normal variant but most commonly occurs in association with infrequent menstrual periods (oligomenorrhoea) as a result of infrequent and impaired ovarian follicular maturation and oestrogen production. Rarely it is due to endometrial fibrosis and partial obliteration of the endometrial cavity (Asherman's syndrome) following traumatic curettage after abortion or childbirth, or due to tuberculosis.

Infrequent menstrual periods (oligomenorrhoea)

See Chapter 15.

Absent menstrual periods (amenorrhoea)

See Chapter 15.

Inappropriate menstrual bleeding

Menstrual bleeding is abnormal before the age of 10 years (precocious puberty; see Chapter 14), after 60 years (delayed menopause) or more than 6 months after a normal menopause. In the last case the isolated resurgence of ovarian activity may be normal, but it is usually impossible to distinguish with certainty from bleeding due to endometrial carcinoma, so that hysteroscopy and biopsy or diagnostic curettage is necessary. With delayed menopause there is some concern about possible endometrial carcinoma due to prolonged (albeit cyclical) oestrogen stimulation unopposed by progesterone, anovulation being presumed. Although the risk is small, diagnostic hysteroscopy and curettage is a wise precaution.

NON-MENSTRUAL BLEEDING

This is non-cyclical, patternless vaginal bleeding which is usually referred to, purely descriptively, as postcoital (PCB), intermenstrual (IMB) or postmenopausal (PMB). IMB and PMB are mutually exclusive, obviously, but either may occur in addition to PCB. (The term metrorrhagia is often used for non-menstrual bleeding but is an inappropriate choice because its meaning – uterine bleeding – is too general.) The implication of non-menstrual bleeding is an anatomical lesion, which must be assumed to be a carcinoma until proved

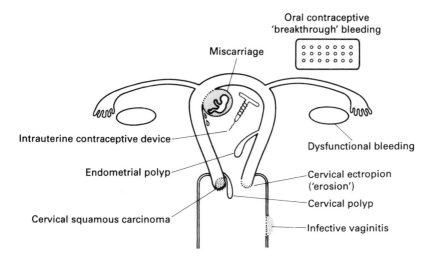

Fig. 16.1 Common and important causes of intermenstrual bleeding.

Table 16.1 Causes of non-menstrual bleeding

Site	Cause	Comments	Chapter reference
Vulva	Carcinoma	Usually postmenopausal	24
Vagina	Vaginitis		
	Infective		18
	Atrophic		23
	Carcinoma		24
	Squamous		
	Adenocarcinoma	Rare but often adolescent	
Cervix	Mucosal ectopy (erosion)		
	Ectropion		24
	Cervicitis		18
	Polyps	Common at all ages	
	Carcinoma		24
	Squamous	Top priority at all ages	
	Adenocarcinoma		
Uterine	Miscarriage	Common	13
body	IUCD	Common	11
	Endometrial polyps		
	Endometrial hyperplasia		
	Endometrial carcinoma	Top priority after menopause	24
	Choriocarcinoma		
Fallopian			
tubes	Carcinoma	Rare	24
Ovaries	Oestogenic tumours		24
	Dysfunction (dysfunctional bleeding)	Common	16
Exogenous			
hormones	Oral contraceptives (breakthrough bleeding)	Common	11
	Oestrogen replacement		23

IUCD = Intrauterine contraceptive device.

otherwise. Bleeding after coital contact suggests a cervical rather than endometrial lesion, whereas IMB or PMB suggests the reverse, but this is not an infallible guide. The causes to consider are shown in Table 16.1 and illustrated in Figures 16.1 and 16.2.

Non-menstrual bleeding is not always due to a lesion. Indeed the commonest cause in young women is miscarriage (Chapter 13), which will be suggested by preceding amenorrhoea and perhaps pain. Ovarian endocrine disorder sometimes causes totally irregular or prolonged dysfunctional bleeding. Oral contraceptives, parti-

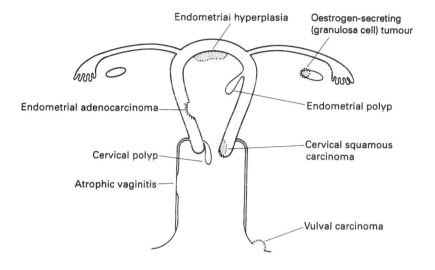

Fig. 16.2 Common and important causes of postmenopausal bleeding.

cularly the progestogen-only pill, sometimes fail to inhibit properly endometrial bleeding, which is then called breakthrough bleeding (see Chapter 11).

Investigation

Non-menstrual bleeding always requires investigation. This involves inspection, diagnostic hysteroscopy or curettage and, if there is a visible lesion, biopsy. Remember that cytology is no substitute for careful visualization of the cervix, because false-negative cytology is commoner with invasive carcinoma than intraepithelial carcinoma, which is symptomless in any case. Diagnostic curettage (but not inspection) can reasonably be postponed in young women when the bleeding has lasted less than a month. Dysfunctional or breakthrough bleeding may persist throughout a disordered cycle and need only be investigated if it occurs in more than one cycle.

The finding on diagnostic curettage of proliferative endometrium after the menopause necessitates looking at the ovaries for the rare possibility of an oestrogen-secreting tumour if there has not been exogenous oestrogen administration to account for it.

When bleeding persists after a miscarriage or childbirth for more than 6 weeks the possibility of a choriocarcinoma should never be overlooked. Although rare, it is truly curable.

Treatment

The treatment is of the cause (see the appropriate chapter reference in Table 16.1).

FURTHER READING

Bayer, S.R. and DeCherney, A.H. (1993) Clinical manifestations and treatment of dysfunctional uterine bleeding. *Journal of the American Medical Association* **269**:1823–1828.

Drife, J.O. (ed.) (1989) *Dysfunctional Uterine Bleeding and Menorrhagia. Clinical Obstetrics and Gynaecology*, vol. 3. Baillière Tindall: London.

Rees, M.C.P. (1992) Modern management of menorrhagia. *Hospital Update* **18**:353–361.

17

Endometriosis and adenomyosis

Endometriosis is one of the most common benign gynaecological disorders. It may be defined as the presence of endometrium-like tissue in ectopic locations outside the uterine cavity. It is mostly found on the peritoneal surfaces of the pelvic organs and deep in the ovaries. Adenomyosis, which used to be called endometriosis interna, means endometrium-like tissue present in the myometrium.

The definition of endometriosis refers to endometrium-like tissue because the glandular and stromal elements, though appearing typical of endometrium, show different responses to the cyclical changes in ovarian hormones. The aetiology, clinical features and management of endometriosis and adenomyosis are different and should be considered separately.

ENDOMETRIOSIS

Aetiology

The aetiology of endometriosis is unknown. Although a number of theories have been proposed, none of these alone can explain the development of the disease in all the sites which have been reported. The main postulated theories are:

1 Implantation of endometrial cells shed into the peritoneal cavity by retrograde menstruation. The viability of menstrual endometrial cells is well recognized and the most common sites of endometriotic deposits are in dependent areas of the pelvis where retrogradely menstruated blood would collect. Retrograde menstruation is however a common normal occurrence; why only some women go on to develop endometriosis is not clear. The intraperitoneal hormonal environment or some degree of immunological deficiency may be important facilitating factors for implantation.

2 Metaplasia of coelomic derivatives. Pelvic peritoneum and ovarian coelomic epithelium are derived embryologically from the same coelomic tissue which forms the Müllerian ducts and uterus. Metaplasia may be induced by infectious or hormonal stimuli or by secretory products released from degenerating endometrial cells reaching the peritoneal cavity by retrograde menstruation.

3 Venous embolization and dissemination. Haematogenous spread of malignant tumours frequently leads to metastatic deposits in the lungs. In a similar way, pulmonary endometriosis (presenting with cyclical haemoptysis at the time of menstruation) may arise by vascular dissemination of endometrial or decidual tissue forced into venous channels by uterine contractions during menstruation or labour.

4 Lymphatic dissemination. Endometrial cells and endometriotic lesions have been reported in both lymphatic vessels and lymph nodes. Lymphatic dissemination is probably responsible for most cases of umbilical endometriosis and is likely to account for some lesions at sites close to the common channels of uterine lymphatic drainage (e.g. kidneys, pleura and retroperitoneal space).

5 Iatrogenic mechanical implantation. Endometrial cells may be accidentally transplanted into surgical incisions. Though rare, the occurrence of endometriomas is most frequent in abdominal scars following caesarean section, hysterotomy or surgical treatment of endometriosis, and in episiotomy scars.

In addition to these aetiological theories there are a number of factors which appear to predispose to endometriosis:

1 *Race*: Although it has traditionally been taught that endometriosis is rare in black women, this only seems to be the case in Africa where younger age at first pregnancy, more frequent pregnancies and a higher incidence of tubal occlusion due to pelvic inflammatory disease reduce the prevalence of retrograde menstruation. There is no difference in the frequency of the disease in black and Caucasian women in the USA. The prevalence of endometriosis in Japanese women is twice that in Caucasian women but there are no clear data on other oriental racial groups.

2 *Genetic and familial factors*: Sisters and mothers of patients with endometriosis are more likely to be affected by the disease themselves. The severity of the disease also seems to be increased in women with an affected first-degree relative. A polygenic or multifactorial maternal inheritance pattern seems the most likely explanation.

3 *Menstrual factors*: Endometriosis is more common in women with Müllerian abnormalities which restrict or obstruct normal menstrual flow, such as lower vaginal atresia (intact hymen). However, there is no apparent risk from the use of tampons or the cervical cap for contraception.

On average, women with endometriosis have had an earlier age of menarche, shorter cycle lengths and longer menstrual flow. Conversely, the lighter menstrual flow associated with combined oral contraceptive use reduces the risk and severity of the disease.

Endometriosis is dependent on the hormonal changes of the normal ovarian cycle. It does not occur before puberty and almost invariably regresses after the menopause. Pregnancy leads to some regression of endometriotic tissue which may be due to the predominance of progesterone, followed by the hypo-oestrogenism during subsequent breast-feeding.

Prevalence

The true prevalence of endometriosis in the general population is unknown. Most disease is diagnosed at laparoscopy but the majority of reports preceded the recent recognition of the more active but non-pigmented lesions (see below) which can easily be missed and the true rate is likely to have been underestimated. Estimates of prevalence vary widely and according to the indication for laparoscopy: up to 80% in women with subfertility, a similar percentage in women with pelvic pain and/or a pelvic mass, and 20% in asymptomatic fertile women undergoing laparoscopic sterilization.

Sites and pathology

Endometrial deposits may be found in various parts of the body but are usually confined to the pelvis, as shown in Figure 17.1. The ovary is the commonest site. The pelvic peritoneum, especially in the pouch of Douglas, and the uterosacral ligaments are also frequently involved. Endometriosis may occur in the bowel, usually in the wall, resulting in stricture or cyclical gastrointestinal bleeding. If the bladder is involved cyclical haematuria may occur. Deposits of endometriosis may be found in the vagina and in scars of the abdominal wall, perineum or uterus. Abdominal wall scars are more likely to be at risk if the endometrial cavity has been opened during surgery (e.g. at myomectomy). An endometriotic deposit at the umbilicus may cause cyclical bleeding externally. Cyclical haemoptysis as well as bleeding from the arm and leg have been reported, but these are extremely rare sites for endometriosis.

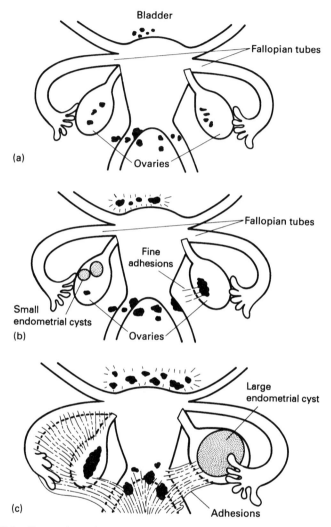

Fig. 17.1   Examples of (a) mild, (b) moderate and (c) severe endo-metriosis in typical sites.

The deposits of endometriosis can vary from minute pinhead-sized spots, typically blackened by haemosiderin, to large cysts filled with old altered blood which becomes thick and brown. These cysts are called chocolate cysts and most commonly develop in the ovary. However, old blood in any cyst has this appearance and both endometrial glands and stroma need to be seen histologically to make the diagnosis of endometriosis.

Recently, atypical non-pigmented lesions have been recognized which may be red, flame-like, white and opacified or simply have the appearance of colourless blisters. These are particularly important because they are more active than pigmented lesions, which seem merely to represent the burnt-out end-stage of disease in those deposits.

The ectopic endometrium usually bleeds when the patient menstruates as most lesions will respond to ovarian hormones in a similar way to normal endometrium. The shed blood can cause an intense fibrous reaction resulting in dense adhesions and cyst formation. Fibrosis may be much worse if a chocolate cyst leaks or ruptures. Endometriosis is relatively commonly associated with fibroids, adenomyosis and endometrial hyperplasia.

Clinical features

The symptoms are very variable and unrelated to the extent of the disease. The most extensive endometriosis may be asymptomatic and discovered incidentally, while small lesions may produce marked symptoms. Infertility may be the main and even the only complaint. The outstanding features are pelvic pain, deep dyspareunia and congestive dysmenorrhoea, which may be caused by small deposits of endometriosis, typically on the uterosacral ligaments and in the pouch of Douglas. Menorrhagia is a frequent symptom due to vascular congestion and, occasionally, associated adenomyosis. If ovarian function is disturbed by direct involvement in endometriosis, the cycle may also alter, usually becoming shorter.

On examination tender nodules (like lead-shot) may be felt along the uterosacral ligaments and in the pouch of Douglas due to endometrial deposits. Tender ovarian masses may be adherent to the uterus, which may, as a result, be fixed, tender and retroverted. Occasionally rupture of an ovarian endometriotic cyst can mimic the signs of a ruptured ectopic pregnancy.

Diagnosis

At best, endometriosis can only be suspected from presenting symptoms and physical signs and there is no reliable serological marker for the disease. The diagnosis should always be confirmed by laparoscopy and if the appearance of the lesions is not characteristic a biopsy should be taken. The main differential diagnosis is pelvic inflammatory disease and, more rarely, pelvic neoplasms. At laparoscopy a very careful and thorough inspection is necessary if endometriosis is suspected. The ovaries need to be lifted up with a probe to check the blind sides (where endometriosis is often hidden) and occasionally it is necessary to needle the ovaries to aspirate a possible deep endometriotic cyst.

Treatment of endometriosis

There are two approaches to treatment, either conservative or radical. Conservative treatment may be hormonal, surgical or a combination of the two. Radical treatment to get rid of the disease is always surgical; hormonal treatment can only suppress it. The choice depends on the severity of symptoms, the site, extent and nature of the endometriotic lesions, and on the age and parity of the patient, and her future desire for pregnancy.

Hormonal therapy

This avoids the risks of surgery and subsequent postoperative adhesions. It is the initial treatment of choice in younger symptomatic women who are concerned about their future fertility. For most hormonal treatments the aim is to interrupt normal hormonal stimulation of endometrial tissue by inducing temporary ovarian inactivity or a pseudopregnancy state

It is important to appreciate that all hormonal therapies suppress but will not eradicate the disease. It is recognized that active endometriotic lesions, like normal endometrium, contain a basement membrane and basal cell layer which will allow deposits to regenerate once treatment is stopped. A range of hormonal treatments are available, as shown in Table 17.1.

Prostaglandin synthetase inhibitors (e.g. naproxen 1000 mg/day) or fenamates, which block prostaglandin receptors as well as inhibiting synthesis, are generally less effective than other hormonal treatments but may be useful for some women who either get no symptomatic benefit or are unable to tolerate other conservative medical approaches.

Table 17.1   Medical treatments for endometriosis

Prostaglandin synthetase inhibitors
Pregnancy (lactation)
Continuous combined oestrogen/progestogen
Continuous progestogens
Danazol
Gestrinone
GnRH (LHRH) agonists

GnRH = Gonodotrophin-releasing hormone; LHRH = luteinizing hormone-releasing hormone.

Pregnancy was once thought to be beneficial as a natural treatment but this has now been shown not to be the case. Any improvement in symptoms following pregnancy is more likely to be related to the hypo-oestrogenic state associated with lactational amenorrhoea.

Continuous use of a combined oral contraceptive pill is generally poorly tolerated due to breakthrough bleeding but may be useful for longer-term pain relief in young women.

Comparative studies of continuous progestogen therapy (e.g. medroxyprogesterone acetate 50 mg daily), danazol, gestrinone and gonadotrophin-releasing hormone (GnRH) agonists suggest that all four hormonal approaches are equally effective for the relief of pain and equally ineffective at improving natural fertility. These treatments are usually given for 6–9 months, based on the duration of pregnancy and the ill-founded belief that pregnancy cured endometriosis. Histologically, the activity of endometriotic implants is fully suppressed by 2–3 months' hormonal therapy and treatment is continued longer as required to maintain pain relief. However, repeated 3–4-month courses are probably as effective for symptom relief as longer durations of treatment and minimize the risk of side-effects that can be a problem with some therapies.

In the treatment of otherwise asymptomatic infertility more prolonged treatment used to be given. It is now clear, however, that hormonal suppression of endometriosis (and ovulation) only delays the opportunity to conceive.

As all hormonal treatments are equally effective in relieving pain, the choice of preparation should depend, logically, on side-effects and relative cost. Progestogens are considerably cheaper than danazol or gestrinone which are, in turn, less expensive than GnRH analogues.

Progestogens counteract the stimulatory proliferative action of oestrogen on endometrial tissue and induce a secretory change similar to the decidual reaction seen in pregnancy. Their major side-effects are breakthrough bleeding, fluid retention and seborrhoea.

Danazol is an androgenic steroid related to testosterone which suppresses gonadotrophin secretion but also has direct actions on ovarian function and endometrial development. Treatment is given orally in a dose of 400–800 mg daily. Side-effects are similar to those of progestogens but, in addition, some women may develop hirsutism, deepening of the voice, clitoromegaly and increased muscularity. These side-effects are related to duration and not necessarily the dosage of danazol treatment.

Gestrinone is also an androgenic steroid with direct antiprogesterone as well as gonadotrophin suppressing actions, and is of high potency. It is given orally in a twice-weekly dosage of 2.5 mg and has a range and incidence of side-effects which are similar to danazol.

GnRH agonists induce profound ovarian inactivity and the resulting oestrogen deficiency is responsible for the majority of their side-effects. These include vasomotor symptoms (hot flushes and night sweats), vaginal dryness and headaches. In addition, there is concern about osteoporosis in the long term, bone loss being evident even within 6 months' treatment. GnRH agonists may be given by nasal spray two to four times daily or by monthly depot injection or subcutaneous implant. These latter two routes have the advantage of achieving the most profound and therefore most rapid suppression of endometriotic activity, but treatment must be switched to steroids for prolonged therapy.

Conservative surgery

This is indicated where a woman still desires fertility but where discrete cystic endometriomas or pelvic adhesions are present which will not usually respond to hormonal therapy.

Conservative surgery is increasingly being undertaken laparoscopically, in some cases at the time of initial diagnostic laparoscopy as a primary treatment. Deposits of endometriosis may be burned with diathermy or vaporized by laser but there is no evidence that this is any more effective than medical therapy for pain relief.

The only evidence for improvement of fertility is from adhesiolysis and excision of ovarian endometriomas which interfere structurally with normal oocyte transport. Laparotomy, using appropriate microsurgical techniques, is usually necessary to deal with dense adhesions and large endometriotic cysts. The results of conservative laser laparoscopy and laparotomy using microsurgical or macrosurgical techniques in the treatment of infertility associated with severe endometriosis (causing structural damage) are illustrated in Figure 17.2.

Recurrence after conservative hormonal or surgical treatment is a common problem. Whether it is truly a recurrence or merely regeneration of original disease remains controversial. Approximately 10% of patients will develop recurrent symptoms within 1 year and 50% within 5 years of any conservative treatment, whether medical or surgical. Patients undergoing conservative surgery have at least a 50% chance of requiring further conservative or radical surgery within 10 years.

Radical surgery

The only curative therapy for endometriosis is radical surgery. This

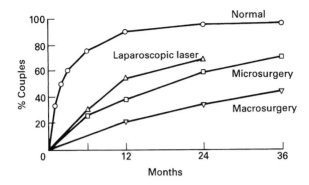

Fig. 17.2 Conception rates after different types of conservative surgery for severe endometriosis.

means total abdominal hysterectomy, bilateral salpingo-oophorectomy and removal of all visible endometriotic lesions. Hysterectomy alone is inadequate as up to 30% of women will require further surgery for recurrent disease within 2 years if the ovaries are conserved.

Oestrogen replacement therapy is not contraindicated after radical surgery as continuous oestrogen does not in practice aggravate any residual endometriosis for most patients. For the few in whom this is a problem, hormone replacement with a continuous combined oestrogen and progestogen may be more appropriate.

ADENOMYOSIS

Although this condition is sometimes referred to as endometriosis interna, this almost certainly misunderstands the condition as adenomyosis generally affects fertile women of an older age grup than endometriosis.

A diagnosis of adenomyosis is usually made by the pathologist following histological assessment of the uterus after hysterectomy for heavy painful periods of unknown cause. The condition may be suspected from this history preoperatively and on examination there may be tender, uniform or localized enlargement of the uterus. Adenomyomas may occasionally be seen on investigation by vaginal ultrasound scanning.

Histologically, endometrial glands and stroma will be seen as islands of tissue with surrounding scarring and evidence of previous haemorrhage deep within the myometrium. It is thought that the lesions develop from decidual fragments passing into venous sinuses after childbirth, or from endometrial overstimulation due to unopposed or excessive oestrogen levels.

The frequency with which the diagnosis is made depends on the assiduity with which the pathologist sections each uterus. Adenomyosis produces a fibrous reaction and lumps known as adenomyomas develop with many clinical similarities to fibroids. Adenomyosis may be associated with fibroids, endometrial hyperplasia, endometriosis and endometrial carcinoma.

The differential diagnosis includes pelvic inflammatory disease, endometrial carcinoma and fibroids.

Treatment of adenomyosis is usually by hysterectomy since hormonal treatment is generally unsatisfactory.

FURTHER READING

Brosens, I. (ed.) (1993) *Endometriosis. Clinical Obstetrics and Gynaecology*, vol. 7.4. Ballière Tindall, London.

18

Genital infections, pruritus and discharge

Infection in the genital tract may result in sterility, chronic pelvic pain, menstrual disorders, dyspareunia (painful intercourse) and general ill health. It is a common cause of death in the developing world, although rarely so in the UK. Prompt diagnosis and treatment are important to minimize damage and the consequent serious long-term problems. The agents responsible are often sexually transmitted but not invariably so.

Some infections and inflammations may affect only the lower genital tract, e.g. vulvovaginitis or vulvitis alone. Other infections may involve the upper genital tract by spreading via the cervix (cervicitis), uterus (endometritis) and parametrium (parametritis) or fallopian tubes (salpingitis) to the ovaries (salpingo-oophoritis) and pelvic peritoneum (peritonitis). Eventually the whole pelvis may be involved (pelvic inflammatory disease, or PID) by acute suppuration (acute PID), abscess formation in the tubes (pyosalpinx) or involving the ovaries as well (tubo-ovarian abscess), later leading to restrictive and/or painful adhesions (chronic PID). A pyosalpinx causing fibrotic occlusion of the fimbrial end of the tube will lead to permanent fluid collection in the tube and distension (hydrosalpinx) although active infection has resolved. Acute PID may also lead to blood-borne spread (septicaemia) and death.

It is important to distinguish between lower and upper genital tract infection. Lower genital tract infections can cause extreme discomfort and distress. They may be recurrent and difficult to eradicate. However, although some viral infections are linked to risk of cervical cancer there are generally no long-term complications.

However the same is not true for upper genital tract infections involving pelvic peritonitis (PID), which are still a major cause of death worldwide, particularly puerperal sepsis (i.e. after childbirth) and postabortal sepsis. Such ascending infections often fail to cause any lower genital tract symptoms. Indeed some PID, like the current scourge due to *Chlamydia trachomatis*, can often be symptomless although causing devastating silent tubal damage with consequent sterility. It also causes what was (and often still is) called non-specific urethritis (NSU) in men. It used to be assumed that gonorrhoea was the main cause of PID and tubal infertility but it is now recognized that *C. trachomatis* is the most frequent cause and is by far the most common sexually transmitted disease in the western world. It is sometimes called the silent scarifier of Fallopian tubes.

In any case of suspected PID the presence of *Chlamydia* should be carefully sought in a swab from the cervical canal (and from the pelvis if laparoscopy is done). Special medium is required for culture but that is unreliable and specific antigen testing is preferred. In symptomless women presenting with infertility *Chlamydia* antibody serology should be done to check for evidence of past infection likely to have caused tubal damage. In acute cases prompt treatment is required to minimize such damage.

The specific treatments of choice for *Chlamydia* are the tetracyclines, and the quinolone antibiotic ofloxacin, and the macrolides, erythromycin and azithromycin. These should be combined with broad-spectrum antibiotics in cases of acute PID on the assumption that *Chlamydia* may be complicated by secondary infecting organisms. Therapy should be started without waiting for confirmation of the organism, to minimize the damaging effects of the infection.

The sexual partner(s) should also be traced and treated as an essential part of effective treatment; this is often forgotten by gynaecologists to whom the woman frequently presents alone. Sensitive discussion with the patient and close liaison with the specialist department dealing with sexually transmitted diseases (STDs) is advisable, and usually more acceptable to the partner(s).

In cases of lower genital infection, in which the organism may be readily identified such as *Trichomonas vaginalis* (see below), it is common practice simply to treat the male partner for the same condition without further consideration. It should be remembered, however, that one sexually transmitted organism is often accompanied by others and every effort should be made to search for all the common organisms, particularly those like *Chlamydia* which can cause silent pelvic infection and damage.

LOWER GENITAL TRACT PROBLEMS

Inflammations and infections of the vulva, vagina and cervix cause much misery because of:

1 Itching, called pruritus vulvae.
2 Discharge.

These symptoms will be considered as problems for management before dealing systematically with the many causes.

Pruritus vulvae

Pruritus vulvae or vulval itching is often chronic, can disrupt sleep and interfere with most activities. The cause is often elusive, which is frustrating for both sufferer and doctor (Table 18.1). In obscure and resistant cases collaboration between a gynaecologist and dermatologist can be helpful; indeed, in some centres a joint clinic is held for vulval diseases. The first priority in management of this condition is to exclude carcinoma or precancerous conditions of the vulva by biopsy of any abnormal area of skin.

Table 18.1 Systematic summary of types of cause of pruritis vulvae (specific causes will be discussed later)

Vulvovaginal	*Systemic disease*
Infections	Uraemia
Infestations	Hepatitis
Discharge without infection	Hodgkin's disease
Chemical – direct or allergic	Pernicious anaemia
Mechanical	
Urinary	*Psychosomatic*
Incontinence	Sexual frustration
Glycosuria	
Pyuria	
Anal	*Malignancy*
Haemorrhoids	
Threadworms	
Skin disease (generalized or localized)	
Dermatitis	
Dermatoses, e.g. psoriasis, lichen sclerosis	

Identifiable causes (see later) should be sought and treated specifically. Often no infection or other cause is found, in which case empirical palliative treatment with 1% hydrocortisone cream twice daily is frequently effective but may need to be repeated if pruritus returns. Avoidance of hot baths and thick nightwear is advised, and the wearing of gloves at night may reduce the trauma caused by scratching. Cotton underwear, stockings and skirts are to be preferred to synthetic materials, tights and tight jeans.

Vaginal discharge

This is a common problem. Pertinent queries about the discharge include:

1 Is it blood stained?
2 What colour is it?
3 What is its consistency?
4 How much is there?
5 Is protection needed? If so, what (e.g. sanitary pads) and how often?

Questions about its background and possible aetiology:

1 How long does it last?
2 What started it?
3 Is it related to the menstrual cycle?
4 Does it vary during the day?
5 Is medication being taken (e.g. antibiotics or oral contraceptive pill)?
6 Has it occurred before?
7 Does her partner have a urethral discharge?
8 Are there associated symptoms, e.g. pruritus, pain, odour?
9 Does she use tampons, douches or any other vaginal device (of which there can be an imaginative variety!)

Before examination:

1 Does she have the discharge at present or has she washed, bathed or douched so as to be 'clean' for the clinic visit?
2 All the equipment likely to be needed should be available: all types of swabs and media, various specula, a good light source, and a slide and microscope to examine a wet preparation immediately in saline.

The patient should be positioned in such a way that the vulva, introitus and perineum can be inspected, and swabs, scrapings or superficial punch biopsies as appropriate can be taken. The use of a colposcope to examine the vulva with magnification may also be helpful.

Swabs from the anal canal, perineum, lower vagina, upper vagina, cervical canal and urethra may all be necessary. A slide for Gram staining may be relevant if gonorrhoea is suspected. The swabs should be placed in appropriate media and forwarded to the laboratory at once.

Treatment depends on the causes, discussed in the specific sections that follow.

VULVITIS

The vulva is remarkably resistant to bacterial infection in spite of constant contact with urine, vaginal secretions and faecal organisms. Poor hygiene reduces the vulva's natural resistance. Inflammation of the vulva (vulvitis) may occur alone, or in conjunction with inflammation of the vagina (vulvovaginitis).

Clinical features of vulvitis are severe irritation (pruritus vulvae) with intense burning pain which is exacerbated by micturition. On examination the labia may be tense and swollen, and there may be accompanying vulval or vaginal discharge. The introitus can be so tender that vaginal examination and coitus are impossible. Specific causes to be considered are as follows.

Mechanical trauma

If pruritus is present the patient may be unable to stop herself scratching particularly at night and the vulvitis will be aggravated by the mechanical trauma.

Chemical agents

The use of chemical agents such as antiseptics (commonly TCP or Dettol) in the bath-water, vaginal deodorants or biological washing powders may cause chemical or allergic reactions; various over-the-counter medicaments including herbals and oils used to treat or alleviate the vulvitis may themselves cause adverse reactions and further aggravate the condition. Nylon underwear which fails to absorb moisture, particularly if worn in association with tights and tight jeans, adds to maceration of vulval skin, predisposing to vulvitis. Poor hygiene may be a contributory factor, for example in elderly obese women who are unable to carry out personal toilet adequately after defecation.

Infections

Candidiasis (*Monilia* or thrush) due to the yeast *Candida albicans* may cause acute vulvitis alone but more commonly vulvovaginitis. However, it is also often found without symptoms at routine examination. Candidiasis can cause redness of the vulva and strawberry appearance of the vagina with a thick, white, cheesy discharge (see below). Exacerbation of the infection is found in association with pregnancy, diabetes mellitus and antibiotic therapy. There is no evidence that infection with candida is associated with or exacerbated by oral contraceptive therapy. This is a myth based on work often since refuted but unfortunately perpetuated; neither is recurrence more likely in women taking oral contraception.

Trichomoniasis of the vagina due to the protozoon *Trichomonas vaginalis* (see below) causes a secondary vulvitis and severe pruritus, so the vagina must always be examined. A profuse, frothy, yellow-green discharge may be apparent at the introitus bathing the vulva.

Herpes infection of the vulva (herpes genitalis) due to herpesvirus hominis type 2 is sexually transmitted and is characterized by groups of small vesicles with surrounding erythema and oedema, producing an intense localized vulvitis and sometimes vaginitis and cervicitis too. Acyclovir cream used topically or tablets taken orally at the earliest stages of the eruption can counter the infection. However, the diagnosis is not usually made until later when there is no effective treatment. Herpesvirus type 2 may be implicated in the genesis of cervical dysplasia and carcinoma (see Chapter 24).

Condylomata acuminata (or venereal warts) are papillary warty growths of the vulva, vagina, perineum and occasionally cervix caused by the human papillomavirus (HPV). The warts have a narrow base (unlike the broad-based condylomata lata of syphilis: see below). They produce a profuse irritant discharge and often coexist with *T. vaginalis*. Treatment is with topical podophyllin 10% in tincture of benzoin for smaller lesions. It is important to protect the surrounding skin with petroleum jelly before painting with podophyllin. Since podophyllin is absorbed and is teratogenetic it should not be used in pregnancy. Cautery, cryosurgery, laser ablation or surgical excision may be needed for larger lesions. The vagina and cervix may also be involved and HPV has been implicated in the genesis of cervical dysplasia and carcinoma (see Chapter 24).

Folliculitis of the hair follicles of the vulva due to bacterial infection is common particularly with diabetes and may become chronic. It is treated with antibiotics in the early stages, but if an abscess forms it requires incision. Sebaceous cysts are common and if secondarily infected may also form abscesses.

Bartholinitis and Bartholin's cyst and abscess. The gonococcus may infect Bartholin's gland and duct bilaterally, emitting a bead of pus at each opening (see Fig. 4.2), but acute bartholinitis rarely presents in this way clinically. Usually, unnoticed infection blocks one of the ducts which then fills with secretion from the gland and forms a cyst, as shown in Figure 18.1. The swelling may be noticed but a Bartholin's cyst is otherwise asymptomatic unless it becomes infected, forming a very painful abscess. Treatment is by marsupialization – eversion of the cyst or abscess wall and suturing

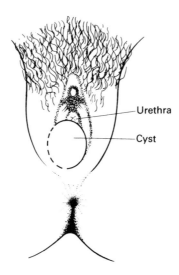

Fig. 18.1   A right-sided Bartholin's cyst (of the duct: see Fig. 4.2) presenting as a characteristic ovoid swelling of the labia at the postero-lateral aspect of the vulva.

it to the overlying skin to allow passage of the secretions. Recurrence of an abscess may necessitate excision given antibiotic cover. Staphylococci, streptococci and *Escherichia coli* are the common organisms involved. Recurrent infection in the older woman may be due to unsuspected diabetes or, very rarely, carcinoma of the gland (see Chapter 24).

Pediculosis pubis due to lice causing irritation in the pubic hair region is transmitted by intimate bodily contact. Various insecticides can be used, such as malathion, and may need to be changed due to resistance. Lotions remain longer and are therefore more effective than shampoos. All members of the affected household should be treated. Another infestation causing pubic irritation is scabies, which also requires treatment of all the family – benzyl benzoate or lindane for the adults, and a less irritant preparation such as mono-sulfiram for the children.

Threadworm infestation usually occurs in children. The worms migrate from the anus at night causing severe irritation. The trauma of scratching produces lesions which are further readily infected. Treatment is with piperazine sulphate.

Skin diseases

The vulval skin may be involved along with a generalized skin disease such as a dermatitis or a dermatosis like psoriasis, lichen sclerosis or eczema, or the vulva may be affected alone. In the obese, intertrigo is common due to moisture of the labial and inguinal regions. Specific localized vulval dystrophies which are potentially cancerous (see Chapter 24) present with pruritus and appear as thickened white or thin red areas, sometimes with cracking. Clinical diagnosis is difficult and any abnormal vulval skin should be examined with a colposcope (for magnification) and biopsied to detect possible malignancy.

VAGINITIS

Vaginitis may occur if the protective physiological environment of the vagina is altered. To maintain its normal bacterial flora the vagina has to be oestrogenized and consequently thickened, moist and acidic. The glycogen produced in the squamous epithelial cells in response to oestrogen is converted to hydrogen peroxide and lactic acid by lactobacilli (Döderlein's bacillus), keeping the pH of the adult vagina at about 4. This acidity provides protection against invasion by microorganisms such as staphylococci and streptococci. The protective acidity and thickness of the squamous epithelium of the vagina are optimal during reproductive life, but can be impaired in some circumstances. Vaginal acidity is reduced during menstruation and sometimes by excessive secretion of cervical mucus, which is alkaline. Vaginal douches and deodorants may also disturb vaginal pH. Antibiotics disturb the normal vaginal flora and lactobacilli are particularly sensitive to broad-spectrum antibiotics. Low oestrogen states as during lactation and before puberty and after the menopause result in a thin vaginal epithelium with low glycogen content which is susceptible to bacterial infection but may also cause a non-infective atrophic vulvovaginitis.

The symptoms of vaginitis of any cause include vaginal itching or soreness, superficial dyspareunia and usually a discharge. The nature of the discharge varies with the cause of the vaginitis, usually in a characteristic way. Table 18.2 summarizes the causes of vaginitis and vaginal discharge.

Infections

Trichomoniasis

Trichomoniasis due to the protozoon *Trichomonas vaginalis* causes a typical thin, greenish-yellow foamy discharge with an unpleasant,

Table 18.2 Systematic summary of causes of vaginitis and vaginal discharge

Infective Trichomonas vaginalis Candida albicans Chlamydia trachomatis Gardnerella vaginalis	*Secretions* Cervicitis Excessive cervical mucus Carcinoma – cervix, vagina Necrotic polyp – cervical, or extruded uterine fibroid
Atrophic Postmenopausal Prepubertal	*Excretions* Urinary fistula Faecal fistula
Mechanical Foreign body Trauma	
Chemical Douches Pessaries Deodorants	

characteristic smell, and usually a constant vulvovaginal irritation. There may also be a strawberry-like punctate reddening of the vagina and/or cervix. The diagnosis can be made in the clinic by examining a drop of the discharge mixed with saline under the microscope to see the pear-shaped protozoan moving with its undulatory membrane and long flagellum (Fig. 18.2). Treatment is with oral metronidazole 200 mg t.d.s for 7 days, for both the patient and her partner at the same time, since the organism is transmitted sexually and harboured asymptomatically in the male. Alcohol

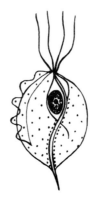

Fig. 18.2 *Trichomonas vaginalis.*

324   Undergraduate Obstetrics and Gynaecology

should be avoided during treatment since metronidazole has a disulfiram (Antabuse)-like action. Metronidazole can be given safely in pregnancy but, as with most drugs, should be avoided in the first trimester.

An appreciable number of women with trichomonal vaginitis will also have other sexually transmitted organisms, particularly *Chlamydia* and sometimes the gonococcus. These should be sought by taking swabs from the urethra, cervical canal and vaginal vault for appropriate culture, Gram staining and *Chlamydia* antigen testing.

Fungal infections

Candidiasis (*Monilia* or thrush) due to the yeast *Candida albicans* is the commonest and frequently also involves the vulva. The discharge is thick, white and cheesy. It is not offensive but is intensely pruritic and also causes soreness and dyspareunia. Treatment is with antifungal vaginal pessaries or creams, of which there are numerous varieties and dose regimens, e.g. nystatin 100 000 units in a vaginal tablet pessary nightly for 14 nights, or clotrimazole 500 mg vaginal tablet pessary as a single dose at night. Application of matching antifungal cream to the vulva facilitates the insertion of the pessary and aids treatment. There is also a single-dose oral preparation, difluconazole, which is effective and well-accepted but expensive. Because reinfection is common, more prolonged and repeated courses of standard antifungal treatment are often necessary. Common asymptomatic sources of reinfection are the gastrointestinal tract and sometimes under the partner's prepuce. Systemic antifungal therapy, and cream applied to the penis, may help break the cycle of recurrence.

Bacterial vaginosis

Bacterial vaginosis is a syndrome caused by disturbance of the normal vaginal flora and an overgrowth of anaerobic bacteria, mainly *Gardnerella vaginalis* and *Mycoplasma hominis*, replacing the favourable types of lactobacilli which produce hydrogen peroxide and lactic acid. The condition is characterized by a thin milky, some-times copious, vaginal discharge accompanied by an unpleasant fishy smell due to excess amines produced by the anaerobic bacteria. It is not clear what causes the disturbance of the normal vaginal bacterial flora but it may be associated with antibiotics, douching, new sexual partners, increased sexual activity, intrauterine contra-ceptive device usage, a debilitating illness or gynaecological surgery. The diagnosis is made by testing for lack of acidity of the vagina and identifying 'clue cells' in the discharge, in association with the distinctive fishy odour amplified by a positive 'whiff test' after adding potassium hydroxide to a sample of the discharge. Clue cells are bacteria-covered cells from the vaginal wall with borders that are obscured, indistinct or roughened. Treatment is by metronidazole pessaries or oral tablets, and the partner should be treated too as for trichomoniasis, but greater dosage and duration may be needed, e.g. 400 mg t.d.s. for 10 days.

Chlamydial infection

Chlamydia trachomatis is one of three *Chlamydia* species (the others being *C. psittaci* and *C. pneumoniae*) of small specialized bacteria which depend on intracellular existence in the host. As previously emphasized, chlamydial infection is of major importance in gynaecology, being the main cause of tubal infertility in the western world, often after silent infection, and a frequent cause of chronic pain and other problems due to pelvic adhesions. In obstetric practice chlamydial conjunctivitis of the newborn is now far more common than gonococcal but is fortunately not as serious. The cervix is the reservoir for the organism, which often causes minimal symptoms. Special transport media are needed for culture but that is unreliable. The organism is best detected by antigen testing using an immunoassay. (By contrast, antibody serology relates to infection in the past.) Specific treatment is by tetracyclines but must be prolonged to 3–4 weeks, or the quinolone antibiotics, oflaxacin or the macrolides, erythromycin and azithromycin. If vaginitis is associated with acute PID, treatment should be combined with broad-spectrum antibiotic therapy because of likely secondary bacterial infection. If vaginitis presents in pregnancy, and *Chlamydia* organisms are found (acute PID would not occur), erythromycin should be preferred as specific treatment. It is also critical that the male partner is treated, as described earlier.

Atrophic vaginitis

In postmenopausal women the vaginal skin is thin, the pH alkaline and the protective lactobacilli lacking. Irritation, soreness and dyspareunia are common. Discharge is not a prominent feature, rather dryness, but bleeding may be. If the postmenopausal woman complains of bleeding, whether just spotting or frank blood, a full examination including assessment of the endometrium by hysteroscopy and biopsy or curettage is mandatory, to look for endometrial carcinoma even if atrophic vaginitis is present as the likely cause. Oestrogen therapy, local or systemic, will overcome atrophic vaginitis. A short course may need to be repeated regularly because of returning symptoms, and long-term needs should be considered in the wider context of oestrogen replacement therapy, as discussed in Chapter 23. Alternatively lactic acid jelly or pessaries may be helpful.

Vaginitis due to foreign body

In children a small object may be inserted exploratively into the vagina, or fluff or toilet tissue may accumulate due to poor hygiene, and form a nidus for infection. In young women a tampon may be forgotten, and there are many reports of extraordinary items removed from the vagina, ranging from champagne corks and wine glasses to bicycle pumps and milk bottles. In the postmenopausal woman a forgotten ring pessary is common. In all cases a profuse offensive discharge is produced, which is cured by removal of the object, although postmenopausal women may also benefit from a short course of oestrogen cream or lactic acid jelly.

Chemical vaginitis

Direct or allergic reactions may occur in the vagina due to chemicals contained in douches, deodorants, bath salts, antiseptics and biological washing powders, and rarely to condoms or even semen. Vaginal soreness is the predominant symptom, rather than discharge. The vagina looks red and inflamed. Careful questioning is necessary to discover the cause.

Secretions causing discharge

Excessive cervical secretion may occur in pelvic congestion syndrome or due to excessive cervical mucosal ectopy. The discharge will not cause any vulvovaginal soreness or irritation, nor any blood-staining. Frequently, however, the patient complains of its offensive odour, although this is often not detected by anyone else, and contamination may irritate the perivulval area. The discharge produces a mixed growth of normal vaginal bacterial flora when cultured.

It is also not uncommon for women, early in their coital experience, to complain of a discharge after intercourse, which is semen. That is simply distinguished by the history and lack of pathological characteristics. Simple explanation is needed about the volume of semen and that only a tiny fraction being sperm leaves the vagina by penetrating the cervix.

Excretions causing vaginitis

Contamination of the vagina with urine from a vesicovaginal fistula or faeces from a rectovaginal fistula (as a result of cancer or obstetric injury, for example) causes secondary vulvovaginitis. The treatment is to deal with the underlying cause if possible, but barrier creams and antiseptic vaginal douches may help.

CERVICITIS

Acute cervicitis

Acute inflammation of the cervix is rare and is usually gonococcal or herpetic in origin, and usually asymptomatic.

Chronic cervicitis

Chronic inflammation of the cervix is a more common cause of symptoms. It is often associated with pelvic pain, discharge and dyspareunia. On examination the cervix is enlarged by multiple mucosal retention cysts, or Nabothian follicles (see Chapter 24), which have become secondarily infected, usually with a mixed bacterial flora. Of the specific causes of chronic cervicitis, *Chlamydia* is the most common. Its detection and treatment were discussed above. Tuberculosis is rare.

Management

A cervical smear should be sent for cytological examination to detect cellular changes due to infection, and cervical and vaginal swabs for bacteriological culture and *Chlamydia* antigen detection. A specific organism is seldom found, however, and antibiotic therapy is therefore seldom needed.

Treatment is usually empirical, aimed at destroying the chronically inflamed Nabothian follicles by cauterization This may be done by cryocautery or electrocautery in the outpatient clinic, but more extensive lesions requiring deeper electrocautery or conization (excision) need to be treated under general anaesthesia. Cautery will cause a marked discharge for 7–10 days and may be associated with secondary haemorrhage around the 10th day as the slough is shed. Rarely, cautery leads to cervical stenosis.

UPPER GENITAL TRACT INFECTIONS

These are of major importance as they can cause death and sterility.

The uterus

Infection of the cervix is common, but spread of infection to the uterus is inhibited by the cervical mucus. The upper part of the cervical canal and the endometrial cavity usually remain sterile. The endometrium is remarkably resistant to infection and, while salpingitis is common, **endometritis** is rare. Infection virtually only occurs when the endometrium is damaged following abortion, miscarriage or parturition. After the menopause secretions may collect in the endometrial cavity if the internal cervical os is stenosed and occluded by atrophy, carcinoma or associated radiotherapy. This collection may become infected and is called a **pyometra**. The symptoms are commonly a purulent or serosanguinous discharge and sometimes abdominal pain and fever. On examination the uterus is enlarged and may be tender, softened and cystic. Treatment is dilatation of the cervical canal to drain the uterus and diagnostic curettage to look for an underlying carcinoma.

Pelvic inflammatory disease

This broad term covers infection involving the tubes, ovaries, parametrium and pelvic peritoneum. Gut may also be involved by adhesions. PID may be acute or chronic.

Causes

1 Sexually transmitted infections ascending through the genital tract, particularly *Chlamydia trachomatis* or, less frequently, *Neisseria gonorrhoeae*, and sometimes other organisms.
2 Direct infection due to trauma, usually related to surgically induced abortion or to delivery of a baby. Infection is by gut or vaginal commensals, quite commonly anaerobic organisms (e.g. *Bacteroides*).
3 Blood-borne infection, classically tuberculosis, usually at the time of puberty, which produces a silent chronic salpingitis and endometritis. Fibrosis can cause severe functional mural damage to the tubes apart from occlusion, and occasionally complete obliteration of the endometrial cavity.
4 Transperitoneal infection from, for example, appendicitis or diverticulitis.

Acute pelvic inflammatory disease

In **salpingitis** the fallopian tubes are congested and oedematous and on microscopy are found to be infiltrated by polymorphonuclear leukocytes. The endotubal mucosa exudes seropurulent fluid and the mucosal folds may be destroyed or agglutinated by fibrinous adhesions. The tubal lumen may become occluded and the wall eventually thickened by fibrosis. Initially pus escapes from the abdominal ostium but this usually becomes quickly occluded to confine the pus, and the tubes become distended and typically retort-shaped. This collection of pus in the tube is known as a **pyosalpinx**. When infection is eventually overcome the blocked tube remains filled with serous fluid, called a **hydrosalpinx**. The initial leakage of pus into the peritoneal cavity may cause **acute pelvic peritonitis**. Spread of infection to the ovary usually binds it closely to the tube and is called **salpingo-oophoritis**, and may result in the formation of a combined **tubo-ovarian abscess**. A collection of pus in the pouch of Douglas is called a pelvic abscess.

Clinical features

The usual symptoms are bilateral lower abdominal pain and fever, deep dyspareunia (if there is any coital activity at all while the patient is ill), and sometimes vaginal discharge.

Abdominal examination in the acute phase characteristically reveals rebound suprapubic tenderness in both iliac fossae. Vaginally, there is bilateral adnexal tenderness, but as yet no swelling. Moving the cervix produces pain (so-called cervical excitation pain). The differential diagnosis is from other causes of acute abdominal pain such as appendicitis, ectopic pregnancy and a twisted ovarian cyst. In all those cases the features are usually unilateral. Salpingitis is never unilateral unless one tube has been removed. After several days, pyosalpinges or tubo-ovarian abscesses may be palpated as bilateral tense, tender, fixed masses. It is imperative that examination at this stage is carried out with utmost gentleness to prevent rupture of the masses leading to generalized peritonitis.

The diagnosis can often only be made definitively by laparoscopy, which also affords the opportunity to take swabs from the fimbrial ends of the tubes and from the pouch of Douglas. The swabs must be transported urgently to the laboratory in the appropriate media for aerobic and anaerobic culture, for *Chlamydia* antigen identification, and a slide sent for Gram staining. Swabs from the lower genital tract are often unhelpful, but should nevertheless be cultured, particularly for *Neisseria gonorrhoeae*, and tested for *Chlamydia* antigen. For that reason swabs should be taken not only from the vagina but also from the cervical canal and urethra.

Treatment

Acute salpingitis is treated with high doses of broad-spectrum antibiotics, including an antichlamydial agent, bed rest and analgesia. Treatment should be started without waiting for bacteriological confirmation of the causative organisms. Early diagnosis and treatment are vital to preserve the function of the fallopian tubes. Once an exudate starts to form, the mucosal folds and fimbria become oedematous, lose their cilia, fuse and may eventually block the tubal lumen or ostium. Even if the tube remains patent, subsequent fertility is grossly impaired due to irreversible functional damage to the mucosa and fimbria.

Severe acute PID with pelvic abscess can cause death, although this is unusual in the UK. Surgical drainage of the pus may be required.

Chronic pelvic inflammatory disease

If treatment of the acute stage is delayed or is inadequate then fibrous damage and adhesions between tube, ovary and surrounding structures usually follow, and the uterus may be drawn into fixed retroversion. The mucosal folds and cilia of the tubes may be largely destroyed, and the tubal lumen may be blocked, most commonly at the fimbrial (distal) end, less often at the proximal end, and infrequently near the middle. Chlamydial infection of the pelvis may bring about all these changes, however, without any apparent acute illness.

Clinical features and management

Fibrosis of the fallopian tubes and inactive adhesions involving other pelvic organs are often, but not always, associated with persistent lower abdominal pain, which is usually bilateral, and deep dyspareunia. There may also be persistent vaginal discharge or menorrhagia. Active chronic inflammation is uncommon but would be suggested by a low-grade fever. There is generalized lower abdominal tenderness, which may now be worse on one side, but there is no rebound tenderness. On pelvic examination, unilateral or bilateral firm tender adnexal masses may be palpable, often adherent to both the uterus and the pelvic side wall.

Acute exacerbations are common and should initially be treated conservatively (i.e. with antibiotics, rest and analgesics) but may eventually require surgical intervention. Total hysterectomy and bilateral salpingo-oophorectomy ('pelvic clearance') followed by oestrogen replacement therapy is the treatment of choice if the patient is prepared to accept loss of her fertility. It may be possible to conserve one or both ovaries in some cases. Operations to restore fertility, by restoring tubal patency and tubo-ovarian anatomy, have limited success (see Chapter 12). Such operations must be done in a quiescent phase of the disease under antibiotic cover.

Differential diagnosis of PID – a cautionary note

The diagnosis of chronic PID is not clear-cut. It is one of the most frequently pronounced, unconfirmed and erroneous gynaecological diagnoses made. The initials PID might well often stand for poorly investigated diagnosis! Be careful not to hang the label of pelvic inflammatory disease round the neck of every woman who complains of lower abdominal pain and is tender on examination. Once done, for ever after any episode of pain will be passed off as 'a flare-up of PID' and treated with antibiotics, often pointlessly. The diagnosis should remain open until laparoscopy is undertaken along with careful bacteriological examination of swabs taken from the pouch of Douglas, the fimbrial ends of the tubes and of any free fluid in the peritoneal cavity, together with triple swabs (high vaginal, cervical and urethral). Chronic pelvic discomfort may result from inactive adhesions, or the pelvic organs may be found to appear completely healthy, in which case psychosexual dysfunction may be the underlying problem (see Chapter 21).

Sexually transmitted diseases

STDs must be seen in relation to customs, attitudes, mores and behaviour, both individual and communal. Society and culture influence the spread of STDs. Some are endemic in almost every part of the world, whilst others, like syphilis, have become sporadic in some countries. STDs tend to become epidemic during times of strife, and particular epidemics may occur in connection with sexual promiscuity, prostitution and homosexual practices.

   In the UK the law outdatedly recognizes only three infections as venereal: gonorrhoea, syphilis and 'non-specific urethritis, NSU'. In fact, *Chlamydia trachomatis* is far more frequent and is now known to account for most cases of NSU. Other STDs have also assumed greater importance, namely herpes and acquired immunodeficiency syndrome (AIDS). Other conditions, though rare, such as chancroid, granuloma inguinale and lymphogranuloma venereum, are mostly transmitted sexually. These last three are usually described together, all causing genital sores. They tend to be limited to seaboard cities with warmer climates than the UK.

   Herpes, papillomavirus and *Chlamydia* infections have been mentioned previously. Gonorrhoea, syphilis and AIDS will be discussed here. Reference to a textbook of genitourinary medicine is more appropriate to cover other STDs which rarely present to a gynaecologist.

Gonorrhoea

During the years 1946–55 the incidence of gonorrhoea and syphilis fell dramatically in nearly all countries as a result of antibiotic therapy, and those diseases were thought to be dying out. Since then, however, there has been a steady increase and the World Health Organization has now declared gonorrhoea to be out of control. Apart from the common cold it is the most prevalent infectious disease. The increase has occurred in females rather than males, and in adolescents rather than adults. Indeed, a quarter of all female cases now occur in women under 20 years old. The explanations for this continuing rise in incidence are development of drug-resistant gonococci, shifting populations and increased promiscuity among the young. The last is the most important and is creating serious medicosocial problems.

The causative organism is *Neisseria gonorrhoeae*, a Gram-negative diplococcus. Infection is by sexual contact, including oral and anal. The incubation period is usually 2–5 days with a virulent organism and low host resistance, but may be as long as 8 weeks with low virulence and high host resistance. The sites of infection are tissues not covered with stratified squamous epithelium, i.e. commonly the urethra, including the paraurethral tubules, Bartholin's glands and the endocervix. The buccal and anal mucosa may also be involved.

Clinical features

Infected women are frequently symptomless. Otherwise the initial complaints are of dysuria, urinary frequency and vaginal discharge. The discharge causes soreness but not pruritus unless there is an associated trichomonal infection. In severe cases, the whole vulva becomes reddened and swollen; inguinal adenitis, general malaise and fever are then likely. Cystitis is a possible development. Untreated gonorrhoea persists as a chronic and contagious disease for many years. The organisms linger in the endocervix, Bartholin's glands and periurethral tubules. Remote lesions may involve joints, tendons and ligaments (probably due to associated non-gonococcal infection). Complications include endometritis, salpingitis and pelvic peritonitis. It is probably the commonest cause of tubal occlusion. The fetus can be infected during delivery and ophthalmia neonatorum (gonococcal conjunctivitis) was a major cause of blindness in the past. It is essential that the gonococcus is eradicated in pregnancy.

The diagnosis is suggested by the history of contact and the acuteness of onset of a purulent discharge with associated urethritis, and is made by demonstrating the gonococcus by Gram stain and culture. Failure to culture the organism often occurs if proper transport medium and plating procedures are not used. When gonorrhoea is diagnosed or suspected it is essential to consider coexistent syphilis, *Trichomonas* and *Chlamydia*, one or more of which is also present in more than half of the cases. Unfortunately, gonococcal infection in women may be symptomless, and it may be worth doing the same tests routinely in high-risk cases such as young women with an unwanted pregnancy.

Treatment

Penicillin is the treatment of choice, usually given as one or two large, long-acting doses by injection to ensure that adequate treatment is completed. It is vital that sexual contacts are sought and treated. Tracing contacts is a major part of any specialist STD clinic service. Follow-up of the primary patient is probably also best carried out in the STD clinic.

Syphilis

Routine blood testing in antenatal clinics has led to detection of syphilis in its symptomless latent phase, which may be anything from 2 to 20 years, and reduction in the incidence of congenital syphilis. If the disease is undetected in a pregnant woman it may infect the fetus, which may die *in utero* or be born with the disease, but treatment of the infected woman in the first half of pregnancy prevents the stigmata of congenital syphilis (Hutchinson's teeth, collapsed nose, etc.). A history of fetal death should always raise the suspicion of syphilis, especially if the placenta was large, suggesting inflammatory response to infection.

Although much syphilis is diagnosed at the latent stage by antenatal screening, it may present at the secondary stage as an ulcer on any part of the female lower genital tract from the vulva to the cervix. Condylomata lata may also be found; these are moist flat warts around the vulval area. Exudate taken or scraped from the ulcerated lesion will reveal *Treponema pallidum* on dark-ground examination. These manifestations of secondary syphilis are usually associated with generalized lymphadenopathy and sometimes a non-irritative skin rash. Any such lesion should be examined with extreme care because they teem with live spirochaetes (*Treponema*) and without protective gloves an examiner may be infected through any minute skin abrasion. When syphilis is diagnosed the patient should be referred to a department of genitourinary medicine because, although treatment with penicillin is usually both simple and effective, extensive investigation and prolonged follow-up are required.

Acquired immunodeficiency syndrome

This disease complex, due to the human immunodeficiency virus (HIV), has reached epidemic proportions in parts of the world, and has profound implications in obstetric and gynaecological practice. Although it came to prominence amongst homosexual men, intravenous drug abuse accounts for most affected women in the UK so far, and in other parts of the world transmission is mainly heterosexual. Female prostitution is a major factor in the AIDS epidemic in Central and East Africa. HIV infection remains latent for several years, although seroconversion occurs within a few months, and its true prevalence in the UK is as yet undetermined. Accurate data are required urgently.

At present serological screening without permission in the UK is considered unethical and individual consent to test for HIV antibodies must be sought. Such consent should be requested from those deemed to be at high risk, e.g. intravenous drug users, prostitutes, sexual contacts of bisexual men or men from Africa, or anyone from those parts of the world with a known high infection rate such as Central and East Africa and the Far East.

Untested patients at high risk of HIV infection must be treated with the same precautions as if they were known to be infected, in order to protect the carers. The use of eye protectors, double gloves and full gowns is particularly important in surgical practice such as obstetrics and gynaecology. In addition there may be fundamental ethical objections to treating infertile HIV-infected patients to assist them to have a child because of the high risk of passage of the virus to the fetus and subsequent AIDS in the child.

Pregnancy and HIV infection

The virus crosses the placenta and can infect the fetus, and the neonate can be infected from the mother's milk. However, the mother's disease does not seem to be accelerated by pregnancy. HIV infection is already a major cause of infant death in many parts of the world and is likely to increase as the epidemic increases. At least one in four babies will be infected in the uterus. Maternal antibody also crosses the placenta and may be present in the baby for several months without indicating infection. It is important to screen an HIV-infected mother for other infectious diseases, such as

Toxoplasmosis, Rubella, Cytomegalovirus and Herpes (TORCH), tuberculosis and other STDs. Sympathetic sensitive counselling is as important when considering testing as it is when discussing evident infection in pregnancy.

FURTHER READING

Gilbert, G.L. (ed.) (1993) *Infectious Diseases: Challenges for the 1990s. Baillière's Clinical Obstetrics and Gynaecology*, vol. 7. Baillière Tindall, London.

Johnstone, F.D. (ed.) (1992) *HIV Infection in Obstetrics and Gynaecology. Baillière's Clinical Obstetrics and Gynaecology*, vol. 6. Baillière Tindall, London.

Shaw, R.W., Soutter, W.P. and Stanton, S.L. (eds) (1997) *Gynaecology*, 3rd edn. Churchill Livingstone, Edinburgh, pp. 707–742.

19
Chronic pelvic pain

Chronic pelvic pain is a cause of misery, disruptive of personal and family life, a common complaint encountered with increasing frequency in gynaecological outpatients where approximately a third of women attending present with this symptom. Chronic pelvic pain is a problem predominantly of women in their reproductive years and over 50% of diagnostic laparoscopies are done to investigate these problems.

The cause of chronic pelvic pain is frequently obscure and not identified, adding to the woman's frustration. The difficulty in precise diagnosis is compounded because chronic pelvic pain may be generated or aggravated by a variety of conditions which may interrelate, as shown in Figure 19.1.

MANAGEMENT

1 Detailed history.
2 General physical examination.
3 Pelvic examination.
4 Investigations:
    a. Full blood count.
    b. High vaginal swab.
    c. Cervical swab.
    d. *Chlamydia* swab.
    e. Serum *Chlamydia* antibodies.
    f. Cervical smear.
    g. Laparoscopy.
5 Treatment:
    a. Involve partner.
    b. Be supportive.
    c. Be specific.

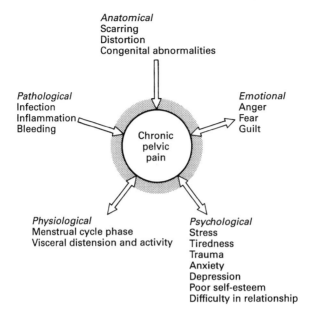

Anatomical
Scarring
Distortion
Congenital abnormalities

Pathological
Infection
Inflammation
Bleeding

Emotional
Anger
Fear
Guilt

Chronic
pelvic
pain

Physiological
Menstrual cycle phase
Visceral distension and activity

Psychological
Stress
Tiredness
Trauma
Anxiety
Depression
Poor self-esteem
Difficulty in relationship

Fig. 19.1   Factors influencing chronic pelvic pain.

A detailed history which not only defines the relationship of the pain to menstruation, sexual relations and other activities, but also takes account of pressure at home and at work, is a prerequisite to attempting to identify the underlying cause. Pelvic pain may be intermittent and related to a specific event such as menstruation (when it is termed dysmenorrhoea) or sexual intercourse (when it is termed dyspareunia) or it may be chronic and associated with pathology such as pelvic inflammatory disease (PID) or irritable bowel syndrome (IBS).

Any assessment of pain has to take account of a variety of factors which modify the severity, extent or perception of pain, including general ill health, lack of sleep, low endorphin levels and poor self-esteem.

Pain may be visceral, somatic or referred:

1 Visceral pain:
   a. From uterus.
   b. From tubes.
   c. From ovaries.
via autonomic nervous system T10–L1 + S2–4.

2 Somatic pain:
   a. From vulva.
   b. From perineum.
   c. From lower vagina.
via pudendal nerves S2–4.
3 Referred pain: from overlying peritoneum to dermatomes supplied by same nerve root.

CLASSIFICATION

1 Dysmenorrhoea (painful menstruation):
   a. Primary or spasmodic – exacerbation of normal cramps.
   b. Secondary or congestive:
      i. Pelvic pathology: endometriosis, adenomyosis, PID.
      ii. Pelvic pain syndrome (PPS).
      iii. Psychosexual.
2 Mittelschmerz (ovulation pain).
3 Dyspareunia (painful intercourse):
   a. Superficial:
      i. Pathological: infectious, e.g. *Candida*; scars, e.g. episiotomy; atrophic vaginitis.
      ii. Psychosexual: vaginismus.
   b. Deep:
      i. Pathological: PID; endometriosis; adenomyosis; IBS; cervicitis.
      ii. Anatomical: ovaries prolapsed in pouch of Douglas; fundus of retroverted retroflexed uterus.
      iii. Psychosexual.
      iv. PPS.
4 Backache:
   a. Skeletal:
      i. Postural.
      ii. Arthritis.
      iii. Osteoporosis.
      iv. Prolapsed intervertebral disc.
   b. Gynaecological:
      i. Sacral dysmenorrhoea.
      ii. Some uterine prolapse.
5 Iliac fossa/lower abdomen:
   a. Gastrointestinal:
      i. IBS.
      ii. Constipation.
      iii. Diverticulitis.
   b. Psychosomatic.

DYSMENORRHOEA

Normal menstruation in the majority of women with ovulatory cycles is associated with discomfort in the pelvis and also commonly the groins, tops of the thighs and sacral region. The discomfort is of a colicky nature, most noticeable on the first day, and is aptly termed menstrual cramps in North America. Most women tolerate this discomfort and only occasionally need a mild analgesic. Dysmenorrhoea however may cause more severe symptoms and can cause much time off from school and work.

Dysmenorrhoea is often described as primary or secondary, which is ambiguous and potentially misleading. Secondary is used meaning secondary to a pathological condition rather than secondary in terms of when it develops in a woman's life.

Primary (or spasmodic) dysmenorrhoea

This form of dysmenorrhoea starts a year or so after the menarche when ovulatory cycles begin. It is colicky in nature, hence the term spasmodic, and is located deep in the suprapubic region, sacral area, groins and thighs, although not always in all sites in the same patient. Primary dysmenorrhoea starts a few hours before or just as menstruation begins and is usually limited to the first day.

Aetiology

The pain is generally associated with ovulatory cycles and is produced by strong frequent uterine contractions. This hypercontractility causes painful ischaemia and may be due to an increase of prostaglandin $F_{2\alpha}$ in menstrual blood. An autonomic nervous disturbance resulting in diarrhoea is a frequent accompaniment. There is a large psychological element in many cases, and the dysmenorrhoeic mother who fails to inform her daughter about menstruation or who hints at the 'sufferings' of women due to 'the curse' and 'being unwell' will tend to produce a dysmenorrhoeic daughter. The incidence of severe spasmodic dysmenorrhoea has decreased greatly with a more educated and sensible approach to menstruation by women. Primary dysmenorrhoea is essentially a severe form of the normal cramps and not due to any organic lesion.

Treatment

Treatment is most effective when ovulation is suppressed with oral contraceptive preparations (and contraceptive requirements should always be reviewed when treating gynaecological problems).

Explanation and reassurance about normality should be given in every case. Mild analgesia taken regularly (e.g. paracetamol 0.5–1 g 4–6 hourly, maximum dose 4 g daily), the first dose anticipating the onset of the cramps if possible, may be all that is necessary.

Some mothers are reluctant to consider the oral contraceptive pill for daughters in their early teens and alternative therapy is required. Prostaglandin synthetase inhibitors such as mefenamic acid in doses of 250–500 mg 8-hourly for the duration of the pain is effective in more severe cases. The greater efficacy of mefenamic acid compared to other prostaglandin synthetase inhibitors may be due to the additional actions of fenemates as prostaglandin receptor blockers. Alternatively progestogen alone may also be effective given from day 5 to 25 of the cycle (e.g. norethisterone 5 mg three times daily or dydrogesterone 10 mg twice daily).

Surgical treatment

Dilatation of the cervix carries the risk of producing cervical incompetence and its effect in pain relief is at best transient. Open surgical treatment such a presacral neurectomy is infrequently undertaken but with the recent increasing interest in laparoscopic surgery the procedure of uterosacral ligament division, transecting the somatic and visceral nerves within them, is being increasingly used under the acronym LUNA (laparoscopic uterosacral nerve ablation). However, this method of treatment remains of unproven benefit.

Summary of treatment

1 Give explanation and reassurance.
2 Provide simple analgesia, e.g. paracetamol, aspirin.
3 Prescribe the combined oral contraceptive pill.
4 Administer prostaglandin synthase inhibitors, e.g. mefenamic acid.
5 Give progestogens on days 5–25, e.g. norethisterone, dydrogesterone.

Secondary (or congestive) dysmenorrhoea

This condition, which begins in adult life, is secondary to acquired pathology or is of organic or psychosexual origin. It is also called congestive dysmenorrhoea, being thought to be associated with pelvic vascular disturbance. The pain starts many days before menstruation approaches. It is more constant in nature and situated in the pelvis and back. It may be secondary to endometriosis or PID and treatment is of that condition. However, laparoscopy reveals no such lesion in about half the women with congestive dysmenor-rhoea and related symptoms; the condition is then called PPS (see below) and is often associated with psychosexual problems.

MITTELSCHMERZ (OR OVULATION PAIN)

This pain occurs cyclically in the middle (*mittel*) of the cycle. It is felt low in the abdomen, often more on one side than the other. There may be associated slight vaginal blood loss caused by the changes in oestrogen level around the time of ovulation. It is wise to ask the woman to keep a careful diary of pain, periods and any other loss so one may be certain that the pain and bleeding are occurring around the time of ovulation.

DYSPAREUNIA

The term dyspareunia means painful intercourse. It may be due to organic or psychological causes, but those with a clear organic aetiology may develop psychological features as well.

Superficial dyspareunia

This term means pain confined to the introitus and perineum. The commonest organic cause is infection, or atrophy in the older woman. An episiotomy scar may sometimes cause pain because of uneven scarring or sometimes thorough obstruction of the flow of secretion from the right Bartholin's gland (most episiotomies are made on the right side). Very rarely there is a congenital abnormality. If, on examination, pathology is excluded, vaginismus with levator spasm and failure of the vagina to lubricate is the usual cause of such complaints as 'My vagina is too small' or 'His penis is too big'. Fear, inadequate sex education and previous painful inter-course, together with poor sexual stimulation and unskilled tech-niques, make for superficial dyspareunia. Education of both partners, reassurance and self-examination and a simple lubricant are often all that is needed. Plastic operations and artificial dilators have a very limited place unless an anatomical abnormality is present.

Deep dyspareunia

In these cases the pain is felt deep in the pelvis or abdominally during intercourse and may be related to position. The pain usually subsides quickly after withdrawal. Deep dyspareunia may be due to pelvic pathology, particularly endometriosis, PID or cervicitis. If the ovaries are prolapsed in the pouch of Douglas in association with a retroverted uterus, collision dyspareunia may occur due to compression of the ovaries during thrusting. This pain usually ceases on withdrawal. Deep dyspareunia may have a psychosexual origin and in these cases often lasts 24 or 48 hours after intercourse. Nevertheless, it must not be assumed that dyspareunia persisting postcoitally is psychosexual until organic cause, especially PID, has been excluded.

Treatment of dyspareunia depends on the underlying pathology, and the collaboration of a skilled psychosexual counsellor can be invaluable for the majority of cases, not just those with more psychosexual problems, since sexual dysfunction resulting from chronic pelvic pain inevitably evokes psychosexual problems too.

PELVIC PAIN SYNDROME (PELVIC CONGESTION SYNDROME)

The patient complains of congestive dysmenorrhoea and deep dyspareunia, often together, with symptoms of fluid retention similar to the premenstrual tension syndrome. There is often excessive cervical secretion leading to the complaint of vaginal discharge, lack of libido and failure to achieve orgasm. The multiplicity of complaints suggests a psychosomatic origin. Pain of psychosomatic origin rarely disturbs sleep, whereas pain due to pelvic pathology may do so. Examination is often difficult, with the patient unable to relax. The uterus is frequently retroverted, bulky and tender. The entire pelvis is tender on examination. Laparoscopy will exclude PID and endometriosis and may reveal grossly distended pelvic veins. Treatment with high-dose progestogens (medroxyprogesterone acetate tablets 100 mg/day) may reduce congestion in these veins and alleviate the symptoms, but they are likely to recur unless attention is paid to background stress factors. Psychosexual counselling is an invaluable adjunct. Hysterectomy may be carried out as a last resort, when congested pelvic veins and thickened fibrosed uterosacral ligaments may be found. The bulky uterus may look mottled but histologically reveal no abnormality. Pelvic pain may continue even after total hysterectomy and bilateral salpingo-oophorectomy, and the psychologically pain-dependent patient must be recognized before being subjected to unnecessary gynaecological procedures. Laparoscopic exclusion of serious organic disease may be sufficient to relieve symptoms in some anxious patients.

RETROVERSION OF THE UTERUS

Retroversion means the leaning backwards in the pelvis of the whole uterus, body and cervix, on the supporting ligaments.

On vaginal examination the cervix points forwards and upwards and the body of the uterus is felt through the posterior vaginal fornix in the pouch of Douglas.

Retroflexion means that the body of the uterus is tilted backwards on the cervix; this is a less common finding (Fig. 19.2).

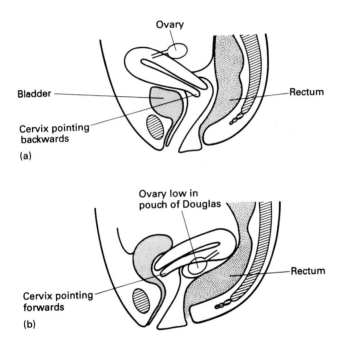

Fig. 19.2   (a) Anteverted and (b) retroverted positions of the uterus.

The diagnosis of retroversion is made on bimanual examination. The differential diagnosis is from other masses in the pouch of Douglas. The passage of a uterine sound will define the position of the uterus if confusion persists.

Mobile (congenital) retroversion of the uterus is a normal finding in about 25% of women and is almost always asymptomatic. A fixed retroversion of the uterus is associated with pathology (usually PID or endometriosis) that causes the fixity.

Retroversion of the uterus in pregnancy

When a woman with a mobile retroverted uterus becomes pregnant the uterus fills the pelvis by 12 weeks, becoming anteverted and easily palpable abdominally by 14 weeks. Very rarely the uterine fundus may be trapped in the pelvis below the sacral promontory and is then termed an incarcerated retroverted gravid uterus (Fig. 19.3). As the uterus grows the urethra is elongated and compressed, causing urinary disturbance, first frequency, then strangury and finally retention. Miscarriage may also be precipitated.

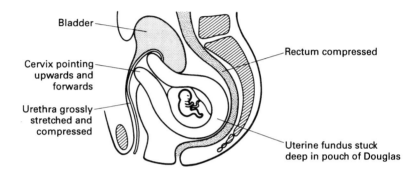

Fig. 19.3   Retroverted gravid uterus causing retention of urine at 14 weeks due to stretching and compression of the urethra.

Management of retroversion

The very large majority of women with a mobile retroverted uterus are symptom-free and need no treatment. If retroversion is associated with deep dyspareunia, the uterine position may be corrected bimanually and a ring pessary inserted. If symptoms are relieved and return after removal of the pessary, the uterus can be permanently placed in an anteverted position by the operation called ventrosuspension.

Ventrosuspension involves shortening the round ligaments and suturing them to the rectus sheath, and may be done at laparotomy or laparoscopy. Plication of the round ligaments alone holds the uterus forwards temporarily and is often done as an adjunct to surgery for some other condition to avoid postoperative adhesions binding the uterus down in the pouch of Douglas.

Incarcerated retroverted gravid uterus

This is usually simply corrected by inserting a Foley catheter and nursing the woman in a prone position.

Discussion of retroversion has been included here since PID and endometriosis, both causes of fixed retroversion of the uterus, are primary causes of chronic pelvic pain. However it must be emphasized that a mobile retroverted uterus is not a cause of chronic pelvic pain and ventrosuspension will not alleviate the pelvic pain.

Chronic pain involves complex interactions concerning the whole person and these interactions must be remembered whenever pelvic pain is considered (see Fig. 16.1).

FURTHER READING

Frappell, J. and Stanton, S.L. (1991) Chronic pelvic pain. In: *Progress in Obstetrics and Gynaecology*, vol. 9, edited by Studd, J. Churchill Livingstone, Edinburgh.

20

Premenstrual syndrome

The premenstrual syndrome (PMS) is a poorly understood condition which has been defined by Magos and Studd (1984) as 'distressing physical and psychological symptoms, not caused by organic disease, which regularly recur during the same phase of each ovarian (or menstrual) cycle, and which significantly regress or disappear during the remainder of the cycle'. The range of symptoms is wide, their severity may fluctuate from one cycle to another and their duration and time of onset in relation to the menstrual and ovarian cycle can vary considerably, although they develop typically during the secretory/luteal phase. Menstruation itself is not critical for the diagnosis to be made, as in premenopausal women symptoms persist after hysterectomy if the ovaries are conserved. For this reason it has been suggested that the condition should be called more correctly postovulatory syndrome. The importance of cyclical ovarian activity is clear from the absence of symptoms before puberty, remission during pregnancy and resolution of the syndrome after the menopause. Postmenopausal women may develop PMS-type symptoms if given cyclical hormone replacement therapy, specifically during the phase of treatment where they are taking a progestogen in addition to oestrogen. It is not uncommon for PMS to present initially following pregnancy or after stopping a combined-preparation oral contraceptive pill and symptoms will usually increase in severity with age up to the time of the menopause.

HISTORICAL AND LEGAL ASPECTS

Observations of excessive behavioural, psychological and physical changes which resolve at the onset of menstruation date back 2500 years to the time of Hippocrates. The term premenstrual tension was first used in the 1930s to describe a complex of symptoms which included cyclical depression, irritability and tension in the 7 days before menstruation and relieved in the first 24 hours of the menstrual loss. However, it became recognized that a much wider range of physical as well as psychological symptoms and behavioural changes affected some women to an abnormal degree and the term premenstrual syndrome, introduced in the 1950s, is more appropriate to take account of the more than 150 symptoms which may arise with this condition.

Recognition of PMS by the medical profession has lagged well behind its recognition by the legal profession, which dates back to the mid 19th century. In 1845, Martha Brixey, a domestic servant, was acquitted of the charge of murdering one of her employer's children on the grounds of insanity arising from 'obstructed menstruation'. There was a considerable public reaction to this verdict but a legal precedent was established and 6 years later, at Maidstone Assizes, Amelia Snoswell was acquitted of the impulsive murder of her baby niece, whom she strangled, on the grounds of 'insanity due to disordered menstruation'. She was reported to have committed impulsive acts of violence previously without being able to recall them and these had been documented to occur before delayed menstruation. Although there are no recent cases of acquittal of murder charges, there have been several occasions where charges of murder have been reduced to manslaughter by reason of diminished responsibility on the grounds of PMS.

Far more frequently, PMS has been used as a defence for impulsive crimes such as shop-lifting and those of aggressive behaviour such as assaults on the police or public officials. Recognition that crimes of this type are more frequently committed in the perimenstrual phase dates from French, German and Italian reports as long ago as 1890. Such a defence is not infrequently accepted in mitigation and has led to reduction in the severity of sentences imposed by the courts in some cases. More recently, there have been a number of British and American studies based on women's prison populations showing a higher than expected proportion of crimes of violence, theft, burglary, embezzlement, forgery and drunkenness to have been committed in the pre-menstrual or early menstrual phase.

SYMPTOMS

Symptoms of PMS may be broadly classified into three groups: physical, psychological and behavioural.

Physical symptoms

One of the major problems with physical symptoms of PMS is that an extremely wide range of hormonal and metabolic parameters fluctuate during the course of a normal menstrual cycle. These affect virtually every system within the body, from activity of the sebaceous glands to gastric acid concentration and from the sensitivity of the blinking reflex to the quality of the voice. In addition, many diseases are more prevalent in the premenstrual phase of a woman's cycle. For example, more appendicectomies in women are undertaken in the second half of their cycles where evidence of inflammation is also more likely to be confirmed histologically and, in asthmatics, acute exacerbations are more prevalent and peak expiratory flow rates are reduced in the premenstrual and early menstrual phase.

Most women who suffer from PMS do complain of some physical symptoms. In the majority of cases these probably represent an abnormal or pathological accentuation of normal physiological changes. The commonest physical symptoms are breast tenderness and swelling, abdominal bloating, peripheral oedema, weight gain, headache, altered bowel habit, pelvic pain and skin disorders. The syndrome needs to be differentiated from less severe premenstrual symptoms that are not considered abnormal or distressing and which are experienced by most women. Dysmenorrhoea must be excluded from the definition, as should any symptoms which are secondary to organic disease.

Psychological symptoms

These may cause significant morbidity and have a considerable effect on the woman's quality of life. The commonest symptoms are depression, tension, irritability, sleep disturbance, loss of libido, increased appetite and thirst.

Behavioural symptoms

In many cases behavioural symptoms may be considered to be secondary to psychological changes. The most common features are a reduced tolerance to stress of any type, lowered intellectual and cognitive performance, impulsive acts, forgetfulness, outbursts of temper and proneness to accidents.

These behavioural symptoms are the ones which most frequently draw the attention of relatives and friends to the condition and may be the factor which precipitates the woman presenting to her doctor.

PREVALENCE

There is a very wide variation in the reported prevalence of PMS, from 5 to 95% of postpubertal, premenopausal women. This wide variation is due to a number of factors: the lack of a universally accepted definition, the difficulty in objectively defining whether symptoms are of a physiological or pathological severity and the wide range of symptoms which may occur. There is no evidence that the prevalence of PMS is related to age, race, class or parity. It is estimated that 5–15% of women suffer from PMS symptoms that are severe enough to be considered life-disrupting.

AETIOLOGY

The aetiology of PMS remains obscure. Many of the hypotheses which have been suggested are poorly substantiated or contradictory. The wide range of symptoms makes it likely that more than one mechanism may be involved.

As PMS is related to the luteal phase of the ovarian cycle, a lot of attention has focused on oestrogen and progesterone levels. There is no evidence to implicate oestrogen and there are conflicting results on whether progesterone levels are reduced or not. In postmenopausal women taking hormone replacement therapy, PMS-type symptoms occur when progestogens are taken in addition to oestrogen but not when oestrogen is taken alone. This may not be a good model for PMS as synthetic progestogens have different effects to progesterone itself.

Concentrations of a vast number of hormones have been assessed in many studies. These include prolactin, cortisol, follicle-stimulating hormone, luteinizing hormone, sex hormone-binding globulin, prostaglandins E_2 and $F_{2\alpha}$, serotonin and β-endorphins. No consistent reproducible pattern of hormone deficiency or excess has been shown to correlate with the symptoms or severity of PMS.

Deficiencies of minerals such as magnesium and zinc or vitamins A, B, B_6 and E have been proposed as causes of PMS. There is no scientific evidence to support these hypotheses and it seems unlikely that deficiency of these substances could be cyclical to match the pattern of symptoms.

Genetic factors may be involved, as the prevalence of PMS symptoms is twice as high in the adolescent daughters of women who have PMS themselves compared with daughters of asymptomatic women. However, this may be due to social or environmental factors as there is also an increased incidence of a personal or family history of psychological problems in women with PMS.

DIAGNOSIS

The absence of any hormonal or biochemical marker for the condition makes the diagnosis of PMS difficult. Some doctors even doubt the existence of the syndrome for this reason. A careful and detailed history is essential to establish which are the major symptoms, their severity, the degree to which they disrupt the patient's life and their relationship to the woman's menstrual cycle. However, a history suggestive of PMS is insufficient in itself to diagnose the condition. Having determined the major symptoms for an individual woman, she should be asked to chart the severity of these prospectively on a menstrual calendar for 3 months. Alternatively, there are a variety of self-assessment questionnaires and visual analogue scales which may be used over the same period of time. On review, up to 50% of women with a history suggestive of PMS will be found to have symptoms that are either non-cyclical or which are not related specifically to their premenstrual phase.

At initial assessment it is essential to consider and exclude other possible diagnoses such as primary or secondary dysmenorrhoea, anxiety states, psychosexual problems and depression.

MANAGEMENT AND TREATMENT

A sensitive and sympathetic approach to the patient is an important aspect of management of PMS It is important to assess whether the severity of symptoms justify the use of medication or whether other measures such as alteration of lifestyle, stress-reduction therapy or supportive counselling may be equally effective.

In the absence of a defined cause of PMS no specific therapy is possible but a wide range of empirical treatments is available. Double-blind studies have repeatedly shown a very high placebo response rate, generally of about 50% but as high as 80–90% in some cases. The majority of empirical treatments which have been advocated or shown to be of benefit in uncontrolled studies have usually been found to be no more effective than placebo when subjected to prospective double-blind trials.

Natural progesterone by suppository, pessary or injection is probably the most widely prescribed treatment but its therapeutic effect is no greater than placebo. Synthetic progestogens have not been shown to be any more effective than natural progesterone.

Suppression of ovulation appears logical as symptoms are confined to the luteal phase but combined-preparation (oestrogen and progestogen) oral contraceptives deliver progestogen from the start of the cycle and may increase the severity and duration of symptoms in some women. Oestrogen given by subcutaneous implant also suppresses ovulation and has been shown to be effective for women with severe PMS. However, symptoms recur when cyclical progestogen is given in addition, which is necessary for protection against endometrial hyperplasia in women who have not had a hysterectomy. Gonadotrophin-releasing hormone (GnRH) agonists induce a pseudo prepubertal state and are more effective than placebo. Unfortunately, GnRH agonists produce side-effects due to oestrogen deficiency and should not be used for long-term treatment. Although concurrent oestrogen replacement therapy can be given to prevent these side-effects, cyclical progestogen will then be necessary as well to prevent endometrial hyperplasia.

Continuous treatment with low-dose danazol (100–200 mg daily) has been claimed to be effective in some cases but has not been adequately assessed in prospective randomized controlled trials. The potentially serious side-effects of danazol (hirsutism and voice change) appear to be related to the duration of treatment rather than its dose and, in addition, it is unreliable as a contraceptive at this low dose. If conception occurred whilst the woman was on treatment there would be the risk of masculinization of a female fetus. For these reasons it is probably best avoided as a treatment for PMS.

Vitamin B_6 (pyridoxine) therapy has been found to be effective in the treatment of the depression which sometimes occurs in women using an oestrogen–progestogen contraceptive pill, due to pyridoxine deficiency. However, it is no more effective than placebo in treating women with PMS.

Bromocriptine, a dopamine agonist which suppresses prolactin secretion, may be particularly effective for patients with premenstrual breast tenderness and swelling. Unfortunately, some women are unable to tolerate the drug because of side-effects.

The prostaglandin synthetase inhibitor mefenamic acid has been shown to relieve many PMS symptoms in placebo-controlled trials. In addition its beneficial effects on menorrhagia and dysmenorrhoea may be useful for some patients. Oil of evening primrose also affects prostaglandin production as it contains linoleic and γ-linoleic acid which are prostaglandin precursors. Reduced levels of γ-linoleic acid have been found in some women with PMS and a recent controlled study has shown oil of evening primrose to be more effective than placebo for relieving symptoms. The dosage required for treatment of PMS is 240 mg of gamolenic acid twice daily.

In addition to other empirical treatments such as diuretics and opiate antagonists (e.g. naltrexone), simple measures such as small frequent meals to prevent subclinical hypoglycaemia may be helpful. Some women with intractable symptoms whose family is

complete may be considered for surgical treatment (total hysterectomy and bilateral salpingo-oophorectomy) followed by hormone
replacement therapy using oestrogen alone. This should only be
considered as a last resort for women with severe life-disrupting
symptoms and where all other medical treatments have failed.

REFERENCE

Magos, A. and Studd, J. (1984) The premenstrual syndrome. In:
    Progress in Obstetrics and Gynaecology, vol. 4, edited by Studd, J.
    Churchill Livingstone, Edinburgh, pp. 334–350.

FURTHER READING

Lachelin, G. (1991) Premenstrual (postovulatory) syndrome. In:
    Introduction to Clinical Reproductive Endocrinology, by Lachelin, G.
    Butterworth-Heinemann, Oxford, pp. 89–100.
O'Brien, P.M.S. (1993) Helping women with premenstrual
    syndrome. *British Medical Journal* 307:1471–1475.

21

Sexual problems

Sexuality is an integral part of each human being and satisfactory sexual function is a component of well-being for most people. Just as dysfunction of the alimentary system may result in generalized problems and malfunction in other systems, so sexual dysfunction may have repercussions generally or disrupt normal functioning in other systems.

Teachers place emphasis on the importance of taking a complete detailed history of function system by system, and this should include sexual function. Obviously, in gynaecology and obstetrics no history is complete without details of sexual function, but it is a difficult and delicate task to accomplish this adequately with ease and lack of self-consciousness. The woman (her partner if present) and the history-taker must be comfortable about such discussions and a good rapport is essential.

No consideration of sexual function should look at anatomical and physiological features in isolation, as the psychological and emotional responses are the prime keys to sexual relation and activities. Having established a good rapport with the woman with earlier history-taking, questions relating to intercourse can be introduced naturally and logically, particularly following the obstetric and contraceptive history. Obviously a couple seeking advice about infertility will be asked different questions from the 70-year-old woman who wants her prolapse repaired. For example, the couple will be questioned about the timing and frequency of intercourse, and whether erection, penetration and intravaginal ejaculation occur. The older woman will be asked whether she wants to have a functioning vagina; whether she has an active sexual relationship – not whether she *still* has intercourse!

LOVING RELATIONSHIP

Sexual contacts and coitus are only part – and for many a minor part – of a loving relationship which involves physical and emotional

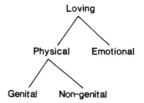

Fig. 21.1   Sexual function in a loving relationship.

aspects (Fig. 21.1), but sexual dysfunction may disrupt and destroy that loving relationship.

Before discussing sexual problems it is important to understand the physiological response to sexual stimulation, which follows the same pattern in the male and the female – a four-stage response described by Masters and Johnson (1966) as excitement, plateau, orgasm and resolution. The length of each phase and the progression to the next depends on the efficacy of the stimulation, on both the physical and emotional plane. The female is potentially multi-orgasmic, that is she can return from the early resolution phase to the orgasmic repeatedly, provided stimulation is adequate. The male, however, is refractory to stimulation after orgasm and cannot return to orgasm until the refractory period has passed – a variable time which increases with age and varies with the individual from a few minutes to several hours.

Each phase is accompanied by general body and specific genital changes. Briefly the major changes are as follows (Fig. 21.2).

During the excitement phase there is general vasocongestion with erection of the penis and lubrication of the vagina. During the plateau phase there is engorgement of the lower third of the vagina and ballooning (or barrelling) of the upper two-thirds. During male and female orgasm there are marked cardiorespiratory changes with the respiratory rate rising, pulse rates up to 180 beats/min, and an increase in blood pressure of about 20 mmHg or more. At this time passive myotonic contractions of the buttocks and limbs occur, and the pelvic floor contracts involuntarily at 0.8-second intervals involving the anal sphincter, the vagina and urethra. A red mottling appears over the upper chest and neck, which may be associated with perspiration. This is the sex flush which varies with the intensity of the orgasm and fades very gradually during the resolution phase as the other changes subside.

Normal sexual intercourse may be defined as any sexual contact giving pleasure to both participants, and defined thus will include homosexual and lesbian relationships. The sources of sexual stimulation are very varied. For some, indulging in fetishes, that is, acting out fantasies with leather, plastic and clothing, or in sadism and

PLATEAU PHASE

Female

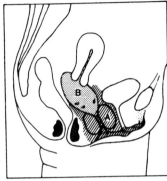

A Engorged perivaginal tissues
B Ballooned vagina and transudate

Male

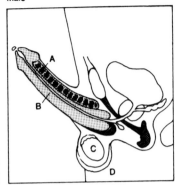

A Corpora cavernosa ⎫ Engorged
B Corpus spongiosum ⎭
C Testes enlarge, engorge and rise
D Dartos muscle thickened and contracted

ORGASM

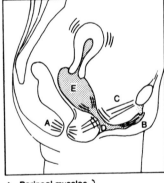

A Perineal muscles ⎫
B Bulbocavernosus ⎪ 0.8 sec
C Pubococcygeus ⎬ contractions
D Outer ⅓ vagina ⎪
E Upper ⅔ vagina ⎭

Emission
A Prostate ⎫
B Vas deferens ⎬ Contract
C Seminal vesicle ⎭
D Urethral bulb collects ejaculate
Expulsion
E Perineal ⎫ Contract 0.8 sec
F Bulbocavernosus ⎭
G Penile urethra contracts and ejaculates

Fig. 21.2 Plateau and orgasmic male and female organs. (Redrawn from H.S Kaplan's *The New Sex Therapy* by kind permission of Baillière Tindall, London, 1974).

masochism, that is, production of pain to one's partner and/or oneself, may play a major part in providing sexual stimulation. The increasing desire for these practices by one partner when the other finds them unacceptable presents the greatest of problems in attempting to decide where 'normality' lies and where adjustments can be made. The doctor must always keep in mind the vast range of normality and the many factors influencing sexual function when faced with sexual problems.

MASTURBATION

The response follows the same pattern regardless of the source of stimulation. The orgasm achieved by masturbation is identical in physiological terms to that achieved by hetero- or homosexual coitus, although the emotional content may alter the way orgasm is perceived. Masturbation is a normal sexual function releasing sexual tensions and in a modified degree it is an almost universal infancy and childhood experience. Only a minority of persons do not masturbate by the time they reach the age of 20. Women are slower to discover masturbation and it is not until their forties that numbers begin to equilibrate, but the Kinsey report and others have shown that at all ages more men than women masturbate.

Masturbation is completely harmless and unrelated to blindness, venereal disease, sterility and any infirmity. There is no evidence to suggest that it causes labial hypertrophy any more than that it makes the penis drop off! It may be important to determine whether the woman who is anorgasmic with her partner can climax with self-masturbation, and likewise whether the man who fails to ejaculate in the vagina can do so during self-masturbation.

FACTORS AFFECTING SEXUAL FUNCTION

Cultural, racial and religious factors all exert influence through upbringing and peer group pressures:

1 *Childhood experience*: Adult sexuality is influenced by parental attitudes and events in childhood; the sexually abused child or adolescent is very likely to have difficulties achieving satisfactory sexual function. Indeed, it is important to ascertain whether there is a history of sexual abuse in most cases where the complaint is of a sexual problem.
2 *Partner rejection*: An unsuitable relationship with partner rejection and failure to communicate is clearly unlikely to be associated with good sexual function.

3 *Ignorance and inadequate techniques*: Satisfactory sexual function depends on both partners receiving adequate stimulation and being free to respond to this. Ignorance may lead to sexual anxiety and fears of failure. In the male this may cause premature ejaculation which enhances the fear of failure and may lead to impotence; in the female such fears, often allied to inadequate understanding of clitoral stimulation and communication about this in a partnership, cause a dry vagina, dyspareunia and eventually frigidity.

4 *Disease*: General ill health and chronic pain decrease libido in both sexes. Long-standing uncontrolled diabetes mellitus may be associated with partial impotence; vaginal or pelvic pathology may cause dyspareunia, and the pain experienced during intercourse leads to fear and rejection of coitus. Many other disorders alter sexual function, from the rigid limbs of the spastic to the problems following ileostomy. Chronic and progressive disease such as multiple sclerosis poses a special problem because genital sensation disappears in the female. A couple may be helped to understand the pleasure of oral sex and so prolong a happy sexual relationship.

5 *Pregnancy*: Many women find intercourse more enjoyable during pregnancy and achieve orgasm more readily at this time. Women should have intercourse during pregnancy whenever they wish. It is, however, usual practice to ask the woman who has a history of recurrent abortion to refrain from intercourse around the time that she usually miscarries and also to advise abstinence in patients who have recurrent bleeding during the pregnancy. There is some suggestion that the uterine contractions provoked as a result of orgasm could be related to the onset of premature labour, and a woman with a history of premature labour may be advised to refrain from intercourse around her danger time.

6 *Drugs*: Drugs usually diminish rather than enhance sexual pleasure, and most aphrodisiacs are pharmacologically inactive. If they do enhance erotic behaviour it is by placebo effects. Small doses of alcohol, barbiturates and amphetamines may release inhibitions and apparently enhance sexuality, but chronic abuse of all of them causes sexual depression. Impotence is a frequent complication of methyldopa and β-blockers, and many other drugs also depress sexual function.

SEXUAL DYSFUNCTION

The expectation of the patient with a sexual problem attending the doctor is that there will be a physical cause found for which there will be a definitive remedy. The reality is that the majority of sexual problems have a psychological cause, and even if there is a physical cause there is almost inevitably a psychological component, especially if the problem is a long-standing one. The patient is often reluctant to accept that there may be a psychological component.

Male

Male sexual dysfunction falls into three main groups: impotence, premature ejaculation and retardation or failure of ejaculation. Impotence and premature ejaculation are such common problems that they may be regarded as part of normal male sexuality, provided that they do not persist.

Impotence

Rarely, this may be of pathological or physiological origin. The prerequisites of erection are intact erectile tissue with an adequate blood supply and intact innervation to the penis. Pathological impotence results from faults at these points. Psychological factors are the cause of failure of erection, or loss of erection at any time during the excitement or plateau phase. Such problems often apply to a man only in a specific partnership; he may find himself entirely normal in a casual rather than committed (or long-term) relationship.

Premature ejaculation

This is an extremely common problem which resolves spontaneously in most cases but not infrequently requires special therapy. The attitude of the partner is all-important in order to prevent persistent premature ejaculation developing into impotence.

Retardation or failure of ejaculation

Fears regarding performance and fears regarding pregnancy may prevent ejaculation. In later middle age pleasurable satisfactory intercourse without ejaculation is not uncommon. The number of times intercourse ends with ejaculation becomes fewer.

Female

Female sexual dysfunction is less obvious, but probably even more common. Fear of frigidity enhances and may even produce dysfunction.

General sexual dysfunction

The woman may be averse to sexual approaches. She will then fail to lubricate and show no genital engorgement. There is little or no vasocongestion in response to sexual stimulation.

Orgasmic dysfunction

Here lubrication occurs and there is evidence of vasocongestion, but there is failure to enjoy the responses to sexual stimulation and/or failure to reach orgasm. In some cases this may be regarded as a type of defence mechanism, with the woman being afraid to 'let go' It is important to differentiate between general sexual dysfunction and orgasmic dysfunction, as different therapies are required for treatment.

Treatment and referral

Psychosexual disorders are very common and probably affect one in five of the population at some time. The clinician must listen to what is said and not said, must give the impression of having unlimited time, must never show disapproval or censure. Pathology must be excluded before assuming that the causative factors are psychological. Unless the family practitioner has special training, the patient and partner should be directed to a properly trained psychosexual counsellor for advice and treatment. The majority of problems can be resolved over time by expert counselling.

Family planning clinics

Usually one or more doctors in any such clinic have had special training and hold special sessions during which psychosexual counselling is undertaken. Such special training is available to all doctors through the Institute of Psychosexual Medicine.

Relate (formerly known as the Marriage Guidance Council)

This also offers the help of trained counsellors – usually not medically qualified but with some special training and virtually unlimited time.

Outpatient clinics

A general gynaecological or psychiatric clinic is *not* a place to which these patients should be referred unless there is specific gynaecological or psychiatric pathology. Psychosexual counselling sessions may be carried out by gynaecologists or psychiatrists who are specially interested and trained in psychosexual therapy.

Sexual activity is just one of many normal body functions. You are trained to take a history about body functions so do not omit a history of sexual function. Give patients the opportunity to discuss their sexual function and problems; listen sympathetically and know where help may be obtained in your community.

HEALTH EDUCATION

Whenever the topic of sexual function is discussed with a young person the emotional and physical risks need to be made clear. The inadvisability of unprotected intercourse, unwanted pregnancy, early intercourse and repeated partners should be spelt out. The young person and the partner should be reminded at every opportunity of the risks of unwanted pregnancy, sexually transmitted diseases and acquired immunodeficiency syndrome (AIDS), pelvic inflammatory disease and carcinoma of the cervix. There may be concern that such reminders may invoke sexual dysfunction; however, it is to be hoped that some unwanted pregnancies, episodes of genital tract infection and subsequent sterility and perhaps carcinoma of the cervix may be prevented if more emphasis is placed on the adverse aspects of coitus. Sexual activity is a normal bodily function but one that requires a degree of self-discipline and carries responsibility.

REFERENCE

Masters, W.H. and Johnson, V.E. (1966) *Human Sexual Response.* Little, Brown, Boston.

FURTHER READING

Bancroft, J. (1989) *Human Sexuality and its Problems.* Churchill Livingstone, Edinburgh.
Fleming, C. and Crowley, T. (1995) How to help patients talk about sex. *Student British Medical Journal* 3:9–11.
Skrine, R.L. (ed.) (1989) *Introduction to Psychosexual Medicine.* Montana Press, Carlisle.

22

Prolapse, urinary problems and retroversion

PROLAPSE

Prolapse is the downward displacement of the uterus or vaginal wall towards or out of the introitus. The remarkable thing about uterine prolapse in the human is not that it occurs commonly but that it is not universal. Since woman (or her ancestors) assumed the erect posture the weight of pelvic and abdominal contents has had to be supported across an aperture which is large enough to allow the passage of a baby. Obviously the supporting mechanism must be sufficiently elastic to allow this passage to occur. Phylogenetically, woman has achieved this by converting the muscles used by her predecessors to wag their tails into a muscular hammock across the pelvis. This hammock is formed by the levator ani muscles, which are the main support of the vagina acting through their insertion into the perineal body. The main supports of the uterus and vaginal vault are the various condensations of the pelvic fascia, especially the transverse cervical ligaments (see Chapter 3) and uterosacral ligaments.

Vaginal wall prolapse

A prolapse of the lowest third of the anterior vaginal wall involves the urethra and is called a urethrocele. A prolapse of the upper two-thirds of the anterior vaginal wall is a cystocele, since bladder is involved. A prolapse of the pouch of Douglas is an enterocele, and the peritoneal sac of the enterocele may contain gut or omentum. Prolapse of the posterior wall of the vagina is termed a rectocele and is distinct from rectal prolapse, where the rectal mucosa extrudes through the anus, turning the rectum inside out. A rectocele is a bulging forwards of the rectum into the vagina and through the introitus. Vaginal wall prolapse is frequently associated with – and probably caused by – a deficient perineum (Fig. 22.1).

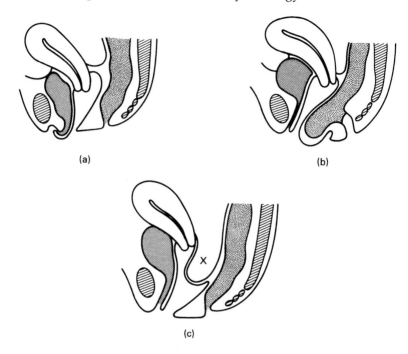

Fig. 22.1 Vaginal wall prolapse. (a) Cystourethrocele; (b) rectocele with deficient perineum; (c) enterocele – the enterocele sac (x) usually contains small bowel.

Uterine prolapse (vault prolapse)

The uterus may prolapse on its own, but usually there is concomitant vaginal wall prolapse. Conversely the vaginal wall may prolapse without uterine or vault descent. Uterine prolapse is divided into three degrees (Fig. 22.2): first-degree descent occurs when the cervix and uterus move down the vagina below the ischial spines. Second-degree descent occurs when the cervix protrudes through the introitus. Third-degree descent, or procidentia is diagnosed when the entire uterus lies outside the introitus. Most prolapse also involves some degree of perineal deficiency.

Aetiology

1 Childbirth.
2 Oestrogen deficiency (postmenopausal atrophy).
3 Chronically raised intra-abdominal pressure.
4 Congenital weakness of the pelvic floor.

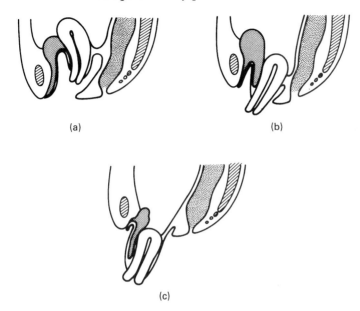

Fig. 22.2   Degrees of uterine prolapse. (a) First-degree; (b) second-degree; (c) third-degree.

Prolapse is very much more common in parous women, particularly those who have had difficult deliveries. Destruction of the perineum and pelvic floor mechanism following difficult or repeated childbirth, or inadequate repair of episiotomy or tear, leaves a gaping introitus with the anterior vaginal wall unsupported. This slips down and the uterus, whose ligaments may have been excessively stretched during delivery, descends too. While it is common to see some element of prolapse in many patients early in the puerperium after normal confinement due to stretching of the perineum and laxity of the pelvic floor, most patients have recovered their pelvic floor tone by 3 months. However, most parous women have some laxity of the anterior vaginal wall in particular and some degree of perineal deficiency.

Prolapse usually presents in the peri- and postmenopausal years, the delay being due to the additional factor of oestrogen deficiency. This affects the strength of the cardinal and uterosacral ligaments, as well as the uterus, vaginal skin and subcutaneous tissue of the external genitalia, and loss of muscle tone in the pelvis and elsewhere.

Raised intra-abdominal pressure stresses the supports of the uterus and vagina, and the mechanism of urinary continence (see below), in the acute situation (e.g. coughing, laughing, sneezing, etc.) and in the chronic situation. It is the latter which helps to produce prolapse. The obese patient, with a chronic cough from smoking or bronchitis, who strains at stool and has done so for years because of constipation, has a chronically stressed pelvic floor. Large pelvic tumours may also be a contributing factor. Many patients with prolapse exhibit one or more of these features, which are ideally best corrected before surgical repair is undertaken.

Clinical features

The typical patient is a parous postmenopausal woman who complains of 'something coming down'. The patient may be aware of a lump protruding from the vulva or simply of a feeling of insecurity and downward pressure. Occasionally prolapse is seen in younger women immediately following delivery or, very rarely, during pregnancy. It is less common in countries where it is customary to squat to defecate.

Pain is not a feature, but backache sometimes occurs and is characteristically worse at the end of the day and relieved by rest. Bleeding due to prolapse is rare and should only be attributed to the prolapse after thorough investigation, including curettage. It is generally associated with visible ulceration on a procidentia. In cases of chronic procidentia there is vascular stasis. The vaginal skin is atrophic, poor perfusion of the tissues increases the vulnerability of the tissues and ulceration due to friction of underclothing is not uncommon.

Many patients with prolapse, and some with procidentia, have no complaints, with the prolapse being an incidental finding, but there may be difficulty with defecation or micturition and this may be relieved in some instances by the patient pushing the prolapse back into the vagina herself.

With virginal (nulliparous or telescopic) prolapse the primary defect is a weakness of the ligamentous supports of the uterus. Because of the weakness the uterus becomes axial to the vagina and the cervix descends to a lower level in the vagina. The vagina may be completely everted but the perineum is intact. Once the uterus and cervix are restored to their normal position, however, there is no cystocele or rectocele to be found.

Examination and demonstration of prolapse are best carried out with the patient in the left lateral position using a Sims speculum to hold back the posterior vaginal wall and a sponge forceps to hold back the anterior vaginal wall, although a procidentia will be apparent in whatever position the patient lies. Inspection of the introitus while the patient coughs may reveal stress incontinence, a urethrocele, cystocele and rectocele. The cervix may become visible too. Examination should be carried out in a systematic manner to observe the various parts that may contribute to prolapse. As all parts of the vaginal skin are seen, an assessment of its oestrogenization is made. First the lower third of the anterior wall is viewed for a urethrocele, then the upper two-thirds. The patient may be asked to cough or bear down. To assess the degree of mobility and descent of the uterus and cervix a single-toothed volsella forceps may be applied to the cervix to demonstrate the degree of uterine prolapse more accurately. However this needs to be done cautiously as it may cause discomfort. Careful bimanual assessment of uterine mobility is vital.

It is important to view the posterior fornix, particularly as the patient coughs, but it can often be difficult to demonstrate an enterocele. As the speculum is withdrawn it is possible to assess the presence of a rectocele by seeing whether the posterior vaginal wall bulges forwards.

Treatment

Although prolapse is not life-threatening and may be asymptomatic, in the majority of cases it causes misery, alters the patient's lifestyle, restricts her activity and requires treatment. Before deciding which form of treatment is appropriate a careful assessment should be made, paying particular attention to the following features:

1 The patient's age and parity, especially her wish for more children.
2 Sexual activity and the need for a functional vagina.
3 The presence of aggravating factors such as obesity, smoking and constipation, which should be eliminated before surgery. Their elimination improves the efficacy of conservative treatment too.
4 Menstrual problems.
5 Urinary symptoms, which must be carefully assessed and sometimes analysed by detailed urodynamic studies (see later).

Prophylactic

Proper attention to the repair of the perineum, together with regular pelvic floor exercises, particularly in the puerperium, will help prevent prolapse. Avoidance of those factors which chronically raise intra-abdominal pressure and the use of hormone replacement therapy may also prevent prolapse.

Conservative

If a patient wants more children, or is unfit for surgery, if there is a long waiting list or she is attending the dietician, it is often possible to control the prolapse and alleviate the symptoms using a pessary. The common type is a ring pessary. These come in different sizes and are made of flexible plastic. Rings should be changed at regular 6–8-monthly intervals and the vagina inspected to exclude any trauma. Rings are only satisfactory for lesser degrees of prolapse. In the postmenopausal woman an oestrogen cream should be used sparingly once or twice a week to prevent atrophy. Shelf pessaries give satisfactory control of major prolapse but are rigid, obstruct the vagina, making coitus impossible and are difficult to fit.

Physiotherapy to the pelvic floor muscles, including faradism, and to the chest for patients with chronic bronchitis, together with weight loss, may cure stress incontinence, or be useful adjuncts to a pessary or preparation for surgery.

Surgery

Preoperative preparation

It is important to define and eradicate, where possible, contributory factors. For instance, the obese patient should be encouraged to lose weight. Overweight patients are an operative hazard in any field of surgery. She should stop smoking for at least 3 months before surgery, and chest physiotherapy may be helpful. Constipation should be eradicated. Local oestrogen creams improve the quality of vaginal skin, and ulcers should be healed before surgery. Prolapse has never killed a patient but surgical repair of prolapse has, so for this elective procedure, which is carried out for the patient's comfort rather than immediate health, she should be as fit as possible. The chance of recurrence of the prolapse postoperatively is also reduced.

Choice of operation

The type of operation carried out depends on what is involved in the prolapse. For instance, anterior vaginal wall repair is appropriate for a cystocele; posterior colpoperineorrhaphy (repair) for a rectocele. If there is uterine (i.e. vaginal vault) prolapse the vault may be best re-supported if the uterus is coincidentally removed (vaginal hysterectomy and repair).

Alternatively the uterus and vault may be supported by shortening the transverse cervical ligaments, which necessitates partial cervical amputation; when combined with anterior and posterior colpoperineorrhaphy, as is often necessary, the whole procedure is called the Manchester (or Fothergill) repair operation. Many gynaecologists now favour vaginal hysterectomy and repair because the long-term results in terms of recurrent prolapse are better, the patients are rarely young and even the younger patients usually desire foolproof contraception, and in any case child-bearing after cervical amputation can be hazardous. For a more detailed description of these procedures see Chapter 25.

URINARY PROBLEMS

Urinary problems present commonly to the gynaecologist, often, but not always, associated with prolapse. Some laxity of the vaginal wall is inevitable after childbirth. The fact that a woman has some prolapse and urinary symptoms does not mean that the prolapse is the cause of the urinary symptoms and that repair of the prolapse will cure these.

It is essential that the urinary problems are carefully investigated on their own. Certainly any associated prolapse must be noted and considered, but not assumed to be involved aetiologically unless proven to be so. Since urinary problems are frequently associated with prolapse or other gynaecological disorders and since they often date from child-bearing, the patient seeks gynaecological rather than urological advice.

Urodynamic studies involving measurement of urethral, vesical and rectal pressure and urine flow-rate, together with video-radiographic visualization of the changes taking place during micturition, have led to the normal mechanisms of continence and micturition being defined more accurately. Consequently more has been learned about incontinence too. The reader should here review the normal mechanism of continence and micturition (see pp. 38–40). The first step in elucidating urinary problems is to take a detailed history with particular regard to frequency, nocturia analysis, dysuria and incontinence.

Frequency

If urine is passed more than 10 times a day, the patient has frequency.

Nocturia

If urine is passed two or more times a night, the patient has nocturia.

Dysuria

If there is infection in the bladder suprapubic pain will be felt during micturition or at the end. If there is local trauma around the urethra or if there is urethral infection there will be a burning sensation during micturition. Infection is associated with frequency and nocturia.

Enuresis

This distressing symptom of bed-wetting is rarely encountered in gynaecology, perhaps because it is not sought. Questions should be asked of the patient relating to her teens and childhood as well as currently, since a positive history may be associated with detrusor instability and may be helpful in elucidating the current complaint.

Retention of urine

This is not uncommon postoperatively or after delivery, especially if there has been periurethral trauma, epidural anaesthesia or recurrent use of a catheter.

Acute retention of urine in the female is a rare event. The causes include a retroverted gravid uterus about 12 weeks' gestation, a uterine fibroid of equivalent size, an ovarian tumour or haemato-colpos (a vagina full of blood). Multiple sclerosis should be considered if there is no evidence of a mass impacted in the pelvis compressing the bladder neck.

Urinary incontinence

Urinary incontinence is a common symptom presented to the gynaecologist and has a number of very different causes, which can be distinguished to a large extent by the exact mode of presentation.

A careful history, comprehensive examination and, in selected cases, the use of urodynamic investigation will define the cause of the incontinence. It must be remembered that other symptoms of lower urinary tract dysfunction, such as frequency, nocturia, hesitancy and urgency and retention of urine may also be present, although urinary incontinence is the most common. Prevalence studies have suggested that 12% of women over 65 years seek medical advice on one or other of these counts. In these cases basic investigation, after neurological testing, should include culture of a midstream specimen of urine to exclude infection, abdominal X-ray to exclude urinary calculi, and occasionally cystoscopy to exclude tumours.

There are five main types of urinary incontinence (Table 22.1).

Table 22.1   Types of urinary incontinence

Type	Cause	Treatment
Stress	Defective urethral sphincter	*Conservative*: Pelvic floor exercises
		Operative: Colposuspension – abdominal Marshall–Marchetti–Krantz procedure – abdominal Sling procedures – abdominal Anterior repair – vaginal Stamey procedure – combined abdominal and vaginal
Urge Sensory	Hypersensitivity to infection or calculi	Antibiotics Surgery Treat cause
Motor	Uninhibited detrusor contraction (Unstable bladder) (CVA, MS)	*Conservative*: Bladder retraining Anticholinergic drugs *Surgery*: Divide nerve supply Increase bladder size
Reflex	Cerebral control lost over local reflex	Indwelling catheter or appliance Reduce sphincter spasm
Overflow	Chronic retention Large residual, e.g. Diabetic neuropathy Post radical pelvic surgery Pelvic mass	Long-term catheterization Removal of pelvic mass where possible
Continuous	*Congenital*: Ectopic ureter Ectopia vesicae *Acquired*: Urethral or vesical fistula	Surgical repair

CVA = Cerebrovascular accident; MS = multiple sclerosis.

The role of urodynamic studies

The cause of the urinary problem may be indicated from the history but the diagnosis may not be clear-cut and there may be mixed symptoms; urge and stress incontinence frequently occur together. It is important to differentiate detrusor instability from genuine stress incontinence and to assess urethral competence so that the most appropriate therapy or surgical approach is adopted.

Pressure is measured in the bladder and the rectum. The intrarectal pressure is equivalent to intra-abdominal pressure so the detrusor pressure is the total pressure minus the intrarectal pressure.

The bladder is filled with water and the volume at which a desire to void first occurs is noted. In the normal bladder this is about 150 ml with a strong desire at 400 ml. There should be no detrusor contractions during filling.

Desire to void at volumes less than 150 ml suggests a sensitive bladder and chronic infection, while detrusor contractions during filling suggest instability and may provoke urge incontinence. Pressure–flow measurements of urethral flow rate in relation to intravesical pressure can indicate if there is bladder neck obstruction.

If there is urethral incompetence there is no voluntary increase in urethral pressure, and a low resting urethral pressure.

Urodynamic studies are of the greatest help in defining the cause and appropriate management in the majority of women with urinary problems.

Stress incontinence

This is defined as involuntary loss of urine when the intra-abdominal pressure is raised, as by coughing, laughing, sneezing, etc., in the absence of any desire to void. The proximal part of the urethra funnels below the level of the pelvic floor and leakage of urine occurs when intravesical pressure exceeds the urethral pressure in the absence of a detrusor contraction. It is associated with a defect of the urethral sphincter. Urodynamic findings include a low resting urethral profile and typical stress urethral pressure in relation to a series of coughs. The patient usually has poor pelvic floor function and is unable to interrupt her stream.

Treatment is aimed at restoring urethral closure pressure. Conservatively this may be achieved by re-education of the pelvic floor muscles by specific training exercises. Alternatively the proximal part of the urethra may be restored surgically above the level of the pelvic floor. This may be done abdominally (a Burch colposuspension where the tissues adjacent to the bladder neck are attached to the pectineal line on each side, or the Marshall–Marchetti–Krantz procedure where these tissues are attached to the back of the symphysis pubis) or vaginally (anterior colporrhaphy/repair). The Stamey procedure and other sling operations use a combined abdominal and vaginal approach.

Urgency and urge incontinence

Urinary urgency is the intense desire to void, which, if overwhelming, leads to incontinence, hence called urge incontinence. There are two distinct types: *sensory* urgency occurs commonly in inflammatory bladder diseases, such as urinary tract infections with trigonitis, and is rarely associated with incontinence. *Motor* urgency is followed by incontinence as it is caused by uninhibited contraction of the detrusor muscle during filling, the contraction pressure exceeding the urethral pressure and urine leakage occurring. This condition is also known as unstable bladder. It may occur in patients who have had a cerebrovascular accident or multiple sclerosis, but in most women the cause is obscure. The patient complains of frequency but may also complain of urgency and urge and stress incontinence. It is diagnosed on urodynamic examination by spikes of increased intravesical pressure causing leakage which may occur spontaneously during bladder filling (or when the patient coughs), and the bladder capacity is functionally reduced. The sphincters of such a patient will be normal and thus the urethral closing pressure will be normal.

Treatment is designed to reduce the activity of the detrusor. This may be achieved with anticholinergic drugs or occasionally with surgery to increase bladder capacity. Bladder habit retraining may prove successful for the highly motivated.

Reflex incontinence

This describes the inefficient voiding pattern and incontinence seen in paraplegics where the cerebral control over the local reflex has been severed. There is often a poor stream and incomplete emptying. Urodynamic studies show a very high urethral pressure and treatment is aimed at reducing sphincter spasm but usually means an appliance or indwelling catheter.

Overflow incontinence

There is a continuous dribble of urine or small amounts leak on effort. There is either chronic retention or a large residual volume of urine due to bladder neck or urethral obstruction. The pool of residual urine in the bladder may act as a focus for repeated infections. The obstruction may be due to urethral stricture or to extrinsic pressure from a pelvic tumour or retroverted gravid uterus. Overflow incontinence may also occur when the bladder becomes atonic and overdistended following radical pelvic surgery (abdominal perineal resection or Wertheim's hysterectomy). Urodynamic findings include a large capacity bladder, no rise in detrusor pressure during voiding, a low flow rate and significant residual urine.

Treatment includes removal of the obstruction, but for those with a denervated bladder long-term catheterization is necessary.

Continuous incontinence

The ureter or bladder may communicate with the uterus or vagina and the patient will have no control over the urinary flow. Fistulae follow radiotherapy, advanced malignant disease, surgical mishaps or major obstetric trauma. Rarely an ectopic ureter may open into the vagina, or the bladder may open directly on to the anterior abdominal wall (ectopia vesicae). Surgical repair is indicated for all forms of continuous incontinence.

The urethral syndrome

The patient experiences dysuria (painful micturition), frequency and urgency and nocturia. Symptoms frequently appear to bear a relationship to intercourse, but may also be associated with oestrogen withdrawal after the menopause. On examination the urethral orifice looks angry, red and inflamed and the anterior vaginal wall is tender to touch. Cystoscopy will reveal a normal bladder and urine culture will be negative. At cystoscopy the urethral orifice is often tight and dilatation of the urethra together with oestrogen therapy, if necessary, is the treatment of choice. It affords immediate relief but occasionally has to be repeated in months or years. The dilatation is carried out under general anaesthesia.

RETROVERSION

In childhood the uterus is a straight upright organ, its body being small in relation to the cervix. As the uterus grows at puberty the body enlarges to a greater extent than the cervix and usually leans forward upon it, causing both angulation of the body on the cervix (anteflexion) and rotation of the whole uterus forward on its supporting ligaments (anteversion). However, the uterus is a mobile active organ contracting throughout reproductive life and can take up many positions. The position of the uterus is altered by changes in adjacent organs, particularly the bladder as it fills and empties. During intercourse in the late excitement phase the uterus is elevated, thus effectively lengthening the vagina. The uterus may be pushed backwards by a mass of fibroids growing from its anterior wall, or forwards by a tumour, usually an ovarian cyst, occupying the pouch of Douglas. A cyst growing from the left ovary may displace the uterus to the right, whereas left adnexal inflammatory disease may draw the uterus across to the left. Although the uterus usually lies in an anteverted, anteflexed position when the bladder is empty, in 25% of women it will be retroverted (but not usually retroflexed). This retroverted position may be quite normal provided the uterus is mobile and it usually presents no problems. Retroversion may be acquired due to pelvic inflammatory disease or endometriosis, in which case it is fixed and cannot be anteverted.

Mobile (congenital) retroversion

This is usually asymptomatic, and it is necessary to assess any symptomatology carefully before attributing it to a mobile retroverted uterus. Backache due to congestion of the uterus as a result of impaired venous drainage may sometimes occur, but backache is much more commonly due to other conditions. Dyspareunia means painful intercourse. Deep dyspareunia, that is, pain felt deep in the pelvis at the top of the vagina during intercourse, may occur if the ovaries are prolapsed in the pouch of Douglas. Dysmenorrhoea, that is, pain due to menstruation, is not related to mobile retroversion, and mobile retroversion is not a cause of infertility.

Fixed retroversion

Fixed acquired retroversion is due to pathology, usually pelvic inflammatory endometriosis or disease, which are discussed in Chapters 17 and 18. The symptoms, signs and management depend on the underlying disease but backache, deep dyspareunia, dysmenorrhoea and infertility may all be present with fixed retroversion being produced by the basic pathology causing the retroversion to be fixed.

Retroversion in pregnancy

When a patient with a mobile retroverted uterus becomes pregnant the uterus fills the pelvis by 12 weeks, becoming anteverted and easily palpable abdominally by 14 weeks. If the uterus is pre- vented from rising out of the pelvis by adhesions, impaction and incarceration may occur, leading to abortion. This set of events is heralded by urinary disturbance, first frequency, then strangury and finally retention. Acute retention in pregnancy is a rare event and is nearly always due to a retroverted uterus impacted in the pelvis, distorting and compressing the bladder neck. It generally occurs at about 14 weeks.

Diagnosis and treatment

The diagnosis of retroversion is made on bimanual examination. The differential diagnosis is from other masses in the pouch of Douglas; the passage of a sound will define the position of the uterus if doubt persists. Surgical correction of the retroversion (ventrosuspension) can be done if the retroverted uterus is causing symptoms. If the retroversion is mobile, manipulation to an anteverted position alone is pointless since the mobile retroverted uterus will return to its usual position. Ventrosuspension involves shortening the round ligaments and suturing them to the rectus sheath, and may be done at laparotomy or laparoscopy. Plication of the round ligaments alone holds the uterus forward temporarily and is often done as an adjunct to surgery for some other condition to avoid postoperative adhesions binding the uterus down in the pouch of Douglas. Acute retention associated with a retroverted gravid uterus is treated by continuous bladder drainage with an indwelling catheter, together with rest in a prone position, which generally allows the uterine position to correct itself.

FURTHER READING

Milton, P.J.D. (1989) Uterovaginal prolapse. In: *Progress in Obstetrics and Gynaecology*, vol. 7, edited by Studd, J. Churchill Livingstone, Edinburgh.

The climacteric, menopause and postmenopause

DEFINITIONS

The *menopause* is the cessation of menstruation at the end of the reproductive phase of life, due to complete and permanent ovarian failure. The *climacteric* is the phase of progressive ovarian failure which commences up to 5 years before, and intermittent ovarian activity which continues up to 1 year after, the menopause. During the climacteric acute severe symptoms often occur due to rising gonadotrophin levels, erratic oestrogen production and intermittent oestrogen deficiency. The *postmenopause* is the remaining phase of life following the menopause. It is important because of the gradual development of chronic symptoms of oestrogen deficiency and other effects leading to debilitating and life-shortening health risks.

Unlike men, where sex-steroid production alters little through adult life and in whom spermatozoa continue to be produced into old age, women are subjected to a major reduction in ovarian hormone production at around the age of 50 (see Fig. 5.7). This follows depletion of primordial follicles in the ovaries to a critical number (about 1000) from the finite number with which she was born (about 1 million; see Chapter 3). Cyclical ovarian activity ceases, and with it menstruation (the menopause). The endometrium atrophies but the basement membrane remains and is capable of regeneration if stimulated by administered oestrogens.

During the last 2–5 years before the menopause the numbers of follicles proceeding to the antral stage, and so available for stimulation to final maturation, decline. As a result circulating levels of inhibin fall, leading to partial elevation of pituitary gonadotrophins, particularly of follicle-stimulating hormone (FSH). As antral follicle numbers fall critically for recruitment, ovulation occurs unpredictably and oestrogen production and menstrual cycles become erratic. This transitional phase of progressive ovarian failure is the climacteric.

A menstrual delay of at least 6 months is required to be sure that complete ovarian failure and the menopause have occurred. There is no reliable hormonal marker which will predict when it will occur. Afterwards there will be gross elevation of serum FSH and luteinizing hormone (LH) and fall in oestradiol. As a biological marker of the end of reproductive function, the menopause is a major milestone in every woman's life. The average age of the menopause in the UK is 51 years, the normal range 48–56 years.

The menopause occurs earlier in women who have previously had an ovary or ovarian tissue removed or who smoke, and ovarian failure occurs earlier in women who have had a hysterectomy. The term premature menopause is used for women whose menopause occurs before the age of 40. Approximately 1% of women will have a premature menopause and for 1 in 1000 this will be before the age of 20.

ACUTE MENOPAUSAL SYNDROME

Table 23.1 summarizes the symptoms which can occur during the climacteric and the complications of oestrogen deficiency which develop postmenopausally. Acute menopausal symptoms often develop several years before the last menstrual period and are probably neuroendocrine in origin, perhaps in response to fluctuating oestrogen levels. In acute experiments hot flushes can be stopped by intravenous naloxone, which blocks opioid action on gonadotrophin-releasing hormone (GnRH) secretion.

Vasomotor flushes and sweats, particularly at night, are the most common symptoms and will be severe in 30% of women. Vasomotor symptoms will persist for more than 5 years after the menopause in 25% of women.

The night sweats disturb normal sleep patterns, disrupt rapid eye movement sleep and produce psychological symptoms similar to sleep-deprivation syndrome. These are similar to the symptoms of sleep deprivation which used to occur in many junior hospital doctors and include difficulty making decisions, poor short-term memory, anxiety, loss of confidence and mood changes, particularly irritability. However, it would be wrong to attribute all midlife psychological symptoms in women to their climacteric hormonal changes. Some will be distressed by the loss of their fertility or unwarranted anxieties about loss of femininity and fears of ageing. At this time too, commonly, her children are leaving home and her own parents are increasingly dependent or may die. These issues need to be carefully explored as underlying endogenous depression almost certainly accounts for the increased incidence of suicide in women at this time.

Table 23.1   Time-scale of climacteric and postmenopausal symptoms and the effects of oestrogen deficiency

Time/duration	System	Symptoms/disease
Acute Months	Neuroendocrine	Hot flushes Sweats Insomnia Psychological Sleep deprivation Oestrogen fluctuation
---------------------- *MENOPAUSE* ----------------------		
Months	Lower genital tract	Genital atrophy Vaginal dryness Dyspareunia
	Urinary tract	Urethral trigone atrophy Frequency/urgency
Years	Skeletal	Osteoporosis
	Arterial	Coronary artery disease Cerebrovascular disease
Chronic		

Daytime hot flushes and sweats may be very embarrassing if frequent and severe. During a flush peripheral cutaneous temperature rises by about 5°C whilst the central body temperature falls by up to 0.7°C. There is intense peripheral vasodilatation particularly of the face, neck and chest which may last a few minutes, whilst the heart rate increases by up to 20 beats/minute. The associated sweating can require a change of clothes. Vasomotor symptoms are completely relieved in over 85% of women by using sex hormone replacement therapy. The severity of the symptoms do not, however, correlate with the degree of oestrogen deficiency, or its long-term consequences.

EARLY CONSEQUENCES OF OESTROGEN DEFICIENCY

After the menopause, ovarian oestradiol production is insignificant. Oestrone becomes the main circulating oestrogen, mainly produced by peripheral adipose tissue from the weak adrenal androgen, androstenedione. Oestrone is a weak oestrogen and usually produced in too small an amount to protect against the oestradiol deficiency. However, very obese women may produce sufficient oestrone to protect against oestrogen deficiency but it may also stimulate endometrial hyperplasia, leading to carcinoma.

In most women the major early effects of oestrogen deficiency are atrophy of the lower genital and urinary tracts which have a common embryological origin. In the vulva and vagina there is loss of skin collagen and tone, and reduced blood flow, and in the vagina there is also shortening, loss of the normal rugae, thinning of the stratified squamous epithelium, and reduced glycogen production leading to an alkaline pH and a consequent higher risk of infections. Reduced vaginal secretions, particularly in response to sexual stimulation, can cause vaginal dryness and superficial dyspareunia. The uterus and cervix also atrophy and shrink in size, the cervix often becoming flush with the vaginal vault. The supporting pelvic ligaments weaken which may result in uterovaginal prolapse. Atrophic changes occur in the urethra and trigone of the bladder which may result in urinary urgency and frequency, whilst loss of tone in the supports of the bladder neck may lead to stress incontinence.

LATE CONSEQUENCES OF OESTROGEN DEFICIENCY

Oestrogen deficiency has effects on bone metabolism which predispose to osteoporosis and increased risk of fractures; on lipid metabolism which predisposes to arterial disease and increased risks of myocardial infarction and stroke; and on skin collagen causing loss which reduces skin resistance to trauma and slows healing of injuries.

OSTEOPOROSIS

Osteoporosis is the commonest metabolic bone disease in the western world. It is characterized by loss of all the constituents of bone, without any imbalance, resulting simply in reduced bone density. Osteoporosis occurs 10 times more commonly in women than men, mostly after the menopause. Women are at increased risk for two reasons. First, the peak bone mass normally achieved late in the third decade of life is 10–15% lower in women than in men, so they start their age-related decline already at a disadvantage. Second, after the menopause bone loss is accelerated for 5–10 years due to oestrogen deficiency.

After more than 30% of bone has been lost, there is a risk of fracture with relatively minor trauma. Trabecular (shock-absorbing) bone is relatively more severely affected than cortical bone. Once individual trabeculae, which provide the supportive connections, are lost they cannot be replaced. The site of any fracture will often depend on the woman's age – of the distal radius (Colles fracture) in her late 50s when she tries to break a fall; of the femoral neck in her 70s when less able to protect herself in the same way; and vertebral crush fractures in her 80s, causing the typical stooped posture (dowager's hump) of old age and often considerable pain and disability. The health risks and social costs of osteoporosis are considerable. Of the women who sustain a fractured neck of femur, 30% will be dead within 6 months, and of those who survive, half will be unable to live independently.

Sex hormone replacement therapy – usually simply called HRT – can maintain bone density for as long as it is given and in some cases it may even cause a small increase. Essentially it is buying time from osteoporosis and its complications for as long as the treatment is given. Once treatment is stopped, bone loss will recommence. The effect of HRT on bone density is illustrated in Figure 23.1. For maximum protection against osteoporosis HRT is best commenced early after the menopause, before significant oestrogen deficiency-related bone loss occurs, and continued long-term. The bone-protecting benefits of HRT can be assessed by measurement of bone mineral density or indicated by the age-specific incidence of fractures, which are reduced by at least 20% after 5 years of HRT and about 50% after 10 years.

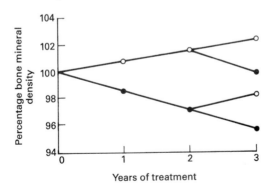

Fig. 23.1 The effect of hormone replacement therapy (HRT; *open circles*) or placebo (filled circles) on bone mineral density. Data summarized from several studies with reassignment of patients' treatment after 2 years. Note the small increase in bone density with HRT and that the rate of bone loss is not increased when HRT is stopped.

CORONARY ARTERY DISEASE

Before the menopause, women appear to be relatively protected against heart disease. Between 35 and 45 years old, death from myocardial infarction is six times more likely in men than women. By the average age of the menopause the difference has fallen to twofold and then reduces progressively. Oestrogens are thought to protect against coronary artery disease by increasing the cardioprotective high-density lipoproteins, and reducing the atherogenic low-density lipoproteins, and also by reducing peripheral resistance, so increasing blood flow. The strongest evidence that it is the menopause which increases the risk of coronary artery disease is that women with a premature menopause, before the age of 40, are at two to four times increased risk of death from myocardial infarction. HRT prevents the excess risk of fatal coronary artery disease, and most studies of HRT in older postmenopausal women show a cardioprotective effect. The reduction in risk of fatal coronary artery disease by HRT is about 20% after 5 years' use and 50% after 10 years.

It is often confusing for women to understand why HRT after the menopause should protect against cardiovascular disease when oestrogen/progestogen contraception in young women is said to increase the risk. The contraceptive pill and HRT are not, however, equivalent. The biological potency of the oestrogens in the two preparations is quite different. The potency of different oestrogens is considered later in this chapter.

CEREBROVASCULAR DISEASE

Strokes are responsible for as many deaths as coronary artery disease in women and together these two causes account for over 60% of deaths in women. A relatively small reduction in the risk of these two conditions occurring prematurely would therefore have a dramatic effect on life expectancy and quality of life. A small but increasing amount of data suggests that after the menopause a woman's risk of a fatal cerebrovascular accident can be reduced by about 30–50% by HRT. The protective mechanisms are likely to be the same as those proposed for coronary artery disease: reduction of low-density lipoproteins, increase in high-density lipoproteins and improvement in peripheral blood flow.

COLLAGEN CHANGES

Oestrogen deficiency causes loss of collagen at various sites, particularly in the skin, with loss of elasticity and an increased tendency to wrinkling. Although these skin changes are often considered trivial, they reflect alterations in the collagen content of many other tissues: bone, articular cartilage, muscle and the ligaments supporting most joints. These may cause musculoskeletal pains, limit mobility and exacerbate arthritic problems. Collagen deficiency in the skin is also more than a cosmetic problem as injuries will heal more slowly and predispose to varicose ulceration, which is almost exclusively a problem of older post-menopausal women.

DIAGNOSIS AND ASSESSMENT FOR HRT

Investigation will rarely be necessary to confirm that a woman is postmenopausal. Only when acute vasomotor symptoms occur in menstruating women, or the last menstrual period occurred only 2 or 3 months ago, would investigations be helpful. A high serum FSH level (>25 iu/l) combined with a low oestradiol level (<110 pmol/l) – the latter to exclude the misleading possibility of a preovulatory FSH, when oestradiol would also be raised – confirm the menopausal transition.

Before commencing HRT, whether for relief of acute symptoms or for protection against the long-term risks of oestrogen deficiency, a careful history, examination and counselling are needed. The range and severity of symptoms and possible contraindications to HRT must be determined. Absolute contraindications to HRT include oestrogen-dependent tumours such as endometrial carcinoma and some breast carcinomas, severe liver disease, undiagnosed abnormal vaginal bleeding and uncontrolled hypertension. Relative contraindications, which may require careful monitoring whilst taking HRT, include gallbladder disease, previous symptomatic endometriosis, previous hypertension whilst taking combined oral contraception or in pregnancy, malignant melanoma and uterine fibroids. Previous deep vein thrombosis or pulmonary embolism may be contraindications if not obviously precipitated by some specific factor at that time such as major surgery, and haemato-logical investigation is advisable to look for any underlying thrombophilic tendency. Natural oestrogens given at the usual low dosage for HRT do not produce any clinically significant effect on coagulation in the absence of a thrombogenic tendency, nor are they diabetogenic.

Thorough counselling about the risks and benefits of HRT, and the different formulations and routes of administration, is valuable. By improving subsequent adherence to treatment and duration of use the patient can maximize the long-term benefits for her health.

HORMONE REPLACEMENT THERAPY

Hormone replacement therapy, or strictly, sex HRT, is the administration primarily of oestrogen to correct and protect against the specific effects of oestrogen deficiency. However, if a woman still has her uterus, unopposed use of oestrogen would stimulate proliferation of her endometrium, leading in time to hyperplasia and increased risk of carcinoma. Therefore additional progestogen is needed for its antioestrogenic – antiproliferative – action on the endometrium. The progestogen may be given cyclically to induce regular endometrial shedding similar to menstruation, or, in older postmenopausal women, continuously, to avoid regular bleeding which at that age often seems a practical nuisance and emotionally unacceptable. Women who have had a hysterectomy may safely take oestrogen replacement alone. Occasionally the addition of a small dose of androgen improves libido.

HRT differs from oestrogen/progestogen oral contraceptive preparations in important ways. Bone is protected by very low oestrogen dosage and often little more is needed to control acute symptoms of oestrogen deficiency, by achieving circulating levels equivalent to the early follicular phase of the ovarian cycle. This can be achieved by various natural oestrogens, often in forms absorbed through the skin (see below) to avoid first passage through the liver. The actual oestrogen level varies between different formulations, as shown in Figure 23.2, but is physiological with respect to normal premenopausal ovulatory women. By contrast, the oral contraceptive dose effect must be much higher to suppress ovulation by feedback on the pituitary, and potent long-acting synthetic oestrogens must be used, taken orally, leading to disproportionate actions on

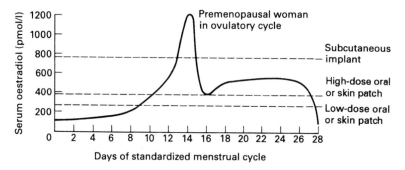

Fig. 23.2 Approximate relative serum oestradiol levels using different hormone replacement therapy preparations compared with the concentrations during a normal menstrual cycle.

liver metabolism. Essentially, HRT is given to mimic normal physiological oestrogen levels whereas the combined oral contraceptive pill is given at pharmacological dosage to override ovarian activity.

Routes and types of preparation

Examples of the more frequently used HRT preparations, their routes of administration and relative advantages and disadvantages, are listed in Tables 23.2 and 23.3. Oral preparations are the most convenient and most frequently used. However, relatively high dosage is needed, partly to maintain 24-hour effectiveness

Table 23.2   Oestrogenic hormone replacement therapy (HRT) routes of administration and their relative advantages and disadvantages

	Advantages	Disadvantages
Oral tablets	Most convenient Easily reversible	Unphysiological oestrogen profile First-pass liver metabolism Effects on liver function
Transdermal patches or gel	Constant hormone level Minimal hepatic effects Convenient Easily reversible	Allergic skin reactions Detachment (not with gel) Cost
Vaginal creams, tablets or rings	As for patches and transdermal creams, but greater local effect	Messy discharge of cream Less effect on systemic symptoms
Subcutaneous implants	Constant hormone level Prolonged effect Ensures compliance Can add testosterone for libido Convenient Inexpensive	Surgical procedure Duration of action if side-effects Supraphysiological oestrogen levels Prolonged effect after HRT is stopped Develop tolerance to higher oestrogen levels

Table 23.3   Examples of commonly used hormone replacement therapy preparations, listed by their route of administration, with or without a progestogen

Route of administration	Oestrogen only	Oestrogen and progestogen
Oral tablets	Premarin (Conjugated equine oestrogens) Progynova (Oestradiol valerate) Climaval (Oestradiol valerate)	Prempak C (with norgestrel) Nuvelle (with levonorgestrel) Climagest (with norethisterone) Trisquens (Oestradiol and oestriol with norethisterone)
Transdermal patches	Estraderm (Oestradiol) Evorel (Oestradiol) Fematrix (Oestradiol)	Estrapak (with oral norethisterone) Estracombi (with patch norethisterone) Evorel-Pak (with oral norethisterone) Evorel Sequi / Evorel Conti (with patch norethisterone)
Transdermal gel	Oestrogel (Oestradiol)	
Vaginal creams, tablets or rings	Dienoestrol cream (Dienoestrol) Premarin cream (Conjugated equine oestrogens) Ovestin cream (Oestriol) Vagifem tablets (Oestradiol) Estring (Oestradiol hemihydrate)	
Subcutaneous implants	Oestradiol	

because levels wane after an initial high, and partly because passage through the liver after absorption from the gastrointestinal tract leads to metabolization to oestrone, which is a relatively weak oestrogen. In addition, passage through the liver can influence the synthesis of, for example, renin substrate, antithrombin III and high- and low-density lipoproteins, increasing the risk of hypertension and venous thrombosis in susceptible individuals, who may therefore benefit from other routes of administration. However, the increase in high-density lipoproteins induced by oral oestrogens is beneficial in protecting against arteriovascular disease.

Transdermal, including vaginal and subcutaneous, preparations of oestradiol avoid first passage through the liver and by direct absorption lead to higher levels of oestradiol than oestrone in the blood, giving greater biological activity. Therefore the total dose of oestrogen needed is relatively low. Application is by adhesive skin patches which need to be changed only once or twice a week, or a gel to be rubbed into the skin daily. Patches occasionally cause an allergic skin reaction. In the case of oestrogen-only preparations, progestogen can be separately prescribed if required (for women with a uterus), either cyclically (e.g. 10–14 days of each calendar month) or continuously. In women with an implant, which may continue to be active for a variable time, progestogen should continue to be used until withdrawal bleeds cease. This is particularly important when implant HRT is stopped, to avoid the risk of unopposed oestrogen stimulating endometrial hyperplasia.

Vaginal creams, tablets or slow-release rings (shaped like a supportive pessary to stay in place) are intended to have a mainly local effect but systemic absorption occurs to a variable extent. They are mainly used to treat atrophic vaginitis and urethritis, particularly in women using a supportive pessary for vaginal prolapse who are unfit for surgery. Because of systemic absorption of oestrogen, if used for more than a few weeks in a woman with a uterus, cyclical progestogen should be prescribed to protect the endometrium.

HRT without cyclical bleeding

One of the commonest reasons why women stop HRT is dissatisfaction because of the continued need for regular withdrawal bleeds if they still have their uterus. However, the frequency can be safely reduced to every 3 months by delaying cyclical progestogen treatment, so long as breakthrough bleeding does not occur earlier. This is only appropriate for women who are truly postmenopausal (at least 1 year past their menopause) or for women who have been on cyclical HRT since before their menopause who reach 54 years – the 90th centile age for ovarian failure. Alternatively, for such women, cyclical bleeding can often be avoided altogether by continuous combined oestrogen and progestogen preparations, such as Kliofem or Premique, or by tibolone (Livial), which is a synthetic oestrogen that also has progestogenic activity. Such continuous progestogenic action on the endometrium keeps it atrophic. Breakthrough bleeding may sometimes be a nuisance but is most likely soon after the menopause due to unpredictable ovarian contribution of oestrogen. Therefore monthly bleeds should be the aim during the first year after the menopause.

Benefits and risks of oestrogenic HRT

These are summarized in Table 23.4. Some of the major health benefits of HRT have already been discussed and there is also some evidence that HRT may reduce the risk of large-bowel cancer. In addition many women gain a welcome improvement in their general sense of well-being through enhanced mood and physical and sexual drive, and enjoy the cosmetic benefit of better skin tone.

The main anxieties about long-term use of oestrogenic HRT are the potential risks of endometrial and breast cancer. Endometrial cancer is oestrogen-dependent and unopposed oestrogen treatment increases the risk 5–15 times depending on dosage and duration. Adding cyclical monthly progestogen protects the endometrium but is only fully protective – indeed, it reduces the risk below that of women who do not take HRT at all - if each course lasts at least 12 days. However, it is safe to extend the interval between courses to up to 3 months for women who are more than 12 months postmenopausal.

A link between HRT and breast cancer is unclear. Many confounding factors influence breast cancer risk, such as family history, age at first live birth, parity, age at menarche and menopause and whether a woman has breast-fed her children. In addition, breast cancer does not behave like a purely oestrogen-dependent tumour as the incidence continues to rise progressively with the woman's age, unlike endometrial cancer which peaks at about 60. Most studies of HRT report no significant increase in breast cancer with up to 9 years' usage. Estimates after longer-term use range widely from zero to a 70% increase but there are insufficient data to be conclusive and it is not possible at present to give unequivocal reassurance. Whilst it seems that HRT does not increase the risk of breast cancer, nor does it seem to reduce it, and women need to be warned that unlike the protective effect on the endometrium, HRT does not protect against breast cancer. However, a reassuring point is that, if a woman is unfortunate and does develop breast cancer whilst taking HRT, the prognosis is much improved.

Table 23.4 Benefits and risks of oestrogenic hormone replacement therapy

Benefits	Risks
Acute symptom relief 85–100% of patients successful No indication of long-term risks of oestrogen deficiency *Sense of well-being* Often improved mood, energy, libido *Osteoporotic fractures* Reduced by 20% after 5 years, 50% after 10 years *Ischaemic heart disease* Fatal myocardial infarction reduced by 20% after 5 years, 50% after 10 years Due to lipid changes and reduced vascular resistance *Cerebrovascular disease* Less well-documented; strokes reduced similarly to myocardial infarction *Large bowel cancer* Colon and rectal cancer reduced by 40% after 10 years ?Due to reduced bile acids *Skin collagen* Improved skin tone ?Reduced risk varicose ulceration	*Endometrial cancer* But protected by cyclical progestogen courses lasting ≥ 12 days *Breast cancer* Risks unclear: no significant increased risk up to at least 9 years' usage Mortality reduced if cancer occurs

CONCLUSION

Female life expectancy has risen steadily since the mid 19th century, from 45 to 82 years. This means that women can now expect to live more than a third of their lives in an oestrogen-deficient state, causing long-term health risks. There are about 10 million post-menopausal women in the UK and the number is predicted to rise considerably in the next two decades. HRT offers them clearly defined preventive health care benefits which greatly exceed the small and poorly defined theoretical risks. The use of HRT should at least be considered in all women and discussed with them at the time of their menopause.

FURTHER READING

Hillier, S.G., Kitchener, H.C., Neilson, J.P. (eds) (1996) *Scientific Essentials of Reproductive Medicine*. W.B. Saunders, London.
Whitehead, M. and Godfree, V. (1992) *Hormone Replacement Therapy – Your Questions Answered*. Churchill Livingstone, Edinburgh.

24

Genital neoplasia and tumours

GENERAL
Prevalence and incidence

Cancer, i.e. any invasive malignant tumour, occurs nearly as often in women (48.5%) as in men (51.5%). Table 24.1 shows that, while cancer of the alimentary tract occurs roughly equally in men and women, men are much more likely to have lung cancer, and women to have cancer of the breast or genital tract. The likelihood of death from cancer in a woman is about 21%, and in a man 23%. Cancer of the breast alone will occur in about 5% of women, and of the genital tract in 4%.

Table 24.1 Proportional incidence (percentage) of the main sites of origin of cancer in women compared with men.

Site	Women	Men
Alimentary tract	27	29
Lungs	5	31
Breast	25	0.2
Genital	18	9

In general, the risk of cancer increases with age. It is rare before 30 years, but thereafter in women the age-specific incidence increases linearly; it accelerates later in men and at about 55 years overtakes the rate in women. The general, i.e. linear, pattern in women applies to cancer of the breast, but not the genital tract. Figure 24.1 shows that the greatest risk of endometrial or ovarian cancer is in the first two decades after the menopause and then falls, whereas the risk of cervical cancer is at a constant high level from about 10 years before the menopause. At the age of 40 years a woman is about four times

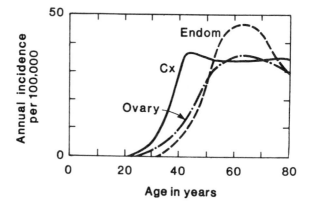

Fig. 24.1 The age-specific incidence of cancer (invasive malignant tumours) in the common sites in the genital tract: cervix (cx), endometrium (Endom) and ovary.

more likely to have cervical than endometrial or ovarian cancer. From 55 years the risk is about the same for all three sites. Figure 24.1 and Table 24.2 show that, although endometrial cancer is rare before the age of 40 years, ovarian cancer is not uncommon between 30 and 40 years.

Table 24.2 Incidence, prevalent age, survival and proportion of deaths in women due to breast and genital cancer, and preinvasive cervical carcinoma.

Site	Life-time incidence* (% of women)	Cause as % of all deaths	Mean age (yr)	Age range (95% limits) (yr)	5-year survival rate † (%)
Breast	5.11	3.94	60	35–86	49
Genital (total)	3.72	2.68	59	34–84	44
Cervix	1.29	0.74	55	33–84	44
Endometrium	1.02	0.37	61	41–83	70
Ovary	0.97	1.24	58	31–82	26
Vulva	0.21	0.15	67	36–89	52
Cervix preinvasive (CIN 3)	?	–	42	25–66	~100

*Calculated from average observed annual age-specific incidence rates and 74-yr life expectancy.
†Survival rate corrected to allow for deaths not due to cancer.
CIN 3 = Cervical intraepithelial neoplasia grade 3.

Cellular dysplasia of increasing severity precedes frank malignant change and the accessibility of the cervix makes it an important
site where cytological screening by regular cervical smears can
detect neoplastic change at a preinvasive and therefore curable
stage. Table 24.2 shows that the most severe form of dysplasia,
cervical intraepithelial neoplasia grade 3 (CIN 3), occurs at a mean
age (which is also the peak age of incidence) about 13 years earlier
than invasive cancer. This suggests that the natural progression
from preinvasive to invasive carcinoma of the cervix takes about this
length of time.

Cancer in other parts of the genital tract is much less common
than in the cervix, endometrium or ovary (Table 24.2). Cancer of
the vulva is next in frequency and occurs in the UK about 10
years later. Cancer of the vagina, fallopian tube or myometrium, or
choriocarcinoma, is extremely rare.

These data are mainly derived from an English midland
population of about 5 million in the 1960s (see Waterhouse, 1974).

Death and survival rates

About 21% of women die from cancer, and about 23% of men.
Amongst women who die from cancer, the tumour originates in the
breast in 20% and the genital tract in 14%. These figures for breast
and genital tract are lower than their relative incidence (Table 24.1)
because survival is generally better than, for instance, alimentary
cancer. Table 24.2 shows, however, that while survival from
endometrial cancer is particularly good, that from ovarian cancer is
particularly bad. The difference is at least partly due to the relatively
early occurrence of symptoms with endometrial cancer (vaginal
bleeding).

Towards earlier diagnosis

The chance of survival is greatly improved by treatment at an early
stage. Early diagnosis will be the main concern of the non-specialist.
The opportunity is unfortunately often missed, for various reasons:

1 Ovarian tumours are commonly asymptomatic. They should
   always be sought by bimanual pelvic examination whenever
   vaginal examination is done for other reasons, such as to take a
   cervical smear or to fit a contraceptive device. However, only
   about 1 in 200 bimanual examinations is likely to detect ovarian
   pathology and the signs of early ovarian carcinoma are often
   subtle and easily missed.
2 Swellings in the pelvis are notoriously difficult to distinguish,

even for experts. The common causes are uterine fibroids, ovarian neoplastic cysts and inflammatory or endometriotic cysts. Abdominal or vaginal ultrasound scanning is extremely useful in determining the origin of a pelvic mass and, by demonstrating its internal structure, can help differentiate benign from malignant ovarian cysts. If there is any doubt, laparoscopic inspection or laparotomy should always be done because of the likelihood and serious implications of ovarian cancer.

3 Non-menstrual (including postmenopausal) bleeding as a sign of uterine cancer is frequently neglected by patients but should always be taken seriously and investigated promptly.
4 Early cancer of the cervix may be missed because of technical failure to expose the cervix to view.
5 Preinvasive carcinoma of the cervix may be missed because of failure to take a cytology smear accurately.
6 Vulval carcinoma may be overlooked in an elderly patient because itching, a common early symptom, may be treated without examination, sometimes for years.

In other words, overcome any inhibitions (often on the part of the patient) about vaginal examination, learn to expose the cervix with facility and to take a good cervical smear, and get specialist opinion on any swelling felt in the pelvis. Remember also that patients often visit their family doctor not expecting to be examined and therefore seem unwilling, but may welcome an offer to return on another day perhaps after bathing.

Advanced genital cancer: management and cause of death

Whatever the exact origin and type of genital cancers, they present the same clinical problems, which include:

1 Pain, especially due to metastatic invasion of bone and damage or pressure to nerve roots.
2 Obstruction of bowel or ureters.
3 Bleeding.
4 Infection due to erosion through the vagina.
5 Urinary or faecal fistulae (connecting with the vagina) due to invasion of bladder or rectum.
6 Cachexia.

The commonest cause of death, in about half the cases, is uraemia resulting from ureteric obstruction – a relatively kind way. Cachexia, anaemia and infection account for most of the remainder.

The major problems to deal with are pain, which is dreaded, and incontinence due to fistulae, which is demoralizing. Radiotherapy may already be spent, and more irradiation may worsen the problem of ulceration by causing further necrosis of both tumour and adjacent normal tissue. Palliative surgery may be useful to divert faeces or urine by colostomy or ureteroileostomy, and if the tumour can be mobilized, exenteration (i.e. removal of rectum and/or bladder with the tumour) may very occasionally be beneficial.

Pain is dreaded but need not be so. Doctors are frequently too inhibited in their use of analgesic drugs, partly because of their unwillingness to concede defeat and accept a short-term outlook. Patients are usually more realistic than many doctors imagine, and can accept approaching death with calm and dignity given proper relief of their physical symptoms. The important objective in treatment is to anticipate pain, as it is much easier to keep it at bay than abolish it once established. The drugs should always be prescribed on a regular basis, not as required. In this way mild analgesics, non-steroidal anti-inflammatory drugs such as diclofenac, or methadone may suffice for a long time before morphine or heroin becomes necessary. Fears about narcotic addiction are out of place in these circumstances, and anyway the dose usually needs little increase once an effective level is reached and regularly maintained. Table 24.3 illustrates the range and potency of drugs which are available for pain relief. Other approaches which may be useful in specific situations include:

1 Local radiotherapy.
2 Epidural steroids where spinal metastases are causing compression of nerves.
3 Occasionally, neurolysis by injection of phenol, cryotherapy or radiofrequency ablation where there is pain from a single nerve root.
4 Carbamazepine or other anticonvulsants for neurogenic pain
5 Amitriptyline for chronic pain which is aching or burning in nature.
6 Local lignocaine infusions.
7 Palliative chemotherapy.

Other distressing symptoms include nausea, which can be relieved by potent antiemetics such as ondansetron, and anorexia, for which glucocorticoids may help by promoting normal anabolic metabolism which has been undermined by the tumour catabolism. Finally, there is no substitute for kind nursing and thoughtful sympathetic doctoring.

Table 24.3 Potency and range of preparations for relief of pain in advanced cancer

---

MILD TO MODERATE PAIN
Non-opioid analgesics
Simple oral agents, e.g. paracetamol

Compound oral agents, e.g. co-proxamol

Non-steroidal anti-inflammatory drugs, especially for bone pain, e.g. diclofenac, either orally or rectally

MODERATE TO SEVERE PAIN
Mild opioid analgesics
Oral, e.g. dihydrocodeine, codeine phosphate, tramadol,
given with a laxative such as co-danthramer to prevent distressing constipation

Parenteral, e.g. dihydrocodeine, tramadol:
   When unable to tolerate oral analgesia
   When sedative effects of strong opioids are not required

SEVERE PAIN
Strong opioid analgesics
Oral morphine solutions or modified-release tablets, e.g. Oramorph, MST Continus

Transcutaneous skin patches, e.g. fentanyl, 72-hour duration of action.
Parenteral:
   When unable to tolerate oral analgesia
   Usually morphine/diamorphine
   Patient-controlled intravenous or subcutaneous infusion
   When too unwell, continuous infusion via syringe driver

VULVAL TUMOURS

Benign vulval tumours

Dermal tumours and cysts

Sebaceous cysts, sweat gland tumours (hidradenomas), lipomas and fibromas occur on the labia majora, as in skin elsewhere.

Bartholin's cysts

This is a soft, unilocular cyst 2–5 cm in diameter, situated postero-laterally just outside the vaginal introitus. It represents the dilated duct of Bartholin's gland, due to obstruction often by past infection, especially gonococcal. It is non-tender but may be a nuisance or worry. It may become secondarily infected, resulting in a Bartholin's abscess. The best treatment is marsupialization, where the cyst is incised, the edges trimmed back to give a wide opening and the base of the cyst is drawn up to the skin by several absorbable sutures. This allows more effective drainage than simple incision. The ostium frequently closes again, however, especially when infected, and recurrence of the cyst is not uncommon.

Venereal warts (condylomata acuminata)

These are viral in origin and may be venereally transmitted, being commonly associated with other venereal infections, notably that caused by *Trichomonas vaginalis*. They are cauliflower-like growths only a few millimetres in diameter, which may be isolated or may cluster over an extensive area. Treatment is by chemical cautery using podophyllin solution or cryocautery or, under anaesthesia, electrocautery, laser ablation or excision.

Syphilis

Syphilis may present as an ulcer on any part of the genital tract between the vulva and cervix, or as condylomata lata, which are moist, flat warts around the vulva. Condylomata lata may be associated with generalized lymphadenopathy and skin rash, being manifestations of secondary syphilis. The lesions teem with *Treponema pallidum*, which should be sought in scrapings by dark-ground microscopy. Genital ulcers and granulomata therefore need to be examined using protective gloves. For a more detailed account of syphilis, see Chapter 18.

Urethral prolapse, caruncle and carcinoma

A sliding prolapse of the posterior urethral mucosa often occurs, to a minor degree, in postmenopausal women and is due to lower urethral atrophy as a result of oestrogen deficiency. Physical exposure can then lead to the development of a granuloma, known as a urethral caruncle. This can cause dysuria and haematuria. It is usually easily recognized by its situation at the posterior margin of the external urinary meatus, but needs to be distinguished from urethral carcinoma and true urethral prolapse.

True urethral prolapse means complete, annular eversion of the mucosa. It usually occurs due to oestrogen deficiency in elderly women, but occasionally in young girls. It may become strangulated and thus greatly swollen and haemorrhagic, and as a result can be confused with a malignant tumour of the vulva or vagina.

Urethral cysts

See the section on vaginal tumours, below.

Vulval dermatoses (dystrophies)

Specific vulval dermatoses, or dystrophies, occur not uncommonly in middle and old age and always cause itching (pruritus vulvae). They must be distinguished from general dermatoses, particularly psoriasis, which can affect the vulva as well as skin elsewhere. Some of the specific dermatoses are potentially malignant and can only be distinguished on biopsy. Diagnostic terminology is both confused and confusing. Common classification, with alternatives, is:

1 Kraurosis or senile atrophy.
2 Lichen sclerosus et atrophicus.
3 Leukoplakia or leukoplakic vulvitis.

The following terminology, however, is preferred.
   Essentially, the lesion may be red because it is thin, or white because of a thick keratinized layer on the surface. It may also be excoriated and cracked due to scratching, but these same features may be due to early invasive carcinoma, which should not go unsuspected. All that can be determined from inspection is whether the vulva is dystrophic. What matters is cellular activity and pleomorphism in the squamous epithelium, which must be determined histologically. And, because the degree of change varies in the whole field of the lesion, which may extend over most of the vulva, multiple biopsies are often required. Histology may show:

1 Atrophy
2 Inflammation   } 90% of cases.
3 Dysplasia
4 Squamous cell hyperplasia   } 10% of cases.
5 Intraepithelial carcinoma

Vulval intraepithelial neoplasia (VIN)

Dysplasia is graded in three degrees of severity according to the depth of epithelial involvement. The most severe degree is VIN 3 which was previously described as intraepithelial carcinoma, carcinoma-*in-situ* or Bowen's disease. The features are malignant change within the squamous cells, especially the nuclei, excess and abnormal mitotic figures, and lack of squamous differentiation in the epithelium, but an intact basal membrane.

These conditions occur in about one-third of cases in areas of chronic vulvitis (see Chapter 18) whatever the cause, including irritant chemicals and venereal granulomata (condylomata). The latter may be syphilitic, for which specific tests should be done, or viral, and, rarely, particularly in Negro immigrants to the UK, granuloma inguinale or lymphogranuloma venereum (see section on sexually transmitted diseases, Chapter 18).

VIN 3 is potentially invasive and must be treated, either by excision or, rarely in the UK, by topical cytotoxic agent (5-fluorouracil). They are often extensive, and total vulvectomy may be required, although without excision of the regional lymph nodes.

Not infrequently, dysplastic changes may also involve the perianal and anal skin (anal intraepithelial neoplasia; AIN), and these tissues should also be inspected in cases of VIN.

Benign dermatoses

Atrophic or inflammatory dystrophies are occasionally due to diabetes mellitus and anaemia (of various causes), which should be sought. Otherwise treatment is symptomatic, the most effective agent being topical glucocorticoids such as 1% hydrocortisone. Oral antihistamines are useful at night for both their antipruritic and sedative action. Vulvectomy is inappropriate because the skin drawn in to cover the area tends to undergo the original change.

Vulval cancer

This is uncommon, accounting for 6% of genital cancer, and in the UK occurs mainly in old age (Table 24.2). It is nearly always squamous. Basal cell, Bartholin's and urethral carcinoma, malignant melanoma and sarcoma are extremely rare.

Squamous carcinoma occurs as a proliferating or ulcerated lesion and presents because of its appearance or bleeding, but if neglected (as often occurs in old age) it may become infected. It spreads initially by local invasion and by lymphatic embolization to the superficial and deep inguinal nodes of both sides (see Fig. 4.5). Its aetiology is unknown, but at least half have been preceded by hyperplastic vulval dystrophy, which occurs on average about 10 years earlier and which in turn may often be due to chronic vulvitis.

Traditionally, treatment at an early stage is by radical vulvectomy, i.e. total vulvectomy and regional lymphadenectomy. The extensive skin loss usually prevents primary wound healing, which largely occurs by granulation, thus requiring prolonged careful nursing. Now it is increasingly common for lesser operations to be undertaken involving removal of the vulva with the central tumour and separate dissection of the lymph nodes. This offers primary closure and improved cosmetic results with similar cure rates. The resulting (corrected) 5-year survival is about 70%, rising to 80% in the absence of lymph node involvement, compared with about 50% for all stages (Table 24.2). Radiotherapy is unsuitable because of the intense inflammatory response in the damaged exposed tissue, including surrounding dystrophic skin.

VAGINAL TUMOURS
Benign vaginal tumours
Urethral cysts

Urethral diverticula and cysts of paraurethral glands, up to 4 cm diameter, occur in the lower anterior vaginal wall. If asymptomatic they are better left alone, because their removal may damage the urethra or lead to blockage of and cyst formation in the ducts of other paraurethral glands. If symptomatic they should not simply be incised; rather, expert help should be sought as their removal can be exceptionally difficult.

Dermal inclusion cysts

These usually occur in the lower posterior vaginal wall due to collected secretions from dermal tissue inadvertently buried when repairing a ragged laceration resulting from childbirth. They can be excised if a nuisance.

Mesonephric duct cysts

Also called Gartner's duct cysts, they occur in remnants of the mesonephric duct and thus occur in the anterolateral aspect of the upper vagina. They may be up to 5 cm in diameter, soft and not usually noticed by the patient. They are better left but can be excised if troublesome.

Vaginal cancer

This is rare, accounting for less than 2% of genital cancer. It is commonly secondary to cervical or endometrial carcinoma. Primary carcinoma of the vagina is usually squamous and occurs after the menopause, most commonly in association with a forgotten ring pessary used for treatment of a prolapse. Of historical interest is the spate of otherwise rare adenocarcinoma in teenage girls (mainly in the USA) which followed maternal treatment in early pregnancy (for threatened abortion) with diethylstilboestrol, a fashion which fortunately passed but should not be forgotten.

Vaginal carcinoma spreads into the paravaginal connective tissues, bladder and rectum, and by lymphatics both upwards to the cervical regional nodes and down to the vulval regional nodes (see Fig. 4.5). It is thus very difficult to treat radically, and the survival rate is low. Radiotherapy (intracavitary and beam) is usually most suitable.

Vaginal intraepithelial neoplasia (VAIN)

As with CIN and VIN, vaginal squamous dysplasia can be graded histologically depending on the depth of epithelial involvement, VAIN grade 3 (formerly described as intraepithelial *in situ* squamous carcinoma) is the most severe. VAIN may occur as a primary change in the vagina, but being invisible to the naked eye it is only recognized in practice when it occurs in association with known cervical squamous, usually preinvasive, carcinoma. It is then seen on colposcopy or exposed by its failure to stain with iodine (see the section on cervical cancer, below).

It occurs in association with 4% of cases of CIN 3. Although found as small isolated lesions, these represent sporadic advances in what is a field change centred on the cervix. The lesions are thus usually found in the vaginal vault, sometimes after cervical conization or hysterectomy done for the cervical lesion, but may extend down to the vulva.

The lesions are potentially invasive and must be treated. Being often multiple, their local excision is impracticable (and some may be missed), and laser vaporization is usually the most effective treatment. When the lesions are confined to a vaginal vault scar after previous hysterectomy, an upper vaginectomy is more appropriate. In some cases, or with recurrent VAIN, treatment is by topical cytotoxic therapy (using 5-fluorouracil), which seeks out all the neoplastic epithelium and causes only temporary inflammation of the normal tissue.

CERVICAL TUMOURS

Benign cervical tumours

Mucous polyp

This is a common pedunculated adenoma, up to 10 mm in diameter, arising from the endocervical mucosa and occurring at any age. It often bleeds, either on sexual intercourse or spontaneously due to congestion or strangulation. If its pedicle can be seen and grasped, the polyp can safely be twisted off when first seen at vaginal examination. The polyp may not be the cause of the bleeding, however, and after the menopause, diagnostic hysteroscopy and curettage are advisable to exclude endometrial carcinoma. Very rarely, the polyp itself may be malignant.

Nabothian follicles

These are mucous retention cysts, usually about 5 mm in diameter, beneath the squamous epithelium of the transitional zone (see below) of the ectocervix. They have resulted from obstruction of gland-like mucosal crypts by squamous metaplasia in what was once surface mucosa. They are of no importance unless associated with chronic cervicitis (see Chapter 18), whilst in the taking of cervical smears they indicate the transitional zone.

Venereal warts and granulomata

Venereal warts (condylomata acuminata) may occur on the cervix (and less commonly in the vagina), as on the vulva (see above).

Granulomata, which sometimes bleed, may also occur on exposed endocervical mucosa when infected by *Trichomonas vaginalis*. They heal when the infection is eradicated.

Cervical intraepithelial neoplasia

Invasive squamous carcinoma of the cervix is preceded by a preinvasive stage lasting some years. Every effort should be made to detect it at this stage when treatment is easy and effective. It usually arises in the epithelium close to the squamocolumnar junction (see Chapter 4). The epithelium here undergoes marked normal changes, but during particular phases it is especially susceptible to carcinogenic stimuli. It is therefore important to understand the normal changes that occur, as well as the dysplastic and neoplastic changes. These are all beautifully illustrated by Burghardt (1973).

The normal cervix, mucosal ectopy, squamous metaplasia and the transitional zone

The squamocolumnar junction is originally situated at the external cervical os. When the cervix grows under the stimulus of oestrogen, differential growth in the underlying parenchyma results in rolling out of the lips of the cervix and thus endocervical mucosa and the squamocolumnar junction are carried out on to the vaginal portion of the cervix. This effect is most marked in adolescence and first pregnancy. The exposure of the endocervical mucosa is called mucosal ectopy (or, wrongly, an erosion, because as columnar epithelium is thinner and more vascular than stratified squamous epithelium, it appears bright red in comparison).

Physical exposure of the ectopic mucosa to the acidity of the vagina leads to its metaplasia to squamous epithelium. This occurs initially by proliferation of reserve cells, i.e. normally isolated cells beneath the columnar epithelium. The proliferated reserve cells form stratified layers which then differentiate into normal squamous epithelium, and the columnar epithelium on the surface is eventually dislodged.

The underlying, gland-like mucosal crypts do not usually undergo squamous metaplasia but continue to secrete mucus via ostia in the surface squamous epithelium. They may become blocked, resulting in retention cysts (Nabothian follicles). These cysts, when they occur, provide the only clue visible to the naked eye of the area of previous mucosa that has undergone squamous metaplasia and is called the transitional zone. This zone is where squamous carcinoma invariably originates, because the metaplastic cellular activity involved in the process of transition seems to render the epithelium particularly susceptible to carcinogenic stimuli. It is therefore imperative that cervical cytology smears are taken from the area straddling the squamocolumnar junction and particularly just outside it, and wherever Nabothian follicles can be seen, which may be over an extensive area.

Dysplasia

Squamous epithelial dysplasia is characterized by basal hyperplasia (i.e. multilayering of the basal cells), nuclear pleomorphism and excessive and abnormal mitotic figures. When these changes occur mainly near the base of the squamous epithelium the condition is called mild dysplasia or, more usually, CIN 1. It usually resolves spontaneously and may, in some cases, be due to infection. When the changes extend close to the surface of the epithelium, the condition is called severe dysplasia or CIN 3. This is very unlikely to revert to normal, and will eventually proceed to invasive carcinoma in many cases. CIN 3 is therefore a form of intraepithelial carcinoma and should be treated accordingly.

The distinction between mild and severe dysplasia is thus of great clinical importance but, being a matter of degree only, can be difficult to make. A third category, moderate dysplasia or CIN 2, is sometimes used to indicate doubt.

It is important to differentiate dysplasia, which is a histological diagnosis made from a tissue biopsy, from dyskaryosis, which is a cytological diagnosis made, for example, from a cervical smear. Dyskaryosis means pleomorphic (i.e. malignant-looking) nuclei set in otherwise normally differentiated (i.e. expanded, typically squamous) cytoplasm. Dysplasia cannot be diagnosed from a cytological preparation such as a smear because it assesses surface and exfoliated cells only, not the full epithelial thickness.

The risk of CIN 3 becoming invasive is high, and spontaneous resolution is very unlikely. There remains some uncertainty about the exact risk, because biopsy for histological diagnosis is likely to interfere excessively (if not completely) with the lesion and its natural development. Nevertheless, it seems clear that invasion would probably occur in nearly all cases eventually, the average time-lag being about 10 years. This means that treatment by local excision is adequate and, although desirable, there is no immediate urgency for it (thus it can be postponed in pregnancy, for instance).

Microinvasive carcinoma

This is characterized by loss of integrity of the basal membrane, at least in parts, of lesions which are otherwise CIN 3 with microscopic

Table 24.4 Clinical staging of cervical squamous carcinoma, required treatment and resulting success.

Clinical stage		Treatment	5-year survival rate (corrected) (%)
0	Intraepithelial	Local excision/ablation	100
1a(i)	Microinvasive		
1a(ii)	Occult (symptomless) invasive		100
1b	Overt, limited to cervix	Radical radiotherapy or surgery	80
2	Involving upper vaginal and/or parametrium not as far as pelvic side walls		60
3	Extending to pelvic side walls and/or lower vagina	Radical radiotherapy	30
4	Extending to bladder, rectum or outside true pelvis	Palliative radiotherapy and/or pelvic exenteration	10

carcinomatous invasion of the underlying stroma. Stage 1a(i) disease is where invasion is virtually unmeasurable and <1 mm deep; 1a(ii) disease is measurable invasion which is <5 mm deep and <7 mm wide. Stage 1a(i) squamous carcinoma (see Table 24.4) can be treated by cone biopsy as for CIN 3 (which is called stage 0).

Table 24.4 shows more clearly the practical divisions between the cervical epithelial dystrophies and carcinoma.

The safety of limited surgical treatment, although proven, is sometimes still doubted and hysterectomy may be preferred in older women with complete families. The safety margin is emphasized by the virtually total survival rate associated also with early (occult) invasive carcinoma (stage 1a(ii): see Table 24.4). Although that is treated radically, the results imply that embolic spread does not occur until the invasive tumour has progressed a further step in size (to stage 1b; see Table 24.4). However, about 5% of 3–5 mm lesions, especially those with involvement of small vessels and lymphatics, will have local lymph metastases even at this early stage. See below for details of treatment.

Diagnosis and treatment of preinvasive carcinoma

Naked-eye examination

Preinvasive (including microinvasive) carcinoma is invisible to the naked eye. Naked-eye examination is, however, an essential part of screening for cervical carcinoma to detect an invasive lesion, because cytology is much more likely to produce a false-negative result with invasive than with preinvasive carcinoma (due to surface necrosis). For this reason, amongst others, there is no place for blind cytology, using aspirate from the vaginal vault, in the diagnosis of cervical lesions.

Cytology

Papanicolaou, an American anatomist, was the first to suggest, in 1943, that the accessibility and small target area made the cervix very suitable for cytological examination. This is best done on a smear made from fresh cells scraped directly from the surface of the cervix (Ayre's smear), in contrast to true exfoliative cytology of posterior fornix aspirate (the original Papanicolaou smear). The latter sometimes affords detection of endometrial and, rarely, ovarian carcinoma but is not reliable for those purposes. It is preferable to concentrate attention on the cervix, using the scrape smear. This must be taken accurately, from the area of the squamo-columnar junction and surrounding transitional zone (see above),

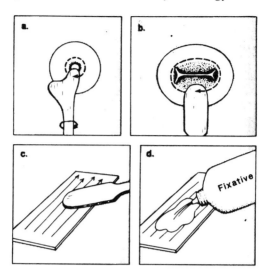

Fig. 24.2   How to take a good cervical smear (the shaded area on the cervix represents mucosa). (a,b) Taking the scrape from around the squamocolumnar junction of a nulliparous cervix with little mucosa visible, or a parous cervix with moderate mucosal ectopy. (c) Speading the smear to achieve a series of thin wedges. (d) Immediate fixing while the cells are fresh.

as demonstrated in Figure 24.2. The smear must be spread so as to achieve ample areas only one cell thick for proper microscopical examination, and must be fixed in a fresh state, as shown in Figure 24.2.

To check that the smear has been taken from the right areas on the cervix, both squamous and columnar cells should be present (and reported) in ample proportions. Malignant and/or dyskaryotic cells are sought, but these are sometimes inappropriately reported in terms which anticipate the histological findings ('CIN 1, 2 or 3'). Incidental findings that are sometimes useful include cellular inflammatory changes, sometimes specifically recognizable as due to herpes or cytomegalovirus; monilial strands and *Trichomonas vaginalis*; and changes indicating oestrogen state.

Cervical cytology may be used to screen healthy women or as a test of cure following local treatment of CIN. The pick-up rate of cytological neoplasia is about 5 per 1000 smears but depends on age and whether the population has been screened before and how often. It is much higher in certain groups of women, for instance those in prison or attending venereology clinics. False-positive findings occur rarely but can cause considerable psychological morbidity. They are usually not false, being explained by technical error in taking the (negative) biopsy, and should be pursued by repeated cytology. The finding of malignant cells in a smear can never be disregarded. False negatives are of great concern. They occur in about 10% of new cases, the majority being due to observer error, which is to be expected when screening. In following up known cases the error occurs in only about 3%. These may be due to inaccurate collection or improper preparation of the smear. A negative smear is sometimes found shortly after a positive one which is then wrongly assumed to have been false because much of the abnormal epithelium may have been scraped off at the original test. A smear should therefore not be repeated in less than 3 months.

In planning cytological screening schedules the false-negative rate must be taken into account as well as the natural history of intraepithelial carcinoma. Repeating the first smear after a year will reduce the false-negative rate to about 1%, which seems acceptable, and thereafter smears every 3–5 years should not overlook any cases prior to invasion.

It remains questionable whether cytological screening actually reduces deaths from cervical cancer. It has been argued that some invasive carcinomas occur with little or no preinvasive stage and are therefore always likely to be missed, but this is improbable. What is true is that the incidence of cervical carcinoma is gradually falling everywhere, which may be unrelated to cytology screening, and may possibly be due to improved socioeconomic conditions. However, the long natural history of preinvasive carcinoma, and further survival after invasive carcinoma has been treated, will require a delay of about 20 years before any effect of cytology screening on cervical cancer mortality might be seen. Unfortunately, women most at risk tend to use the service least. Computerization has resulted in an increased proportion of the female population being screened effectively by automatically generating recall letters at appropriate intervals. Amongst screened women the incidence of invasive cervical carcinoma has undoubtedly been reduced by treatment of preinvasive carcinoma. More worryingly, at present, 60% of women who develop invasive cervical cancer have never been screened. The recently introduced financial incentives to general practitioners for reaching screening targets may, in theory, have a considerable impact on the detection of preinvasive, curable disease. However, inner-city practices with a changing population and where cervical cancer risks are highest (see the section on aetiology, below), may recognize that their target level for screening is unrealistically high and may be deterred from actively trying to achieve it. In addition, increasing teenage coitus and pregnancy (see the section on aetiology, below) are leading to a steady rise in cervical cancer in women in their 20s, although it is still relatively uncommon at this early age.

Colposcopy

The colposcope is a binocular instrument that allows 5–40× magnification of the cervix. It is positioned outside the vagina, making it easy to use, and the view is obtained with the help of an ordinary vaginal speculum.

The colposcope cannot be used to detect cytological detail within the epithelium or invasion from the basal layers. Its usefulness depends on the pattern of the vascular supply that is so closely related to the degree of epithelial neoplasia. The vessels are larger and are carried (in loops) closer to the surface than normal between the rete pegs, giving rise to an appearance of punctation on the surface. In more advanced lesions the punctation occurs in close alignments, giving rise to mosaic patterns. Branching vessels running on the surface suggest invasive carcinoma. (For illustration, see Langley, 1976.)

Colposcopy is relatively time-consuming and therefore not practicable for screening. It is used as an adjunct to cytology once neoplastic cells have been found. It has three major applications:

1 To identify the part of a lesion which shows the most severe changes for diagnostic biopsy. Small punch or diathermy loop biopsies can be taken without anaesthesia.
2 To define the extent of CIN so that surgical excision or destruction can be minimized. If cone biopsy is required its dimensions can be prescribed for the surgeon. (Before colposcopy was available, very large cones were taken, resulting in unfortunate damage risking future fertility; see below.) As an alternative to cone biopsy, a diathermy loop or laser excision of the abnormal area may be undertaken as a diagnostic and (potentially) therapeutic procedure.
3 To observe mild dysplasia (usually associated with mild dyskaryosis on cytology) without treatment until either it regresses or advances to severe dysplasia, needing excision. Observation by colposcopy needs to be repeated every 6–12 months.

Non-specific staining

Iodine

Normal cervical squamous epithelium, whether original or meta-plastic, contains glycogen which is stained by iodine, unlike dysplastic squamous epithelium. Lack of staining does not give any clue to the severity of the lesion, but it provides the surgeon with definition of the area to be excised for cone biopsy in the absence of colposcopy.

Acetic acid

This gives dysplastic squamous epithelium an opaque appearance. It is therefore sometimes used at colposcopy, especially as it removes mucus, but it tends to obscure the vascular pattern.

Treatment

CIN 3 should be treated by local excision and/or ablation, whereas microinvasive carcinoma is best treated by local excision and not ablation (see Table 24.4). Ablation can be by hot or cold cautery or laser but it is essential first to exclude invasion by biopsy. When the lesion is extensive, cone biopsy or large loop diathermy excision of the transformation zone (LLETZ) is necessary, the limits of the biopsy being prescribed by colposcopy and/or iodine staining. Because the severity of the lesion varies in its different parts, histo-logical examination of the cone needs to be comprehensive: 10–20 sections are taken from all parts. If the lesion is seen not to be completely excised in the cone, re-conization can be done.

The immediate risks of cone biopsy are haemorrhage and infec-tion, particularly because the bed of the cone is best left exposed to re-epithelialize (from its edges and from the remaining depths of divided crypts). This is done so that any lesion remaining in the crypts will be exposed for subsequent cytology, which is the test of cure.

Cone biopsy, whether achieved by surgical knife, laser or diathermy loop, also involves particular risks to future fertility, by excessive loss of mucus-secreting crypts (which are mainly situated in the lower part of the cervix), and by incompetence of the internal os in pregnancy. Oddly enough, stenosis of the cervical canal can also be a sequel.

Hysterectomy is sometimes chosen as treatment in older women who have completed their families, especially when there is microinvasion. This does not remove the need, however, to maintain cytological follow-up on the remaining nearby tissues in the vaginal vault, which continue to be at particular risk. National recommendations in the UK are that two negative vault smears 6 months apart are sufficient, but some gynaecologists still advocate indefinite annual vaginal vault cytology.

Cervical cancer

Invasive tumours of the cervix may be:

1 Squamous cell carcinoma (65%).
2 Adenosquamous carcinoma (30%).
3 Adenocarcinoma (5%).
4 Sarcoma (very rare, usually botryoid (i.e. grape-like) sarcoma in children).

They mostly occur on the ectocervix and are usually exophytic or ulcerative, giving rise to bleeding, typically on coitus. Endocervical carcinoma (usually adenocarcinoma) tends to be mainly infiltrative and may expand the cervix without broaching the surface of the ectocervix, which, however, becomes irregular, firm and vascular. In this case bleeding also occurs but not so readily on coitus.

As Figure 24.1 shows, the incidence of cervical cancer is high from the age of 40 years onwards, and not uncommon from 30 to 39 years. Indeed, the incidence in younger women has been steadily increasing, so that cervical cancer is now not rare even in women aged 20–29 years. This change reflects changes in social and sexual behaviour concerned with the aetiology of squamous cell carcinoma.

Squamous carcinoma of cervix

Aetiology

The outstanding aetiological factors in squamous carcinoma of the cervix are coitus and early age of coitus. The actual carcinogenic agent could be sperm DNA, although there is little real evidence for this. Herpesvirus type 2 was, at one time, a hot favourite but now seems less likely a cause. Present interest is on various strains of the human papillomaviruses, which cause the venereal warts found most commonly at the vulva (see above).

Cervical cancer is extremely rare in virgins, shown for instance by studies in nuns. Youth is important, probably because this is when squamous metaplasia in ectopic mucosa is most active and thus the epithelium most susceptible to carcinogenesis. All other demonstrable aetiological associations are probably related to early coitus: low socioeconomic status, early marriage, high parity, promiscuity, prostitution and venereal disease. Ritual male circumcision was once thought to be protective, as in Jews and Muslims, but the relatively low incidence of cervical cancer in these groups is probably related to cultural differences affecting coital behaviour.

Treatment and prognosis

The mode of treatment depends on the way in which the cancer spreads and on the extent of spread (Table 24.4). Cervical cancer spreads initially by local invasion (to the vaginal vault and/or parametrium) and to lymph nodes within the pelvis (internal and external iliac and obturator nodes; see Fig. 4.5). Thus in its early stages it lends itself to radical therapy, i.e. aimed at the tumour and the pelvic lymphatic field. Radical hysterectomy (Wertheim's hysterectomy) is the preferred treatment for stage 1a(ii), 1b and 2, especially in younger women. Radiotherapy is most commonly used worldwide, mainly because of the lack of available surgical expertise, and is more appropriate for more advanced tumours. Intracavitary irradiation (using sources placed in the cervical canal, vaginal vault and uterine cavity) is usually combined with external beam therapy to the lateral lymphatic fields. More advanced cancer is usually treated by beam therapy to the whole pelvis, but palliative surgery is occasionally appropriate (see the section on advanced genital cancer, above). For recurrent and advanced disease, chemotherapy is occasionally used but the response is generally poor.

The prognosis depends on the stage reached by the tumour before treatment (Table 24.4). The staging is, of course, done clinically, and the failure of treatment in some cases at stages 1 and 2 is due to the presence already of clinically undetectable embolization beyond the pelvic lymph nodes. Although the 5-year survival rate of overt stage 1 cervical cancer is 80%, many cases of cervical cancer present much later, resulting in fewer than half of the patients surviving overall (Table 24.2). These poor results are tragic because they would mostly be avoidable if prompt attention were paid to the bleeding that invariably occurs at an early stage.

TUMOURS OF THE UTERINE BODY

Gross enlargement of the uterus is usually due to benign myometrial tumours (fibroids) and may or may not be associated with symptoms (usually menorrhagia). Modest enlargement is commonly due to overall hypertrophy associated with premenopausal anovulatory cycles and menorrhagia, or sometimes to adenomyosis. Rarely it may be due to endometrial carcinoma. Endometrial carcinoma much more commonly presents at an early stage with bleeding, before any uterine enlargement has occurred.

Benign tumours

Fibroids

Fibroids are the commonest uterine tumours. They are leiomyomas, sometimes called fibromyomas, arising in the myometrium. They are firm, round, well-defined tumours with a whorled pattern on the cut surface. They are usually multiple; sometimes there appears to be one alone but close examination usually reveals many other small ones. They are benign and rarely progress to sarcoma. Their origin is uncertain but may be from vascular elements. They are particularly likely to occur in Negro women and in women remaining nulliparous after the age of 30 years. Fibroids are clearly dependent on ovarian hormones because they occur in the reproductive epoch, grow particularly in pregnancy and regress after the menopause. They may outgrow their vascular supply in pregnancy and undergo infarction with internal bleeding (acute or red degeneration). After the menopause gradual hyaline degeneration occurs but occasionally fibroids may calcify post-menopausally, producing 'womb stones' which may be found incidentally on abdominal X-rays.

Fibroids cause symptoms as a result of:

1 Their exact situation in the uterus (Fig. 24.3).
2 Acute accidents to them.
3 Their size.

Very large subserous fibroids causing abdominal swelling may otherwise be symptomless. They may present with urinary symptoms of frequency or stress incontinence through pressure on the bladder. However, fibroids that enlarge or distort the uterine cavity cause painless menorrhagia – the most characteristic feature. Submucous fibroids may interfere with implantation of the blastocyst, causing infertility. Pedunculated submucous fibroids may be extruded through the cervix and become strangulated, causing severe bleeding. Pedunculated subserous fibroids may undergo torsion, causing severe pain. Acute (red) degeneration in pregnancy causes severe pain which tempts surgical exploration but will resolve in a few days if treated conservatively. Fibroids situated in the cervix can obstruct labour but are fortunately rare.

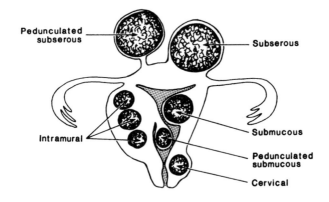

Fig. 24.3   Fibroids – their various situations in the uterus (the related significance is described in the text).

A rare and unexplained association with fibroids is polycythaemia, which in some cases disappears after hysterectomy.

Fibroids need to be removed only if they cause symptoms, although large fibroids are sometimes removed only for fear of the tiny risk of sarcoma. Hysterectomy is the usual choice. Myomectomy (enucleation of the fibroids from the uterus, which is conserved) is done only to preserve fertility because it is usually a more difficult operation, involving the removal of many fibroids, and because it is more dangerous on account of bleeding and associated greater postoperative morbidity. However, the risks of myomectomy can be reduced by preoperative treatment with gonodotrophin-releasing hormone (GnRH) analogues which induce a hypo-oestrogenic state, produce shrinkage of fibroids and allow easier dissection of them from the normal myometrium.

Adenomyoma/adenomyosis

These represent the fibromyomatous reaction to ectopically sited endometrial tissue deep in the myometrium and usually continuous with the normal endometrium. It leads to enlargement of the uterus. The condition may be diffuse (adenomyosis) or localized (adenomyoma). It causes menorrhagia but, unlike a fibroid, an adenomyoma causes pain and is poorly circumscribed. For the latter reason hysterectomy is the only means of treatment. Adenomyosis is discussed in more detail in Chapter 17.

Uterine hypertrophy

Generalized enlargement of the uterus, two- or threefold, sometimes occurs in association with menorrhagia in the last menstrual decade. It is probably due to the effect of oestrogen unopposed by any progesterone, associated with anovulatory cycles. The menorrhagia should be treated as dysfunctional bleeding (see Chapter 16) despite the uterine size.

Endometrial adenoma (benign polyp)

This is a soft, red, fleshy tumour of the endometrium, which may be sessile or pedunculated, and is prone to bleed irregularly. If pedunculated, it may appear through the cervix, and may then become strangulated and bleed profusely. It varies in size from about 1 cm diameter, if it consists only of endometrium, up to 5 cm, if it includes a myometrial or fibrous framework.

The diagnosis may be suspected from a pelvic ultrasound scan or made by curettage, which is done because of irregular bleeding. A hysteroscopy should be undertaken at the time of diagnostic curettage as – paradoxically it may seem – larger polyps are more likely to be missed if curettage alone is undertaken and are usually then discovered only at hysterectomy done for intractable bleeding. Not all endometrial polyps are benign; histological examination must always be made.

Endometrial hyperplasia

There are two different types, one benign and the other with malignant potential. They both tend to occur in the last menstrual decade.

Cystic hyperplasia

This results from prolonged oestrogen stimulation unopposed by any progesterone, i.e. anovulatory menstrual cycles. The cycles are often prolonged and associated with heavy menstrual bleeding, and this syndrome is called metropathia haemorrhagica. The endometrium is thickened and often polypoid. Both the glands and stroma show mitotic activity and many of the glands are markedly dilated, but because of the absence of any progesterone effects, there is no secretory activity. On section the distended glands are visible to the naked eye, giving rise to the description of 'Swiss cheese' appearance.

Cystic hyperplasia affects the whole endometrium. It is a benign condition of no danger and is responsive to progestogens, which when withdrawn result in normal shedding of the endometrium.

Adenomatous (atypical) hyperplasia

This is a focal condition involving only the glands, which become crowded together. It varies in degree. When there is intraluminal folding and tufting of the glandular epithelium with cellular pleomorphism it is sometimes called carcinoma-*in-situ*. It causes bleeding.

Adenomatous hyperplasia depends on oestrogen but, unlike cystic hyperplasia, does not seem to depend on excessive oestrogen and is only partly responsive to progestogens. The risk of progression to invasive carcinoma is about 20%, so treatment is mandatory. A thorough curettage is essential to ensure that all areas of atypia are assessed as treatment will depend on the most severe degree of abnormality. In women under 40 years of age, high-dose progestogens (e.g. medroxyprogesterone acetate 100 mg daily) may be used cyclically for 21 out of every 28 days over 3 months followed by a review curettage and assessment. If the abnormality persists, hysterectomy is the usual choice of treatment. This may be appropriate as primary treatment anyway for women whose family is complete and who are over 40 years of age as the condition is highly likely to recur.

Cancer of the uterine body

Invasive tumours originating in the body of the uterus include:

1 Endometrial:
   a. Adenocarcinoma.
   b. Squamous cell carcinoma.
   c. Stromal sarcoma.
2 Myometrial:
   a. Leiomyosarcoma
3 Trophoblastic (conceptual):
   a. Hydatidiform mole (invasive type).
   b. Choriocarcinoma.

In practice nearly all are endometrial adenocarcinoma. Of the others, the invasive trophoblastic tumours are the most important because they are usually curable (in the true sense). Delay in diagnosis of choriocarcinoma is particularly tragic because it is often a young mother who will die, and that could have been avoided.

Endometrial adenocarcinoma

This may involve the endometrium generally, or focally in the form of a polyp or polyps. Histologically there are usually glandular (tubular) formations typical of endometrium. Invasion of the myometrium occurs to a variable extent, and some bulky tumours expanding the uterus three- or fourfold may invade very little. The tumour is soft and friable, and vaginal bleeding usually occurs at an early stage so that most cases come to light while the uterus is still normal in size and the walls unbroached. Occasionally, tumour obstructs the cervical canal, leading to a painful pyometra (pus-filled uterus).

Aetiology

Endometrial adenocarcinoma occurs most often in the two decades after the menopause and is rare before it (see Fig. 24.1 and Table 24.2). In contrast to cervical squamous cell carcinoma, it is increasing in incidence and is relatively more common in the higher socioeconomic classes. The associated features classically described, of obesity, hypertension, nulliparity and often diabetes mellitus, are open to question. The only clear association is with oestrogen but it does not seem to depend on the amount. The particular oestrogen is possibly the important factor, e.g. oestrone, which is relatively predominant after the menopause as a result of extraglandular conversion (in subcutaneous fat) from adrenocortical precursors. Endometrial cancer is occasionally due to an oestrogen-secreting ovarian tumour, usually a granulosa cell tumour. Progestogens probably protect against endometrial cancer by their antioestrogenic action, and their cyclical inclusion in postmenopausal oestrogen replacement therapy is an important safeguard.

Treatment and prognosis

Adenomatous hyperplasia is a common but not invariable precursor of endometrial cancer. Screening for and treating adenomatous hyperplasia would unfortunately not offer a reliable means of preventing endometrial carcinoma. Endometrial cancer spreads initially by lymphatics and involves the para-aortic nodes directly via the ovarian vascular route (see Fig. 4.5), by seeding to the ovary (through the fallopian tube) in about 10% of cases and to the vagina (through the cervix), and later by embolization in the blood. The tumour tends to be confined to the uterus and does not break through its walls until a late stage. The depth of invasion of the myometrium correlates well with lymph node involvement and provides the best prognostic index.

Primary lymphatic spread beyond the pelvis makes radical therapy (as applied to cervical carcinoma) inappropriate. Endometrial adenocarcinoma is also less sensitive to radiotherapy than cervical squamous cell carcinoma. Treatment (Table 24.5) is thus primarily by hysterectomy and bilateral salpingo-oophorec-

Table 24.5   Clinical staging of endometrial carcinoma, required treatment and resulting success

Stage	Treatment	5-year survival rate (corrected) (%)
1 Confined to uterine body	Surgery with local radiotherapy	90
2 Involves cervix	Surgery with irradiation of whole pelvis	50
3 Extending outside uterus but confined to pelvis	Irradiation of whole pelvis with surgery if possible	25
4 Extending outside pelvis or including bladder or rectum	As for stage 3, plus irradiation of isolated metastases or progestogen therapy	5

tomy. More extensive resection is sometimes done, particularly including removal of the upper vagina, but is of no proven benefit. Additional radiotherapy aimed at the uterus and upper vagina reduces the risk of pelvic recurrence of tumour after operation. It may be given postoperatively to destroy any seeds disseminated by operative manipulation, or preoperatively to inhibit tumour activity and so prevent any operative seeding. Pre- and postoperative irradiation seems equally effective. More extensive radiotherapy may be appropriate in more advanced cases, to the regional lymph nodes and isolated distant metastases. Extensive metastasis can be checked in about a third of cases, and complete regression occasionally achieved, by progestogen therapy in prolonged high dosage. Progestogen therapy while the tumour is confined to the uterus does not seem to improve on the good results of hysterectomy and local radiotherapy (Table 24.5). In general the survival rate with endometrial carcinoma is good (see Table 24.2) because most cases present relatively early, the tumour being slow to spread beyond the uterus.

Trophoblastic tumours and trophoblast disease

The tumours arising from trophoblast are the hydatidiform mole and choriocarcinoma, described below. Choriocarcinomas are mostly highly malignant, whereas hydatidiform moles are mostly benign. The invasive potential and vigour of any individual tumour cannot, however, be distinguished histologically. Normal trophoblast also has the capacity to invade and spread – it is often found deep in the myometrium, and emboli reaching the lungs occasionally cause haemoptysis – but it does not persist. The concept has thus developed of trophoblast disease, i.e. a spectrum of trophoblastic invasiveness and neoplasia ranging from the normal to cancers of extreme malignancy, and whose activity (and size) is best determined by their human chorionic gonodotrophin (hCG) production, which is indicated by levels in blood or urine. Trophoblast disease thus includes:

1 Metastatic normal trophoblast.
2 Hydatidiform mole (1 in 2000 pregnancies).
   a. Benign (90%).
   b. Malignant or invasive mole (10%).
   c. Choriocarcinoma (1 in 20 000 pregnancies).

Aetiology
Trophoblastic tumours occur most commonly in Far Eastern racial groups and more commonly in Negro women than in Europeans. The tumour karyotype appears to be female in most cases. This is possibly due to multiple fertilization of the oocyte or to spermatozoal abnormalities characterized by extra X chromosomes, the latter being suggested by occasional examples of trophoblast tumours occurring in numerous consecutive pregnancies.

Hydatidiform mole
This occurs in about 1 in 2000 pregnancies amongst European women. The tumour consists of distended fluid-filled chorionic villi lacking fetal blood vessels. It forms a grape-like mass of vesicles, each 5 mm in diameter. The clinical features depend on the sometimes excessive mass of the tumour (in relation to the gestational age) and the excessive production of hCG. Thus it usually presents like a threatened miscarriage and with one or more of the following features:

1 Vaginal bleeding.
2 Excessive vomiting.
3 Hypertension (pre-eclampsia).
4 Excessive uterine size.
5 Doughy uterine consistency (instead of cystic).

There are two types of hydatidiform mole – complete and partial. In a complete mole no fetus is present and the pregnancy consists solely of hyperplastic chorionic villi. It usually results from fertilization of an ovum which subsequently loses its nucleus and the chromosome complement is derived solely from the father – either homozygous 46,XX from meiotic duplication of a single haploid sperm (90%), or heterozygous 46,XX or 46,XY from fertilization by two sperm followed by extrusion of the nucleus of the ovum (10%). In a partial mole a fetus is usually present. In this case the chromosome complement of the mole is often triploid (69,XXX or 69,XXY), with the extra set of chromosomes resulting from fertilization by two sperms or failure of the first paternal meiotic division.

The differential diagnoses are multiple pregnancy and acute poly-hydramnios. The diagnostic features are the absent fetal heart, the sonogram which shows the multiple echoes from the vesicles looking like a snowstorm, and abnormally high levels of hCG. An occasional feature is ovarian enlargement by theca-lutein cysts due to excess hCG.

Treatment is by suction evacuation of the uterus (as for vaginal termination of pregnancy). This is better than curettage or induction of abortion using oxytocic agents because these methods increase the likelihood of embolization of the tumour. Usually some tumour, having invaded the myometrium, persists for a while, but spontaneous regression occurs in 90% of cases within 6 months. Until then, the tumour need not be treated so long as hCG levels are declining. These levels need to be measured every 2 weeks at first. hCG provides the test of cure but should remain undetectable for 12 months before the risk of resurgent growth from persisting microscopic invasive tumours can confidently be eliminated. Meanwhile a further pregnancy would cause dangerous confusion and should be avoided. Oral contraceptives delay regression of the tumour and their use should be postponed until hCG is undetectable.

In the UK, surveillance and monitoring of affected women are arranged via three national centres in Sheffield, Dundee and London. All women in whom a hydatidiform mole is diagnosed are registered with their nearest centre which then arranges subsequent monitoring and advises the patient, her general practitioner and her gynaecologist of the results. In this way, cases of incomplete evacuation of a benign mole or diagnosis of invasive mole are recognized early and patients are rarely lost to follow-up.

Persistence, progression or metastasis (indicating malignancy: invasive mole) occurs in 5% of cases and needs to be treated as for choriocarcinoma. A further 5% gives rise to actual choriocarcinoma. Treatment under these circumstances is usually undertaken only at two of the national centres, in London and Sheffield.

Choriocarcinoma

This occurs in about 1 in 20 000 pregnancies, about half following hydatidiform mole and the other half following equally abortion or childbirth. Very rarely, choriocarcinoma may originate in the ovary (as in the testicle). The tumour consists of sheets of syncytio- and cytotrophoblast without villi. It is soft, highly vascular and bleeds readily; indeed, death from choriocarcinoma is most commonly due to bleeding, either at the original site in the pelvis, or from pulmonary or sometimes cerebral metastases.

The presenting symptom is usually vaginal bleeding. Although this often follows a known hydatidiform mole it also often occurs some weeks or months after unremarkable childbirth or abortion. Persistent or irregular bleeding after childbirth or abortion should therefore never be ignored (although it is much more likely to be due to ordinary retained placental tissue). The diagnosis is made by curettage.

Treatment is by intermittent chemotherapy using combinations of cytotoxic agents. The tumour response is monitored by means of hCG levels. There is a high risk of granulocytopenia and consequent infection can be reduced by isolation of the patient in a sterilized 'cell'. Large pelvic tumours may require surgical excision; otherwise complete remission with preservation of normal reproductive function can be expected in 75% of cases. If the tumour is detected early, nearly all patients should be cured.

TUMOURS OF THE FALLOPIAN TUBE

These are extremely rare. Various benign tumours of connective tissue can occur. Malignant tumours (usually adenocarcinoma) represent much less than 1% of genital cancer. They occur after the menopause and present with vaginal bleeding or sanguineous or even watery discharge and/or pelvic mass, and are usually only diagnosed at laparotomy. Spread outside the tube has usually already occurred, and despite surgery and/or radiotherapy, the survival rate is poor.

OVARIAN TUMOURS

The symptoms of ovarian tumours and in some cases the mode of treatment are determined by the histological type and whether benign or malignant. The tumours will therefore be considered under these headings.

Table 24.6   Classification of the majority of ovarian tumours

Origin and type	Malignancy	Remarks
NON-NEOPLASTIC		
Follicular		Common, premenopausal
Non-luteinized follicular cyst		
Corpus luteum cyst		
Theca-lutein cysts		
Endometriotic		
NEOPLASTIC		
Epithelial (i.e. from coelomic epithelium)		
Serous cyst	B or M	Common
Mucinous cyst	B or M	Common
Endometrioid carcinoma	M	
Brenner tumour	B	
Sex-cord tumours (i.e. from cortical mesenchyme)		
Granulosa cell tumour	LM	Usually oestrogenic; thecoma-fibroma fairly common
Theca cell tumour (usually thecoma-fibroma)	B	
Tubular androblastoma (arrhenoblastoma)	LM	Usually androgenic
Hilus cell (Leydig cell) tumour	LM	
Gynandroblastoma	LM	Mixed steroidogenic
Germ cell tumours (i.e. from primordial germ cells or oocytes)		
Embryonic cell types		
Teratoma (benign form = 'dermoid' cyst)	B or M	'Dermoid' cyst common
Extraembryonic cell types		
Endodermal sinus tumour	M	Secretes AFP
Choriocarcinoma	M	Secretes hCG
Undifferentiated dysgerminoma		
Connective tissue tumours		
Fibroma	B or M	
Lipoma		
Metastatic tumour	All M	
Commonly breast or gastrointestinal		

B = Benign; M = malignant; LM = low-grade malignancy; AFP = α-fetoprotein; hCG = human chorionic gonadotrophin.

Histopathological classification of ovarian tumours

There is a very great variety of ovarian tumours, as shown in Table 24.6. Disordered follicular growth resulting in cysts occurs of course only in premenopausal women and accounts for about half of ovarian enlargement in young women. Endometriotic cysts also occur only before the menopause, being dependent on oestrogen, but are uncommon. Of the neoplastic tumours occurring in young women, dermoid cysts and sex-cord tumours are relatively common, although the epithelial (serous and mucinous) cysts are commonest at all ages.

Table 24.7 shows that, of ovarian neoplasms, 80% are cystic (serous, mucinous or dermoid). As serous or mucinous cysts become malignant the proliferative parts contribute greater solidity to the tumour, while malignant teratomata (the malignant counterpart of dermoid cysts, which are benign teratomata) are almost entirely solid. About 20% of ovarian neoplasms are solid and of these the majority are malignant. Many solid tumours secrete sex steroids (the sex-cord tumours).

Table 24.7   The proportionate (percentage) incidence of ovarian neoplasms by cystic or solid state, by individual cystic types and by benign or malignant state

Type of neoplasm	Benign	Malignant	Total
Serous cysts	26	7	33
Mucinous cysts	23	6	29
Dermoid cysts	18		18
Total cysts	67	13	80
Solid tumours	8	12	20
Total	75	25	100

Follicular cysts

These are derived from ovarian follicles. The normal Graafian follicle reaches up to 2.5 cm diameter. Further enlargement up to 5 cm is called a cystic follicle and can be ignored. Enlargement greater than 5 cm is more likely to be due to a neoplastic cyst and can never be ignored (see the section on treatment of ovarian tumours). Their very presence implies disordered ovarian function and they can be associated with temporary menstrual disturbance. However, they are often symptomless, or only cause symptoms suddenly, due to an accidental complication (see the section on clinical features of benign ovarian tumours, below).

Corpus luteum cysts arise as a result of haemorrhage (the blood usually later having been resorbed) into a previously normal corpus luteum. The prominent luteinized granulosa cell layer is characteristic, and these cysts occur singly.

Theca-lutein cysts are uncommon, being associated with trophoblast tumours and due to the high levels of hCG. They are multiple and the theca is prominently luteinized, in contrast to the normal corpus luteum.

Endometriotic cysts

These are relatively uncommon. They are always filled with blood, due to regular menstruation. The blood being partly altered, they represent the typical – but not the only – example of so-called chocolate cysts. Being surrounded by inflammatory reaction they cause pain and fixation as well as swelling of the ovary (see Chapter 17).

Epithelial cysts

These are thought to be derived from the coelomic epithelium of the ovary. Remembering the close embryonic relations of the various structures of the genitourinary tract (see Chapter 3), it is not surprising that the ovarian epithelial tumours bear histological resemblance to the normal epithelia of the fallopian tube (serous cysts), endometrium (endometrioid carcinoma), endocervical mucosa (mucinous cysts) and urinary tract (Brenner tumours).

Serous cysts are usually unilocular and mucinous cysts often multilocular. They are usually thin-walled, lined by the active epithelium and surrounded by a smooth fibrous capsule. Epithelial secretions form within the cyst and lead to its enlargement. Some reach football size. In malignant cysts there is heaping-up of the epithelium, often as cauliflower-like excrescences, which are initially confined within the cyst; at this stage cystectomy is usually curative. Later, the capsule is invaded and tumour excrescences appear on the outer surface of the cyst, and the general tumour structure becomes semisolid. About a quarter of epithelial cysts are malignant. Epithelial carcinomas of the ovary are bilateral in about 20% of cases, often due to metastasis but sometimes originally. Benign tumours are occasionally bilateral; therefore, in practice, when a cyst is found the other ovary should be examined and, if the patient is over 40, removed together with the uterus.

Endometrioid tumours are always malignant and solid. They need to be distinguished from metastatic endometrial carcinoma. Thus, when a solid ovarian tumour is found, diagnostic curettage, in addition to laparotomy, is mandatory.

Brenner tumours (named after the man who first described them) are hard tumours, being composed of tiny islands of transitional or squamous epithelium set in a dense fibrous stroma. They are uncommon and usually benign.

Sex-cord tumours

Sex-cord tumours are so called because in the embryonic differentiation of granulosa and theca cells from the ovarian cortex (see Chapter 3), the cortex first differentiates into radial cords (the sex cords), which later break up into the typical follicular arrangements. The sex cords also involve the primordial medulla, which, although it mostly regresses in the ovary, gives rise to the androgen-secreting hilus cells; these are analogous with the testicular Leydig (interstitial) cells.

The histological variants of sex-cord tumours shown in Table 24.6 should thus be self-evident. These tumours secrete sex hormones which are usually typical of their cell type. The presenting features of these tumours are usually due to their hormone secretion: menstrual disturbances, postmenopausal bleeding associated with proliferative endometrium, or defeminization and virilization. When a tumour is suspected in these circumstances the ovary may need to be visualized by laparoscopy or even split open at laparotomy, because these tumours may be very small (although they vary greatly in size). They are solid and unilateral.

The majority of sex-cord tumours are malignant but not very aggressive, being mainly only locally invasive. The commonest example is, however, benign: the theca cell tumour. This tumour usually includes a prominent fibrous component, hence called a thecoma-fibroma, being dense, hard and rounded.

Germ cell tumours

These tumours show great variety (Table 24.6), being derived from totipotential cells. The commonest example is the benign teratoma. Its most prominent element is dermal, thus forming a cyst filled with sebum and hair (hence called a dermoid cyst), but it commonly includes bone, cartilage and dental structures. Occasionally endocrine tissue, particularly thyroid, can cause hormonal disorder. Dermoid cysts commonly occur in young women. Although they rarely occur in young girls, they account for the majority of ovarian tumours at that age.

All other germ cell tumours are malignant. Amongst this group dysgerminomas are the most common; they need to be distinguished because they are very sensitive to both chemotherapy and radiotherapy. Chemotherapy is preferable in younger women whose family is not complete as it gives a better chance of preserving fertility. Endodermal sinus tumours (of yolk-sac origin) and choriocarcinoma are very rare, but they need to be distinguished because they are highly sensitive to chemotherapy; they also secrete specific substances (α-fetoprotein and hCG, respectively) which can be used as tumour markers to monitor response to treatment.

Connective tissue tumours

These are uncommon. Indeed, most 'fibromas' are probably thecoma-fibromas.

Metastatic tumours

These comprise about 3% of ovarian neoplasms, are often bilateral and usually originate from breast or gastrointestinal carcinomas, being blood-borne.

Clinical features of benign ovarian tumours

Benign ovarian tumours occur at all ages, and of those occurring in young women, about half are follicular cysts. They may remain 'silent' until they reach a very large size, when abdominal swelling and tightness of clothing are noticed. However, they are frequently brought to notice because of complications, which include:

1 *Physical accidents* (commonest), all causing pain:
   a. Torsion.
   b. Haemorrhage (into the tumour).
   c. Rupture (of a cyst), leading to:
      i. Haemoperitoneum.
      ii. Myxoma peritonei (in the case of mucinous cysts).
2 *Pressure symptoms*:
   a. Pelvic discomfort.
   b. Dyspareunia.
   c. Urinary frequency and nocturia.
3 Endocrine/menstrual disturbance.
4 Obstruction of labour.
5 Infection (of the tumour: blood-borne).
6 Malignant change (20%).

Ovarian tumours, especially cysts, are frequently complicated by physical accidents, which all cause sudden pain. Torsion is the commonest and is most likely to affect medium-sized tumours, i.e. about 10 cm in diameter. The whole ovary and fallopian tube twist about the broad ligament, strangulating the ovary and causing sudden severe pain and often vomiting. This may occur intermittently but, if it goes too far, congestion, oedema, haemorrhage and infarction of the ovary and tube occur, causing continuous severe pain and signs of peritonism. Cyst torsion is more likely with benign tumours as malignant ovarian neoplasms develop periovarian adhesions which restrict ovarian mobility. The main differential diagnosis is a bleeding ectopic pregnancy, but the ovarian mass is usually easily distinguished and in either case laparotomy is needed.

Rupture of a cyst causes bleeding and may also lead to widespread peritoneal seeding of neoplastic cells with malignant potential. In the case of mucinous cysts, even when benign, this can lead to a serious condition called myxoma peritonei – a form of mucinous ascites often associated with intestinal adhesions and obstruction.

Abdominal or vaginal ultrasound scanning is very useful in assessing whether an ovarian mass may be malignant by demonstrating its internal structure. Benign tumours are usually cystic, and any papillary or solid components within should increase the suspicion of malignancy. Ascites may also be demonstrated by ultrasound scanning before it becomes clinically apparent.

Treatment

Ovarian tumours should always be excised without delay, for two main reasons: the high risk of malignancy or progression to malignancy, and the even higher risk of accident, particularly torsion, which is likely to disrupt or infarct the ovary and require its surgical sacrifice.

In premenopausal women, a discrete cystic swelling of the ovary up to 8 cm diameter is likely to be follicular, and its removal can be delayed for 6 weeks in the hope of regression.

In pregnancy, removal of a discrete cyst is better postponed until the middle trimester to minimize the risk of causing miscarriage.

In premenopausal women, benign cysts should be enucleated, conserving the ovary. Rupture should be carefully avoided in case neoplastic cells are disseminated in the abdomen.

If there is any doubt whether an ovarian tumour is benign a careful and thorough laparotomy should be undertaken. This should include aspiration of peritoneal fluid for cytology and omental biopsy. The whole ovary should be removed with careful examination and possibly biopsy from the opposite ovary.

After the age of 40, bilateral oophorectomy with hysterectomy may be best, because the tumour is more likely to be malignant than in a young woman and reproductive function is less likely to be required.

Ovarian cancer

Ovarian cancers are mainly of epithelial origin (i.e. carcinoma: serous, mucinous and endometrioid adenocarcinomas). Of the remainder, the most likely types are dysgerminoma and granulosa cell and metastatic tumours.

Ovarian cancer occurs mostly after the menopause but is not uncommon between 30 and 40 years of age (see Fig. 24.1). It will occur in about 1% of all women. It accounts for a quarter of all genital tract cancers but half the associated deaths (see Table 24.2). The relatively poor survival rate is due to the late clinical presentation of ovarian cancer; in about two-thirds of cases it has already spread beyond the pelvis.

Unfortunately there is no reliable means of screening for ovarian cancer. All that can be done towards early detection of neoplasms at their benign stage is to take every opportunity to do bimanual pelvic examination when vaginal examination is being performed, e.g. to take a cervical smear. Potential screening methods for early detection using ultrasonography with or without colour Doppler to assess blood flow and biochemical screening by measurement of the serum tumour marker CA125 are currently under evaluation.

Spread usually occurs in the following order:

1 Local invasion within the pelvis.
2 Peritoneal seeding across the abdominal cavity.
3 Lymphatic embolization (see Fig. 4.5) to:
    a. Para-aortic nodes.
    b. Uterus.
    c. Other ovary.
4 Blood-borne metastasis.

The common presenting features are:

1 Abdominal swelling due to a mass and/or ascites.
2 Abdominal pain.
3 Vaginal bleeding.

It is also not uncommon to find symptomless ovarian cancer accidentally.

Treatment

This depends mainly on the extent of spread of the tumour, as shown in Table 24.8. There remains much controversy, however, about the choice of treatment, and whether to be more or less aggressive. When the tumour capsule is intact (and the diagnosis of cancer may only be made later on histology) excellent results have been claimed for conservative surgery, which is particularly appropriate in young women, but this is not universally accepted. Chemotherapy is of course unpleasant and dangerous, and it is generally agreed that in advanced cancer it only achieves temporary remission, not eradication, of the disease; furthermore, surgical reduction of most of the tumour bulk is essential to give chemotherapy (or radiotherapy) a reasonable chance to be effective. It is therefore a difficult question in advanced ovarian cancer whether to seek the probably limited benefit from aggressive treatment or to take a fatalistic view and merely ease the patient's remaining passage through life.

Table 24.8 Clinical staging of ovarian cancer, required treatment and resulting success

Stage	Treatment	5-year survival rate (corrected) (%)
1 Confined to ovary:		
(i) unilaterial, intact capsule	Cystectomy or unilateral oophorectomy and biopsy of other ovary	60–90
(ii) bilateral, tumour excrescences	BSO, hysterectomy and omentectomy; with or without chemotherapy or intraperitoneal irradiation	
2 Extension within pelvis	As for stage 1, plus pelvic beam irradiation	40
3 Extension to abdominal peritoneum	Chemotherapy after surgery, as possible	10
4 Extension outside abdomen	As for stage 3, plus ?immunotherapy	1

BSO = Bilateral salpingo-oophorectomy.

Causes of death are commonly:

1 Cachexia.
2 Haemorrhage.
3 Intestinal obstruction.
4 Ureteric obstruction and renal failure.

REFERENCES

Burghardt, E. (1973) *Early Histological Diagnosis of Cervical Cancer.* Saunders, Philadelphia.
Hillier, S.G., Kitchener, H.C., Neilson, J.P. (eds) (1996) *Scientific Essentials of Reproductive Medicine.* W.B. Saunders, London.
Langley, F.A. (ed.) (1976) *Cancer of the Vulva, Vagina and Uterus. Clinics in Obstetrics and Gynaecology*, vol. 3. Saunders, Eastbourne.
Waterhouse, J.A.H. (1974) *Cancer Handbook of Epidemiology and Prognosis.* Churchill Livingstone, Edinburgh.

FURTHER READING

Creasman, W.T. (ed.) (1986) *Endometrial Cancer. Clinics in Obstetrics and Gynaecology*, vol 13. Saunders, Eastbourne.
Jones, H.W. (ed.) (1995) *Cervical Intraepithelial Neoplasia. Clinical Obstetrics and Gynaecology*, vol. 9. Baillière Tindall, London.
Williams, C. (1992) Ovarian and cervical cancer. *British Medical Journal* **304**:1501–1504.

25

Obstetric and gynaecological procedures

Although students do not need to know the details of operative technique, it is entirely appropriate to have a broad understanding of the main procedures undertaken in order to be able to describe and explain them to patients (and it may make the hours spent in theatre a little more interesting!). This chapter therefore covers the main obstetric and gynaecological procedures, describing the nature of the operations together with their principal complications.

OBSTETRIC PROCEDURES

Chorionic villus sampling (CVS)

CVS is a technique for obtaining actively growing chorionic material for chromosome analysis or genetic testing. It is performed at 10–12 weeks of pregnancy and results of chromosome analysis can be available within 48 hours. The procedure involves advancing a wide needle into the edge of the developing placenta guided by ultrasound. This may be done through the abdominal wall with local anaesthesia or through the cervical canal. Suction applied to the needle then allows the withdrawal of small fragments of chorionic tissue. The main attraction of the technique is the speed of the chromosome analysis that is possible and the early stage of pregnancy at which it can be done, which together mean that fetal karyotyping can be available at a time when vaginal termination is still possible. The major problem is a miscarriage rate of about 5%. This makes it principally suitable for situations where the likelihood of finding an abnormality is high and the ease of termination may be felt to outweigh the relatively high miscarriage risk. As with other invasive obstetric procedures, there is a risk of sensitization of a rhesus-negative woman and anti-D should be given (see Chapter 7).

Amniocentesis

Amniocentesis is an alternative method of obtaining fetal material for chromosome or genetic analysis. Amniotic fluid is removed (about 10 ml, less than 5% of the volume at 16 weeks) by inserting a fine needle into the amniotic cavity under ultrasound guidance. Exfoliated cells in the fluid are then cultured, and only when they are actively growing can chromosome testing be done. This process means that a result would not usually be available until about 2½ weeks after the amniocentesis. Amniocentesis is not usually performed until 16 weeks. Earlier attempts have been made but have been associated with higher complication rates and failure to establish a cell culture so that no result is obtained. Miscarriage risks are 0.5–1% and rhesus sensitization is also possible. The main draw-back is not getting a result until 19 weeks, with the possible added unpleasantness and risk of a late termination. However the low risk of causing miscarriage makes it the diagnostic method of choice in a low-risk situation (such as a 38-year-old previously infertile patient with a Down's risk of 1 : 200).

Cordocentesis

This technique involves direct needling of umbilical cord vessels under ultrasound direction either to remove blood for diagnostic purposes or to infuse blood or other substances (principally to trans-fuse rhesus-negative blood in cases of severe rhesus disease). The technique is possible from about 18 weeks and carries a small risk of fetal loss (about 1%).

Fetoscopy

Fetoscopy entails introducing a small endoscope into the amniotic cavity through the maternal abdominal and uterine walls in order to inspect the fetus directly. The improved resolution of ultrasound scanners has led to scanning taking over many of the former appli-cations of fetoscopy. Fetoscopy carries a miscarriage risk of a few per cent and is confined to a small number of specialist centres.

Cervical sutures

Cervical suturing was originally described by Shirodkar as a treat-ment of cervical incompetence. His technique involved an incision across the anterior fornix with the bladder being reflected up off the upper cervix. A wide suture was then inserted at this level encircling the uterine isthmus. The knot was tied anteriorly and buried under

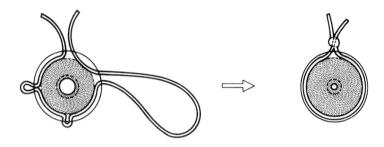

Fig. 25.1   Insertion of a cervical suture.

the bladder as the vaginal incision was repaired. Simpler techniques have been devised and the one now commonly used in this country is the McDonald method. A 3- or 5-mm tape is passed in a subcutaneous plane around the upper cervix without reflecting the bladder and then tied fairly tightly to give support for this region. It is generally done in four bites, as shown in Figure 25.1.

The procedure is commonly undertaken at 12–14 weeks with a general anaesthetic and carries a very small risk of immediate miscarriage – probably under 1%. The stitch is removed without anaesthesia at 38 weeks or sooner if labour starts or the membranes rupture.

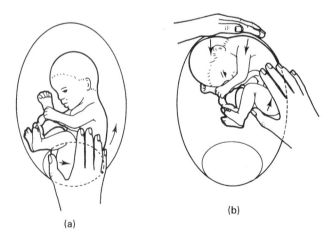

(a)

(b)

Fig. 25.2   External cephalic version. (a) Disimpact baby's bottom from pelvis; (b) the baby is gently pushed nose-first, maintaining a flexed attitude.

External cephalic version (ECV)

This is a procedure for turning a fetus from breech to cephalic presentation by manipulation through the mother's abdominal wall (Fig. 25.2). In the past it was widely practised and, if necessary, with the patient sedated or anaesthetized. It is now only performed with the patient fully awake and then only by relatively few obstetricians as sedation or anaesthesia was shown to increase the risk of complications significantly (placental abruption, cord entanglement, fetal distress, premature labour, rhesus sensitization).

To do an external version the breech has first to be disimpacted from the pelvis. Pressure is then applied to both ends of the fetus in such a way as to maintain the state of flexion of the fetus and to encourage it to turn in a nose-first direction. Following any version or attempted version it is important to check the fetal condition, and to give anti-D if the woman is rhesus-negative.

Artificial rupture of membranes (ARM)

ARM is used widely to induce labour, or to encourage progress in labour (Fig. 25.3). The bulging bag of membranes below the presenting part can usually be ruptured easily with any sharp instrument as long as the cervix is 2 cm dilated or more. This form of membrane rupture is sometimes called a low artificial rupture, in distinction to a high artificial rupture of the membrane. This latter

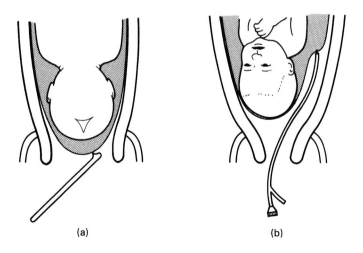

(a)   (b)

Fig. 25.3 Artificial rupture of membranes. (a) Forewater rupture with Amnihook; (b) hindwater rupture with Drew Smythe catheter.

procedure is now largely of historical interest. It was performed with a Drew Smythe catheter – an elongated S-shaped catheter with a wire obturator, which could be slid up between the membranes and the uterine wall to puncture the membranes above the level of the head. It was used in the hope of avoiding cord prolapse and to minimize infection risk, but was less efficient at inducing labour and associated with the occasional disaster due to perforating the placenta with the instrument. Drew Smythe was a Bristol obstetrician in the Second World War and after, and it is sometimes claimed that the design of the catheter is modelled on the road plan outside his old house!

Episiotomy

Episiotomy is the deliberate incision of the perineum to enlarge the introitus and facilitate delivery. It is usually carried out with scissors after infiltration with local anaesthetic Episiotomy may be done electively in some situations (such as fetal distress or shoulder dystocia), but will generally be done when it is judged to be necessary to avoid perineal tearing. The need for episiotomy can be

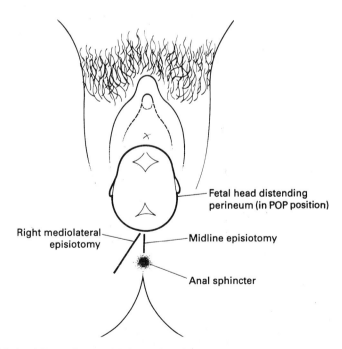

Fig. 25.4   Alternative episiotomy incisions.

assessed by gauging the elasticity of the perineum with a finger tip placed between the perineum and the fetal head as the head descends. If the perineum feels rigid and a significant amount of extra opening is still needed, then tearing or damage to the perineal structure is inevitable if episiotomy is not carried out.

Two main options exist (Fig. 25.4). The right mediolateral episiotomy is most widely used as it carries the incision away from

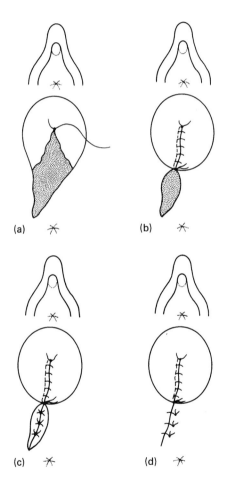

Fig. 25.5 Repair of episiotomy. (a) First stitch at apex of vaginal skin incision; (b) vaginal skin closed with continuous suture; (c) deep tissues of perineum brought together with interrupted sutures; (d) skin edges closed with interrupted sutures.

the region of the anal sphincter. It does, however, cut through muscle fibre, tending to produce a degree of muscle wasting and asymmetrical healing. The midline episiotomy goes through less vascular tissue, is somewhat easier to repair and probably heals with less scarring and distortion. It has the disadvantage that any extension is likely to involve the anal sphincter and rectum. This means it is best reserved for experienced obstetricians who can confidently predict the size of the episiotomy needed.

Episiotomies are repaired in three stages after ensuring adequate local anaesthesia (Fig. 25.5). First the edges of the vaginal skin are brought together with a continuous catgut suture starting from the apex and working down to the fourchette. Second the deep tissues are brought together with interrupted catgut sutures and finally the perineal skin edges are brought together with silk mattress sutures (or occasionally with subcuticular catgut). Accurate apposition of the skin edges is crucial if delayed healing and coital problems are to be avoided. When episiotomy repairs break down it is generally due to poor suturing rather than infection and they are usually best re-sutured rather than waiting for healing to occur by second intention.

Operative delivery

The techniques of forceps, ventouse, breech and caesarean deliveries are described in Chapter 8.

GYNAECOLOGICAL PROCEDURES

Dilatation and curettage (D&C)

For several generations of gynaecologists, a D&C has been the standard means of diagnosing intrauterine pathology, but it is now being largely replaced by hysteroscopy. A D&C is essentially a diagnostic procedure and only rarely is it therapeutic (as, for instance, if a fibroid polyp or a lost coil is removed) but there is a widespread lay feeling that a 'scrape should put your periods straight'. A D&C is generally done with a brief general anaesthetic, although it is possible to do it with a paracervical block. The cervix is dilated gradually to 9 or 10 Hegar (9 or 10 mm dilators designed by Hegar). Greater dilatation risks permanent damage to the cervix and is unnecessary. The cavity is explored with polyp forceps hoping to grasp any polyp (a process a bit like apple-bobbing with your eyes closed!). A curette is then used to remove strips of endometrium from around the cavity for histological examination (or occasionally culture for tuberculosis). The shape and regularity of the cavity are also assessed by 'feeling' its surface with the curette. Complications of D&C are extremely rare, other than the occasional perforation of the uterus.

Hysteroscopy

This involves putting a small endoscope into the uterine cavity to visualize it. The cervix needs minimal dilatation. The cavity is distended with carbon dioxide and its surface can then be inspected minutely so that isolated polyps or other pathology are not missed. Often the cavity will be curetted as well to obtain endometrium for histology (an H&C). Various endoscopic operations are also possible: resecting fibroids or a uterine septum, cannulating tubal openings or destroying all or most of the endometrium (endometrial ablation – see below).

Evacuation of the uterus

It is common for bits of placental material to be retained in the uterine cavity after spontaneous miscarriage, giving rise to risk of haemorrhage or infection. These retained products of conception are generally removed operatively by evacuation of the uterus. The cavity is explored with sponge forceps and a large curette. There is usually no need to dilate the cervix as it will remain open as long as there are retained products. Patients may sometimes report having had a D&C after a miscarriage but the correct term is an evacuation. A degree of care is needed in performing this operation as the softer state of the tissues makes it possible to curette down into the myometrium and give rise to adhesions across the cavity – a complication which appears to be particularly common in Greece, and is known as Asherman's syndrome.

Vaginal termination of pregnancy

A pregnancy may be terminated surgically up to 12 weeks with little risk. Under general anaesthesia or paracervical block the cervix is dilated to 10 Hegar (10 mm) or less for very early pregnancies. The cavity is emptied with a disposable plastic sucker. For pregnancies under 12 weeks this is a surprisingly quick and relatively bloodless procedure. Serious complications are rare, but incomplete emptying of the uterus may lead to problems with bleeding or infection. Infection is more common in those who are carriers of *Chlamydia* or gonococci and checks for these infections should be carried out preoperatively in at-risk cases.

Laparoscopy

This involves the insertion of a rigid endoscope through an umbilical incision to view the pelvic organs (and sometimes other abdominal structures). Diagnostic laparoscopies for infertility, pain or suspected ectopic pregnancy are performed frequently in gynae units and operative procedures are also possible. Sterilization by the application of clips to the medial part of the fallopian tubes is well-established and widely practised. Egg collection for *in vitro* fertilization or gamete intrafallopian transfer may be performed this way but is being replaced by ultrasound-guided techniques. Endometriotic deposits may be cauterized and adhesions divided, or the uterus may be fixed in a permanently anteverted position (a ventrisuspension operation) Many new procedures are being developed in a move to minimally invasive surgery.

Hysterectomy

The uterus may be removed either abdominally or vaginally and with or without tubes and ovaries (although it is difficult to remove the latter structures vaginally). Ovaries will generally be removed at the time of hysterectomy if the indication is cancer of the uterus or ovary, if there is severe endometriosis or if the woman is close to or past the menopause (when the ovaries have no further function).

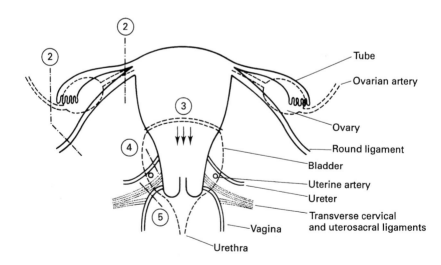

Fig. 25.6 Hysterectomy – principal steps are referred to in the text.

The main steps of a total abdominal hysterectomy are (Fig. 25.6):

1 Abdominal incision – usually a low Pfannenstiel.
2 Divide broad ligament either at side of uterus or lateral to the tube and ovary, if these are to be removed.
3 Divide the bladder peritoneum and push the bladder down off the front of the uterus.
4 Divide the uterine vessels.
5 Cut round the margin of the cervix, separating the uterus from the vagina and supporting the ligaments.
6 Sew it all up.

Vaginal hysterectomy is the same operation done more or less backwards:

1 Incision around the cervix.
2 Separate the bladder anteriorly and push it up; open the peritoneum and pouch of Douglas and the uterovesical pouch.
3 Divide the supporting ligaments (uterosacrals and transverse cervical).
4 Divide the uterine vessels.
5 Divide the upper broad ligament with contained structures (round ligament, tube and ovarian ligament).
6 Sew it all up!

Serious complications are rare following hysterectomy. Venous thrombosis is uncommon except in high-risk women. Bladder disturbance or prolapse of the vaginal vault are occasional late problems, and psychological problems may occur if the woman was not adequately counselled or was pressurized into hysterectomy against her judgement (it is much more common for her to say it was the best decision she had ever made). The occurrence of granulation tissue in the vaginal vault is less serious but relatively common and the main reason for the need for follow-up examination of the patient. Granulation tissue is readily treated by touching with a silver nitrate stick, but if left it will cause discharge and postcoital bleeding, which can persist for years. The removal of ovaries produces abrupt onset of menopausal symptoms unless hormone replacement is given (usually in the form of an implant).

Wertheim's hysterectomy

This is a radical hysterectomy done usually for early stages of invasive carcinoma of the cervix. The uterus, tubes and ovaries are removed together with the upper third of the vagina and the parametrial tissues and the pelvic lymph nodes. This involves laying bare the ureters, the rectum and the major pelvic vessels. Complications are much more likely than with a total hysterectomy, particularly thrombosis, fistula formation (ureter or bladder) and swelling of legs due to lymphatic disruption.

Prolapse operations

The most widely used prolapse operation now is vaginal hysterectomy and pelvic floor repair. The repair part of this procedure consists of separate operations on the anterior vaginal wall and the posterior vaginal wall together with the perineum. These procedures are called anterior and posterior colporrhaphy and are sometimes employed without hysterectomy in the absence of uterine descent. Anterior colporrhaphy consists essentially of taking a tuck in the bulging vaginal wall (Fig. 25.7). Deeper fascial sutures may

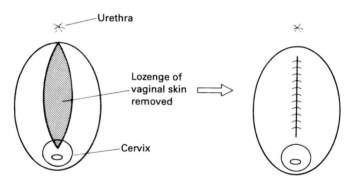

Fig. 25.7   Anterior colporrhaphy.

also be inserted to increase urethral and bladder neck support. Posterior colporrhaphy involves removing redundant vaginal skin and bringing together deep tissues of the perineum so as to lengthen and strengthen the perineum and restore the calibre of the vagina to its pre-delivery state (Fig. 25.8). It can be quite difficult to produce an adequate repair without narrowing the vagina to the point where coitus is difficult, painful or impossible. This is particularly so in the postmenopausal woman not on hormone replacement therapy, whose vagina has a natural tendency to progressive constriction anyway. The use of hormone replacement therapy or local oestrogen cream goes some way to preventing this sort of problem

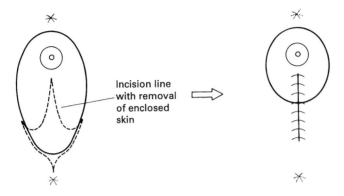

Incision line
with removal
of enclosed
skin

Fig. 25.8   Posterior colporrhaphy.

but occasionally the older woman is faced with the situation of an adequate repair only being possible at the expense of losing sexual function.

The Manchester repair (or Fothergill operation) is now more or less of historical interest only, but involved amputation of the cervix with joining of the transverse cervical ligaments in front of the cervical stump (thus pushing this upwards and backwards). It would normally have been combined with pelvic floor repair.

Myomectomy

This involves the removal of fibroids from the uterus. Quite large fibroids can be removed with uterine function being maintained. The operation is generally done through an abdominal incision, although small intracavity fibroids can be removed hysteroscopically. It generally involves more surgery (i.e. more blood loss and possibly more risk) than a hysterectomy, so that it is usually restricted to those who hope to have further children. The wound heals securely and should not preclude labour and vaginal delivery.

Endometrial ablation techniques

For women with menorrhagia various methods of endometrial ablation have been developed. With hysteroscopic visualization of the endometrial cavity the endometrial layer may be excised with electrocautery (endometrial resection) or destroyed with laser (laser ablation). Alternatively, the endometrium may be destroyed with various heat-producing probes as a blind procedure. These techniques significantly reduce menstrual blood loss for 80% or more of women, but do not generally affect dysmenorrhoea. It is not clear yet whether the benefits will be long-lasting. Such procedures involve less inpatient time than hysterectomy but serious complications have been encountered, particularly in the learning phase for the technique.

Tubal surgery

For normal fertility the fallopian tube needs to be patent, mobile and to have a normal functional tubal lining (endosalpinx). In addition the ovarian surface needs to be bare. Tubal surgery aims to restore these conditions although it cannot influence the state of the endosalpinx. In practice, infections that have produced significant pelvic adhesion or tubal blockage will often have caused significant damage to the endosalpinx and this will limit the subsequent pregnancy rate. *In vitro* fertilization is a better alternative if the underlying tubal state is not relatively normal.

The main components of tubal surgery are adhesolysis and salpingostomy. Adhesolysis involves the careful removal (as atraumatically as possible) of adhesions to lay bare the ovaries and restore tubal mobility. Salpingostomy involves opening the tubal ampulla at the point where the fimbriae have fused together (Fig. 25.9). Small radiating incisions are made and the ends are tacked back like the petals of a flower with fine sutures. This is usually done at open operation but can be achieved laparoscopically. These operations have few immediate complications but there is a significant risk of ectopic pregnancy as a late complication – perhaps 10% of all future conceptions.

Colposuspension

Various operations have been devised to elevate and support the bladder neck in order to cure stress incontinence. The cave of Retzius is opened through a suprapubic incision. In the Marshall–Marchetti operation sutures are placed in the paraurethal spaces (identified with the help of a Foley catheter and a volunteer with his or her fingers in the vagina!) and these are then fixed to the periosteum at the back of the pubic bones. This has the effect of elevating the bladder neck so as to bring the urethra into the abdominal pressure zone, and also of increasing resting urethral pressure. Alternative operations suspend the paraurethral vaginal wall to other structures. All of these operations have a good success rate, both short term and after longer follow-up. Retention of urine and urinary tract infections are common early complications.

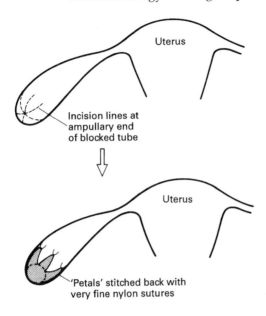

Uterus

Incision lines at
ampullary end
of blocked tube

Uterus

'Petals' stitched back with
very fine nylon sutures

Fig. 25.9   A 'rose' salpingostomy.

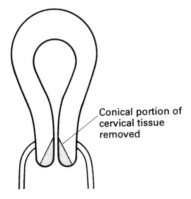

Conical portion of
cervical tissue
removed

Fig. 25.10   Cone biopsy.

Cone biopsy

Smear abnormalities are generally dealt with by colposcopy, biopsy of affected areas and local destruction of abnormal tissue by laser, or controlled hot probe (called cold coagulation) destruction. If the colposcopic abnormality extends up the cervical canal out of view it is sometimes desirable to perform cone biopsy to remove the abnormal tissue. This allows assessment histologically of the nature and extent of the lesion and usually proves to be curative. Under general anaesthetic, a conical portion of the cervix is excised (Fig. 25.10). The excision site is generally vascular and needs cauterizing or suturing for haemostasis. Secondary haemorrhage is a potentially serious early complication and either cervical incompetence or fibrosis and cervical stenosis may complicate future pregnancies. Large loop diathermy excision of the transformation zone is a less damaging means of excising the transformation zone by using a loop diathermy which removes a portion of tissue for histology and prevents haemostasic problems. It is not suitable however for situations where the upper edge of the abnormality is out of sight in the cervical canal.

Abbreviations

We would not want to encourage excessive use of abbreviations but it would be idle to pretend that they are not used widely, so we present here a list of abbreviations used in obstetrics and gynaecology practice. It is a good policy never to use an abbreviation unless you can be quite certain that your audience is familiar with it or in an examination answer unless you have already defined it.

AC	abdominal circumference
AF	amniotic fluid
AFP	α-fetoprotein
AID	artificial insemination by donor – now generally referred to as donor insemination (DI) to avoid confusion with AIDS
amnio	amniocentesis
APH	antepartum haemorrhage
ARM	artificial rupture of membranes
A/V	anteverted
BBA	born before arrival
BC	birth control
βhCG	β human chorionic gonadotrophin
BPD	biparietal diameter
BSO	bilateral salpingo-oophorectomy
BV	bacterial vaginosis
C/C	cystocele
CG	chorionic gonadotrophin
CIN	cervical intraepithelial neoplasia
CL	corpus luteum
COC	combined oral contraceptive
CRL	crown–rump length
CS	caesarean section
CTG	cardiotocograph
CVS	chorionic villus sampling

Cx	cervix
D&C	dilatation and curettage
DHEA(S)	dehydroepiandrosterone (sulphate)
DI	donor insemination
DOA	direct occipitoanterior
DOP	direct occipitoposterior
Dp	dyspareunia
DR	Down's risk
DTA	deep transverse arrest
DUB	dysfunctional uterine bleeding
E/C	enterocele
ECV	external cephalic version
EDD	estimated date of delivery
ERPC	evacuation of retained products of conception
FD	fully dilated
FH(H)	fetal heart (heard)
FHR	fetal heart rate
FM(F)	fetal movements (felt)
FSH	follicle-stimulating hormone
GIFT	gamete intrafallopian transfer
GnRH	gonadotrophin-releasing hormone
HC	head circumference
H&C	hysteroscopy and curettage
hCG	human chorionic gonadotrophin
HELA	hysteroscopic endometrial laser ablation
HIV	human immunodeficiency virus
HPL	human placental lactogen
HSG	hysterosalpingogram
HTB	hydrotubation
HVS	high vaginal swab
I/C	intercourse
ICSI	intracytoplasmic sperm injection
IMB	intermenstrual bleeding
IUCD	intrauterine contraceptive device
IUD	intrauterine death or intrauterine device
IVF	*in vitro* fertilization
K	katamenia = menstrual periods
LARM	low artificial rupture of membrane
LH	luteinizing hormone
LHRH	luteinizing hormone-releasing hormone = GnRH
LLETZ	large loop excision of transformation zone
LMP	last menstrual period
LOA	left occipitoanterior
LOL	left occipitolateral
LOP	left occipitoposterior

L/S	lecithin/sphyngomyelin
LSA	left sacroanterior
LSCS	lower-segment caesarean section
LSL	left sacrolateral
LSP	left sacroposterior
MH	menstrual history
MMK	Marshall–Marchetti–Krantz
NND	neonatal death
OA	occipitoanterior
OC	oral contraceptive
OFD	occipitofrontal diameter
OP	occipitoposterior
para	parity (usually followed by number of pregnancies)
PCB	postcoital bleeding
PCC	postcoital contraception
PCO	polycystic ovaries
PCOD/S	polycystic ovarian disease/syndrome
PCT	postcoital test
PET	preeclamptic toxaemia
PG	prostaglandin
PID	pelvic inflammatory disease or (flippantly) poorly investigated diagnosis
PIH	pregnancy-induced hypertension
PMB	postmenopausal bleeding
PMS	premenstrual syndrome
PMT	premenstrual tension
PNM	perinatal mortality
POP	persistent occipitoposterior or progestogen-only pill
PPH	postpartum haemorrhage
PRL	prolactin
PV	*per vaginam*
R/C	rectocele
RML	right mediolateral
ROA	right occipitoanterior
ROL	right occipitolateral
ROP	right occipitoposterior
RCL	right sacrolateral
RSA	right sacroanterior
RSP	right sacroposterior
R/V	retroverted
SB	stillbirth or stillborn
SHBG	sex hormone-binding globulin
SI	sexual intercourse
STOP	suction termination of pregnancy
SUZI	subzonal injection/insemination

TAH	total abdominal hysterectomy
TCRE	transcervical resection of endometrium
TENS	transcutaneous electrical nerve stimulation
TOP	termination of pregnancy
TOS	trial of (caesarean section) scar
USS	ultrasound scan
VE	vaginal examination
VT(OP)	vaginal termination (of pregnancy)
ZIFT	zygote intrafallopian transfer

Index

Abdominal palpation, 48
Abortion, 234–5, 257–60
  see also miscarriage
  methods of, 234–5
  mid-trimester, 168
Abruption, and clotting defects,
  190
Abscess, Bartholin's, 320–1
Acetic acid, 409
Acquired immunodeficiency
  syndrome (AIDS), 334–5
  see also Human
    immunodeficiency virus
ACTH, *see* Adrenocorticotrophic
  hormone
Acupuncture, 156
Adenocarcinoma, 408, 418
Adenomatous hyperplasia, 413,
  414
Adenomyosis, 313–14, 411
Adhesolysis, 440
Adolescence, 269–75
  see also Puberty
  problems of, 271–5
Adrenal androgen effects, of
  puberty, 268
Adrenal functions, 78–9
Adrenocorticotrophic hormone
  (ACTH), 265
'After-pains', 196
Age, and fertility, 237
Agenesis, 25
AIDS, *see* Acquired
  immunodeficiency syndrome
Albuminuria, 147

Albuminuric pre-eclampsia, 117
Alcohol, 101, 246
Aldosterone, 79
Alpha-feto protein, 98, 108
Ambulation, 209
Amenorrhoea, 276–89, 279(table),
  301
  anatomical causes of, 277
  diabetes and, 289
  endocrine causes of, 277–83
  exercise and, 282
  hyperprolactinaemia in, 282–3
  hypothalamic disorders in, 280–2
  investigation of, 289–90
  and obesity, 289
  and oral contraception, 289
  primary ovarian failure in, 280
  treatment of, 290–1
Amniocentesis, 109, 138, 431
Amnionitis, 169
Amniotic fluid, 88
  see also Polyhydramnios
Amniotomy, *see* Artificial rupture
  of membranes
Anaemia, 300
  in pregnancy, 148–9
Anaerobic streptococci, 207
Anaesthesia, in labour, 211
  examination in postpartum
    haemorrhage, 190
Anal sphincter, 40, 161
Analgesia, in labour, 156
Androgen excess, 28
Anencephaly, 111, 216
Anorexia nervosa, 273, 281

Antenatal care
  see also Pregnancy
  clinical examination, 99–101
  high-risk situations, 135–40
  midwife in, 96
  normal pattern of, 96–7
  objectives of, 95–106
  pregnancy, complications of,
    106–35
  shared, 96
  subsequent visits, 98
Antenatal classes, 150–1
Antepartum haemorrhage (APH),
  96, 119–24
  management of, 121–3
Anterior colporrhaphy, 440(fig.)
Anti-D immunoglobulin, 137, 138
Antibiotics, in pregnancy, 104
Anticoagulants, 105, 209
Antiemetics, 104
Antihistamines, 105
Antithyroid drugs, 104
Antral follicles, 56, 57
Anuria, 191
Anus, 40
Anxiety, 156
Apgar score, 164
APH, see Antepartum haemorrhage
ARM, see Artifical rupture of
  membranes
Arterial blood pressure, in normal
  pregnancy, 80
Artificial insemination, 248
Artificial rupture of membranes
  (ARM; amniotomy), 162, 163,
  433(fig.), 433–4
  procedure for, 167–8
Ascending genital tract infection,
  197
Ascites, 426
Asherman syndrome, 244, 277, 437
Aspiration termination, 235
Aspirin, 158
Assisted conception methods,
  254–5
  conception rates in, 255(fig.)
At-risk cases, for fetal
  abnormalities, 108
Auscultation, 159
Avomine, 104, 107

Ayre's smear, 403
Azoospermia, 238, 241–2, 248–9

Babies
  death/stillbirth, 218
  feeding, 203(fig.)
  survival rate, 87(fig.)
Backache, 338, 373
Bacteriuria, 146
Barrier methods, of contraception,
  230–2
Bartholin's abscess, 320–1
Bartholin's cysts, 320–1, 321(fig.),
  396–7
Bartholin's glands, 30
Bartholinitis, 320–1
Bathing facilities, on admission to
  hospital, 154
Bed-wetting, 368
Bereaved, tending to, 217
Bicornuate uterus, 260
Biochemical screening, for spina
  bifida and Down's syndrome,
  108
Biophysical profiles, fetal, 135
Biopsy of cervix, small punch
  biopsies, 406
Biparietal diameter, fetal, 86(fig.)
Birth, circulatory changes at, 88
Birth injury, 216
Birth weight, 87
Bishop's score, 166
  inducibility rating, 167(table)
Bladder, urinary, 38–40
Blastocyst, implantation of, 55(fig.)
Bleeding
  antepartum, 119–24
  cyclical, and HRT, 387–8
  intermenstrual, 301(fig.)
  non-menstrual, 301–4
  as puerperal complication, 205–6
  menstrual, see Menstrual
    bleeding
  non-menstrual, causes of,
    302(table)
  postmenopausal, causes of,
    303(fig.)
  postpartum, see Postpartum
    haemorrhage
Blood, changes in pregnancy, 200

Blood sugar levels
   diabetes in pregnancy, 142
   fasting, 79
Blood sugar tests, 259
Blood supply, of the pelvic organs,
      36–7
Blood urea, 147
'Blues', in the puerperium, 201
Bonding, in puerperium, 202
Bone mass, 368
Bony pelvis, 43–4, 47(fig.)
Booking clinic, antenatal, 97–8
Bowen's disease, 396
Bradycardia, fetal, 228
Braxton Hicks contractions, 153
Breast cancer, 386
Breast development, 270(fig.)
Breast-feeding, 199, 203(fig.)
   see also Lactation
Breast milk, 202
Breasts
   development of, 77
   in pregnancy, 92
Breech presentation, 100, 113–15
   see also External cephalic version
   management of, 115–16, 176–8
   terms used in, 114(fig.)
Brenner tumours, of ovary, 424
Bromocriptine, 204, 250, 251, 351
Brow presentation, 45, 175(fig.)
Burch colposuspension, 370–1
Burns–Marshall method, 178

Cabergoline, 283
Cachexia, 392
Caesarean section, 89, 122, 166, 173,
      185–7, 186(fig.), 211
   and malpresentation, 176
Cancer, 389
   breast, 386
   cervical, 408
   Fallopian tubes, 418
   ovarian, 425–7
   pain relief in, 397 (table)
   sites of origin, 389 (table)
   uterine body, 413–18
   vaginal, 398–9
   vulval, 397–398
Candida albicans, 319
Candidiasis, 319, 324

Carbimazole, 146
Carbohydrate metabolism, 79
Carbon dioxide, 161
Carcinoma, 395
   microinvasive, 402–3
   preinvasive, 403–8
Cardiotocography, 133
Cardiovascular system, in
      pregnancy, 80
Caruncle, urethural, 395
Case presentation
   gynaecological, 11–13
   obstetric, 7–10
Cellular dysplasia, of cervix, 391
Cephalic presentation, 89, 100
Cephalopelvic disproportion, 126,
      183
Cephalopelvic relationships, 46–9
Cephalosporins, 104
Cerebral anoxia, 117
Cerebral irritation, 184
Cerebral thrombosis, 221
Cerebrovascular disease, 380
Cervical caps, 231
Cervical intraepithelial neoplasia,
      400–8
Cervical mucus, 58, 64, 220, 242
Cervical os, 199(fig.)
Cervical polyp, 121, 302(fig.),
      302(fig.)
Cervical secretion, 326
Cervical smears, 95, 406(fig.)
Cervical sutures, 97, 260, 431–2
   insertion of, 432(fig.)
Cervicitis, 327
Cervix, 34, 192, 402–3
   atresia, 273
   cancer, 392(table), 399–400, 402
      (table), 408
   cytology, 404–5
   dilatation of, 161
   effacement of, 91(fig.)
   intraepithelial neoplasia, 400–3
   microinvasive carcinoma, 402
   mucosal ectopy, 400–1
   preinvasive carcinoma, 403–8
   squamous carcinoma of, 408–9
   'transitional zone', 401
Chemotaxis, 15
Chemotherapy, 426

Childhood, gynaecological
    problems in, 264–6
Chlamydia trachomatis, 315–16
Chocolate cysts, 308
Cholesterol, 221
Choriocarcinoma, 413, 418
Chorionic villus sampling (CVS),
    97, 109, 428
Chorionitis, 169
CIN, *see* Cervical intraepithelial
    neoplasia
Circulatory changes, at birth, 88
Climacteric
    definition of, 375–6
    time scale of, 377(table)
Clinical examination, in antenatal
    care, 99–101
Clitoris, 21, 22, 29
Clomiphene, 248, 250–1
Clotting defects, 188
    in postpartum haemorrhage,
        190–1
Clotting function tests, 123
Coccyx, 43
Coelomic epithelium, 16, 17
Coital history, in subfertility, 245
Coitus interruptus, 231
Cold coagulation, 441
Collagen changes, 380–1
Colostrum, 202
Colporrhaphy
    anterior, 438(fig.)
    posterior, 439(fig.)
Colposcopy, in preinvasive
    carcinoma, 406
Colposuspension, 440
Commensals, 207
Conception, assisted treatment
    methods, 254–5
Conception rates, 236(fig.)
    assisted conception methods,
        255(fig.)
    after endometriosis, 314(fig.)
    in subfertility treatment, 247(fig.)
    in unexplained infertility,
        253(fig.)
Condom, 230
    female, 231
Condylomata acuminata, 320, 395,
    400

Condylomata lata, 333
Cone biopsy, of cervix, 442,
    441(fig.)
*Confidential Enquiries into Maternal
    Deaths*, 213–14
Congestive dysmenorrhoea,
    340–1
Connective tissue tumours, of the
    ovary, 423
Conservative surgery, treatment of
    endometriosis, 312
Conservative treatment, in uterine
    prolapse, 368
Constipation, 200–1
Continence, *see* Incontinence
Contraception, 199, 219–34,
    291
    barrier methods, 230–2
    caps, 231
    chemicals, 232
    coitus interruptus, 231
    depot, *see* Hotmonal
        contraception
    and depression, 222
    hormonal, *see* Hormonal
        contraception
    intrauterine devices, 226–9
    natural family planning, 231
    oral, *see* Hormonal
        contraception
    postcoital, *see* Hormonal
        contraception
    progestogen-only pills, *see*
        Hormonal contraception
    rhythm method, 231
    safe period, 231
    sterilization, 232–4
    withdrawal method, *see* Coitus
        interruptus, 231
Contractions, timing of, 91
Contraindications, in
    oestrogen–progestogen
    combinations, 223
Cord, umbilical
    entanglement, 433
    prolapse, 176
    traction, 189
    velamentous insertion of,
        122(fig.), 122(fig.)
Cordocentesis, 110, 431

Coronary artery disease, 380
Corpus luteum, 54, 74
  cysts, 423
  development, 243
Corticosteroids, 78–9, 79
Cortisol deficiency, 265
Cryptomenorrhoea, 25, 273
Cryptorchidism, 24
CVS, see Chorionic villus
  sampling
Cystic hyperplasia, of
  endometrium, 297, 412
Cystitis, 333
Cystocele, 361
Cysts, 400
  Bartholin's, 320–1, 321(fig.),
    396–7
  chocolate, 300
  dermoid, 420, 422
  endometriotic, 423
  epithelial, 421–2
  follicular, 420–1
  mesonephric duct, 398
Cytology, of the cervix, 403–6
Cytomegalovirus, 404
Cytotoxic drugs, 105

D & C, see Dilation and curettage
Dalkon Shield, 226
Danazol, 311, 351
Debendox, 104
Decidua, 59, 75
Deep transverse arrest, 173
Deep vein thrombosis, 209, 221
Dehydration, 170
Dehydroepiandrosterone (DHA),
  267
Delivery, 163
  breech presentation, 176–8
  face presentation, 174
  forceps, 181–4
  of head, 177–8
  occipitoposterior position,
    172–3
  operative, 436
  options, 151–2
  place of, 95–6
  of twins, 179–81
Dental care, in pregnancy, 102
Depot contraception, 225

Depression, 201, 209–10
  cyclical, 347
  and hormonal contraception,
    222
  neonatal, 105
Dermal inclusion cysts, 398
Dermal tumours, 394
Dermatoses, benign, 397
Dermoid cysts, 420, 422
Desogestrel, 221
Developmental abnormalities,
  25–8, 215
Dexamethasone, 130
Diabetes, 127, 222
  and amenorrhoea, 288
  with polyhydramnios,
    8–10(table)
  in pregnancy, 141–3
Diagnostic curettage, 303
Diagnostic tests, in pregnancy,
  83
Diaphragm, 230
Diathermy, Fallopian tubes, 232
  loop biopsies, of cervix, 406
Diazepam, 105, 118, 119
Diet, in pregnancy, 101
Dihydrotestosterone, 21, 22
Dilation and curettage (D & C),
  434–5
Disproportion, cephalopelvic,
  126–8, 183
Diuresis, 105, 200
Döderlein's bacillus, 322
Domino delivery, 151
Donor insemination, 249
Dopamine antagonist, 204
Doppler studies, 135
Down syndrome, 98, 108
Drew Smythe catheter, 434
Drugs in pregnancy, 104–5
Duchenne muscular dystrophy,
  109
'Dutch cap', 230
Dysgerminoma, 266, 422
Dyskaryosis, 402, 404
Dysmenorrhoea, 338, 339–41
Dyspareunia, 191, 338, 341–2
Dysplasia, 396, 401–2
Dystrophies, 396–7
Dysuria, 208, 368

Eclampsia, 116–19
  emergency treatment of, 118–19
  management of, 117–19
  see also Pre-eclampsia
Ectocervix, 35
Ectopic pregnancy, 229, 261–3
ECV, *see* External cephalic version
EDD, *see* Expected date of
  delivery
EGF, *see* Epidermal growth factor
Ejaculation
  premature, 358
  retardation of, 358
Embryo, 59–60
Endocarditis, 143
Endocervix, 35
Endocrine system
  see also individual hormones
  in amenorrhoea, 277–83
  control of reproduction, 60–8
  disorders of, 276–94, 279(table)
  non-amenorrhoeic disorders, 288
  in puberty, 267–8
Endocrine changes, 78–9
Endodermal sinus tumours, 425
Endometrial cycle, 68–9
  see also Ovulation
Endometrioid tumours, 421
Endometriosis, 252–3, 306–14
  aetiology of, 305–7
  clinical features of, 309
  conception rates in, 252(fig.),
    313(fig.)
  diagnosis of, 309–10
  examples of, 308(fig.)
  medical treatment, 310(table)
  prevalence of, 307
  sites and pathology of, 307–9
  surgery of, 312–13
  treatment of, 310–13
Endometriotic cysts, 423
Endometritis, 169
Endometrium, 35, 68–9, 69
  ablation techniques, 439–41
  adenocarcinoma, 413–15, 414,
    415(table)
  adenoma, 412
  carcinoma, 415
  changes, in menstrual cycle,
    68(fig.)

fibrosis, 276
hyperplasia, 412–13
Endosalpinx, 36
Enema, 154
Enterocele, 361
Entonox, 158
Enuresis, 368
Epidermal growth factor (EGF),
  62
Epididymis, 242
Epidural anaesthesia, 158, 172, 212
Epimenorrhagia, 297
Epimenorrhoea, 297
Epiphyseal closure, 273
Episiotomy, 164–5, 177, 197, 434–6
  incisions for, 165(fig.), 434(fig.)
  repair of, 435(fig.)
  scar, 341
Epithelial cysts, 17, 423–4
Epsikapron (Epsilon-aminocaproic
  acid), 123
Episilon-aminocaproic acid
  (Epsikapron), 123
Ergometrine, 92, 118, 189, 206,
  258
Escherichia coli, 147
Essential hypertension, 223
Ethics, in subfertility practice,
  239–40
Ethinyloestradiol, 220
Exercise
  causing amenorrhoea, 282
  in pregnancy, 102
Expected date of delivery (EDD),
  98
External cephalic version, 115,
  432(fig.), 433
External genitalia, 21(fig.), 21–3
Extrauterine life, preparation for,
  87–8

Face presentation, 173–5, 174(fig.)
Fallopian tubes, 36
  see also Tubal ...
  ectopic pregancy in, 261–2
  surgery, 440
  tumours of, 418
Family planning clinics, 359
Faradism, 466
Fasting blood sugar levels, 79

Feeding
    bottle, 202–4
    breast, 202–4, 203(fig.)
    technique of, 203–4
Female condom, 231
Female examination, in subfertility,
    245
Female history, in subfertility, 244–5
Female life expectancy, 387
Female pseudohermaphroditism,
    265
Female sexual dysfunction, 359
Female sterilization, 232–3
Femshield, 231
Fenamates, 311
Fertility, 145, 146
    definition of, 237–8
    incidental factors, 246
    normal, 237
Fertilization, 58–9, 244
Fetal alcohol syndrome, 101
Fetal head, 45(fig.), 46(fig.)
    crown-rump length, 85(fig.)
    delivery of, 177–8
    'trapping', 89(fig.)
Fetus, 44–6, 84–8
    abnormalities, 100, 107–11
    activity, 132
    adrenal activity, 90
    anaemia, 137
    back, position of, 101
    blood pH, 161
    death, 168
    disproportion, 126–8
    distress, 122, 156, 184, 433, 434
    engagement of, 100
        see also Breech presentation
    head, see Fetal head
    heart rate, in labour, 159–61
    heart rate traces, 133, 160(fig.)
    hypoxia, 131, 159
    indications for Caesarean
        section, 185
    karyotyping, 428
    legs, positions of, 114
    lie, 100
    tachycardia, 130
    transfusion, 139
    weight, 86(fig.)
    well-being, 133–5, 158–61

Fetoscopy, 109–10, 431
Fibrin, 117
Fibrinogen
    concentration, 123
    degradation, 191
Fibrinolysis, 121
Fibroids, 410–11, 411(fig.)
    removal of, 439
Fibromyomas, 410
Fibrosis, of Fallopian tubes, 329,
    330
Folic acid, 113, 149
Follicle-stimulating hormone
    (FSH), 287, 289, 290
Follicles, Nabothian, 402
Follicular cysts, 420–1
Follicular growth
    in the adult, 53–7
    control of, 54–7
Folliculogenesis, 51
Fontanelle, 46, 175
Footling presentation, 114
Forceps
    in common use, 182(fig.)
    rotational, 182–3
Forceps delivery, 181–4
    dangers of, 184
    indications for, 183–4
    prerequisites for, 183
Fothergill repair operation, 367, 439
Fourchette, 191
Frank breech presentation, 114
'French letter', 230
Frigidity, 358
Frusemide, 118
Fungal infections, in vaginitis, 324

Galactorrhoea, 294
Gallstones, 145
Gamete intrafallopian transfer
    (GIFT), 252, 254, 255
    conception rates in, 255(fig.)
Gametes, 50
Gametogenesis, 50–3
Gartner's duct cysts, 400
Gastrointestinal system, 81–2,
    200–1
Gender, 264
Genetic counselling, 110–11
Genital bleeding, see Bleeding

Genital changes, ovarian hormone
    dependent, 64
Genital ducts, 17–20
Genital hair, *see* Pubic hair
Genital neoplasia, 389–94,
    390(table)
    advanced, 392–4
    age-specific incidence of,
        390(fig.)
    death rates, 391
    diagnosis of, 391–2
    prevalence of, 389–91
Genital tract, 31(fig.)
    involution of, 198–9
    lymphatic pathways draining,
        38(fig.)
    in pregnancy, 88–92
Genital tract infection, 207–8
    ascending, 197
    lower, 316–17
    spread of, 208(fig.)
    upper, 327–35
Genitalia
    differentation of, 27(fig.)
        see also Sexual differentiation
    external, 21–3
Germ cell tumours, 424–5
Gestodene, 221
Gestrinone, 311–12
GIFT, *see* Gamete intrafallopian
    transfer
Gingivitis, 102
Glucose, 141
    tolerance tests, 142
Glycogen, 133, 409
Glycosuria, 141
GnRH, *see* Gonadotrophin-
    releasing hormone
Gonadal descent, 23–4, 24(fig.)
Gonadal maldescent, 26
Gonadal oncogenesis, 17
Gonadotrophins, 63(fig.), 65–7, 267,
    268
    see also Follicle–stimulating
        hormone; Luteinizing
        hormone
    adult cycle, 66–7
    and sex steroid cycles, 70–3
Gonadotrophin-releasing hormone
    (GnRH), 65, 67

Gonads, 15–17
Gonococcus, 324
Gonorrhoea, 316, 318, 331, 332–3
GP unit delivery, 151
Graafian follicle, 51, 422
Grand multipara, 136
Granulocytopenia, 418
Granulomata, 400
Granulosa cell tumour, 17
Granulosa cells, 54, 60
Grief, after stillbirth and neonatal
    death, 217
Growth hormone (GH), 267
Gubernaculum testis, 24
Gynaecological case presentation,
    11–13
Gynaecological history taking,
    10–11
Gynaecological problems
    of adolescence, 269–70
    of childhood, 264–6
    of puberty, 266–9
Gynaecological procedures, 436–44

H-Y antigen, 15
Haematological changes, in
    pregnancy, 80
Haemoglobin levels, 148
Haemoglobinopathies, 148, 149
Haemophilia, 109
Haemorrhage, *see* Bleeding,
    abnormal
Haemostasis, 188
Hair
    ambisexual, 293
    pubic and genital development,
        271(fig.)
hCG, *see* Human chorionic
    gonadotrophin
HDL, *see* High-density lipoprotein
Health education, sexual function,
    360
Health risks, of polycystic ovary
    disease, 287
Heart disease, 382
    in pregnancy, 143–4
Heart failure, 143
Hegar's sign, 83
Heparin, 105, 209
Hepatitis, 240

Hermaphroditism, 266
Herpes genitalis, 320, 406
Herpesvirus type 2, 410
High-density lipoprotein (HDL), 221
Hilar cells, 60
Hindwater rupture, 167
Hirsutism, 286, 292–3
  treatment of, 293
Historical perspective, obstetric practice, 211–13
History taking
  gynaecological, 10–11
  obstetric, 6–7
HIV, *see* Human immunodeficiency virus
Home delivery, 151–2
Homosexual relationships, 354
Hookworm infestation, 148–9
Hormonal contraception, 220–6
  depot injection, 225
  hypertension in, 222
  postcoital, 225–6
  metabolic effects in, 221–2
  progestogen-only pills, 224–5
  thromboembolism in, 221
Hormonal disorders, 26–8
Hormonal stimulants, in ovulation, 250–1
Hormonal therapy, in endometriosis, 310–12
Hormone replacement therapy, 379, 382–7
  and cyclical bleeding, 385–6
  diagnostic indications for, 382
  effects of, 379(fig.)
  examples of, 384(table)
  serum oestradiol levels in, 382(fig.)
Hormones, 104–5
  see also Hormonal ...; Endocrine system; *and individual hormones*
  gonadotrophin-releasing, 67
  ovarian, 60–5
  reproductive, 71(fig.), 72(fig.), 74–8
Hot flushes, 280
HPL, *see* Human placental lactogen

HRT, *see* Hormone replacement therapy
Human chorionic gonadotrophin (hCG), 74, 75(fig.), 251, 261, 418
Human chorionic somatomammotrophin (HCS), *see* Human placental lactogen
Human immunodeficiency virus (HIV), 230
  and AIDS, 334–5
Human placental lactogen (HPL), 77(fig.)
Hydatidiform mole, 107, 260–1, 418–19
Hydralazine, 105, 118
Hydramnios, *see* Polyhydramnios
Hydrocephalus, 111, 127, 175, 216
Hyperandrogenism, 286, 293
Hyperemesis, 107
Hyperinsulinaemia, 287
Hyperplastic chorionic villi, 418
Hyperprolactinaemia, 67, 282–3
Hypertension, 102, 116, 147
  and hormonal contraception, 222
  non-pre-eclamptic, 140–1
Hyperthyroidism, 78
Hypertonic uterine action, 170
Hypertonus, of extensor muscles, 174
Hypnosis, 156
Hypofibrinogenaemia, 121, 191
Hypoglossal cyst, 174
Hypomenorrhoea, 301
Hypoplasia, 25
Hyposmia, 278
Hypotension, 228
Hypotensives, 105
Hypothalamus
  and amenorrhoea, 282
  disorders, 280–2
  failure, 278–9
  hormones of, *see* Gonadotrophin-releasing hormone
Hypothalamic gonadotrophin releasing hormone (GnRH), 250, 251, 267, 351, 378
Hypothyroidism, 146, 291

Hypotonic uterine action, 170
Hypovolaemic shock, 191
Hypoxia, 161, 213, 216
Hysterectomy, 300, 409–10,
    438(fig.), 438–9
    Wertheim's, 439–40
Hysterosalpingography (HSG),
    243, 260
Hysteroscopy, 437
Hysterotomy scars, 193

Identical twins, 111
IGF-1, see Insulin-like growth
    factor-1
IgG, see Immunoglobulin G
Iliac fossa, 338
Immunoglobulin G (IgG), 137
Immunological changes, in
    pregnancy, 82
Implantation, 59–60, 244
Impotence, 358
In vitro fertilization (IVF), 59
    conception rates in, 255(fig.)
Incontinence
    continuous, 372
    overflow, 371–2
    reflex, 371
    stress, 370–1
    urgency and urge, 371
    urinary, 368–9
Induction of labour, 166–9
    dangers of, 168–9
    methods for, 166–8
Infertility
    see also Subfertility
    assisted conception treatment
        methods, 254–5
    conception rates in, 253(fig.)
    definition of, 237–8
    unexplained, 253–4
Infundibulopelvic ligaments, 32,
    33
Inhalational analgesia, in labour,
    163
Inhibin, 62, 375
Innervation, of pelvis, 37–8
Insemination, 57–8
    donor, 249
Institute of Psychosexual Medicine,
    359

Insulin, 141
    resistance, 287
Insulin-like growth factor-1
    (IGF-1), 62, 267, 268
Intercourse, sexual
    see also Sexual function
    painful, see Dyspareunia
Intermenstrual bleeding (IMB), 302
Internal pudendal artery, 37
Intersex, 264–6
Interstitial (Leydig) cells, 70
Intracytoplasmic sperm injection
    (ICSI), 248, 249
Intrapartum fetal pneumonia, 169
Intraperitoneal haemorrhage, 262
Intrauterine contraceptive devices,
    226–9
    active, 228–9
    passive, 226–8
Intrauterine fetal asphyxia, 114
Intrauterine fetal death, 168
Intrauterine fetal weight, 86(fig.)
Intrauterine growth retardation,
    131–35
Intrauterine insemination (IUI),
    254, 255
Introital analgesia, 181
Inversion of uterus, 193
Involution of genital tract, 198–9
Iodine, use of, 78, 409
Iron, 113, 148
Irritable bowel syndrome (IBS), 337
Ischial spine, 43, 181
Isoimmunization, 137–40
IUI, see Intrauterine insemination
IVF, see In vitro fertilization

Jaundice, 144–5

Kallmann syndrome, 278
Ketosis, 170
Kidney, see Renal ...
Kjelland's forceps, 182–3
Kyphosis, 278

Labetalol, 105
Labia majora, 21
Labour
    abnormal, 169–79
    active management of, 162–3

brow presentation in, 175–6
carbohydrate metabolism in, 79
diagnosis of, 153–4
episiotomy in, 164–5
face presentation in, 174
fetal heart rate in, 159–61
fetal well-being in, 158–61, 160(fig.)
induction of, 166–9
initiation of, 90
malpresentation in, 176–8
maternal well-being in, 156–8
mechanism of, 154–63, 155(fig.)
multigravidae, 152–3
observations in, 157(fig.)
occipitoposterior position in, 171(fig.), 172
pain relief in, 156–8
partogram in, 162
premature, 129–31
primigravidae, 152–3
stages of, 90–2, 155–6, 155–6, 161–2
trial of, 128
uterine rupture in, 194
Lacerations, in the genital tract at delivery, 188
Lactation, 92, 294
    see also Breast feeding
Lactic acid, 161
Laparoscopy, 243–4, 436
Laparotomy, 194
Laser ablation, enodometrial, 441
Last menstrual period (LMP), 14, 98
Late termination, of pregnancy, 235
Lecithin, 87
Leiomyomas, 410
Leukaemia, 105
Levator ani muscles, 31–2
LH, see Luteinizing hormone
Lice, pubic, 321
Lie, abnormalities in, 126
Lignocaine, 165, 181
Lithotomy, 176
Liver
    disease, in pregnancy, 144–5
    function, in pregnancy, 82
Liver palms (palmar erythema), 82
LMP, see Last menstrual period

Lochia, 197
Løvset manoeuvre, 177
Lower genital tract problems, 317–18
Lungs, in premature babies, 87
Lupus anticoagulant, 259
Luteinizing hormone (LH), 51, 74, 286, 287, 289
Lymphatic dissemination, 307
Lymphatic drainage
    of the vulva, 30
    pelvic organs, 37

McDonald cervical suture method, 430
Magnesium sulphate, 118
Malaria, 149
Male examination, in subfertility, 245
Male pseudohermaphroditism, 265–6
Male sexual dysfunction, 358
Male sterilization, 233
Malignant tumours, see Cancer
Malnourishment, of fetus, 213
Malpresentation, 176–8
Manchester (or Fothergill) repair operation, 367, 439
Mannitol, 118
Marriage Guidance Council, see Relate
Marshall–Marchetti–Krantz procedure, 371
Marsupialization, 321
Masculinization, see Hirsutism
Masturbation, 356
Maternal blood investigations, in neonatal death/stillbirth, 218
Maternal distress, in labour, 183
Maternal mortality, 212(fig.), 213–15, 214(table)
Maternal trauma, 191–5
Maternal weight, 132
Maternal well-being, in labour, 156–8
Maturity assessment, fetal, 98
Mauriceau–Smellie–Veit manoeuvre, 177
Meconium, 159, 161
Medroxyprogesterone acetate, 225

Mefenamic acid, 340
Meiosis, 52
Melatonin, 68
Membranes, fetal
    artificial rupture of, *see* Artificial
        rupture of membranes
    premature rupture of, 130, 131
Menarche, 267, 272
    delayed, 272–4
Meningomyelocele, 216
Menopausal syndrome, acute,
    376–7
Menopause, 73, 375–88
    definition of, 375–6
Menorrhagia, 297, 309, 411
Menses, 69
    excessive, 297–8
    and short cycle, 297
Menstrual bleeding, 69–70
    abnormal, 296–301
Menstrual cycle, 64, 69–70
    endometrium changes in,
        68(fig.)
    short, 297
Menstrual periods, 16
    absent, 300
Menstruation, 69–70
    see also Amenorrhoea; Menarche;
        Menopause; Menstrual ...
Mentoanterior position, 174
Mesenchymal cells, 16, 17
Mesonephric duct, 17
    anomalies of, 25
    cysts, 400
Mestranol, 220
Metabolism, in postnatal care, 201
Methotrexate, 262
Methyldopa, 105
Metoclopramide, 204
Microinvasive carcinoma, of the
    cervix, 402–3, 407
Micturition, 39, 40, 200
    see also Continence; Incontinence
Midwifery services, 96
Mifepristone, 234
Miscarriage, 106
    complete, 258
    first trimester, 257–60
    inevitable, 258
    recurrent, 259–60

second trimester, 260
    septic, 259
    threatened, 257–8
Mitosis, 50, 51
Mittelschmerz, 338, 341
Montgomery's tubercles, 83
Morphine, 158
Mortality
    maternal, 212(fig.), 213–15,
        214(table)
    perinatal, 94, 136, 212(fig.),
        215–17
Mothercraft, 103
Mucinous ascites, 424
Mucosal crypts, of cervix, 401
Mucosal ectopy, of cervix, 400–1
Mucosal retention cysts, of cervix,
    327, 400
Mucous polyp, of cervix, 399–401
Müllerian inhibiting substance, 17,
    19
Müllerian system, 23, 26
Multigravidae, 152–3
Multipara, grand, 136
Multiple pregnancy, 100, 111–13,
    112(fig.), 134(fig.), 179–81
    see also Twins
    complications of, 113
Multiple sclerosis, 368
Myocardial infarction, 221, 380
Myomectomy, 439
    scars, 193
Myometrial stretch, 90
Myometrium, 42, 75
    invasion of, 414
Myxoma peritonei, 424

Nabothian follicles, 327, 400, 401
Nalorphine, 158
National Childbirth Trust (NCT),
    101, 150
Natural family planning, 231
Nausea, in pregnancy, 107
NCT, *see* National Childbirth Trust
Negative feedback, 71
Neonatal deaths
    see also Perinatal mortality
    causes of, 216(table)
    management of, 217–18
    trends, 212(fig.)

Neoplasia
  genital, *see* Genital neoplasia
  and hormonal contraception,
    222–3
Nephritis, 147, 148
Neville Barnes forceps, 181
Niemann–Pick disease, 109
Nifedipine, 105
Night sweats, 376
Nitrogen excretion, 198
Nocturia, 369
Non-pre-eclamptic, hypertension,
    140–1
Non-specific urethritis (NSU), 316,
    332
Norethisterone, 104
Nortestosterone, 104
NSU, *see* Non-specific urethritis

Obesity, 136–7, 290
Obstetric anatomy, 42–9
Obstetric case presentation, 7–10
Obstetric history taking, 6–7
Obstetric procedures, 428–34
Obstetric shock, 194–5
Occipitoanterior position, 47
Occipitofrontal diameter (OFD),
    115
Occipitolateral position, 47
Occipitoposterior position, 170–3
  delivery with, 172–3
Oedema, in pregnancy, 116
Oestradiol, 60, 63, 76
  in hormone replacement therapy,
    384(fig.)
Oestriol, 76
Oestrogens, 56, 76–7, 198
  see also Oestradiol; Oestriol;
    Oestrone
  deficiency, 291, 379–80, 377(table)
  effects of puberty, 268
  metabolism, 76(fig.)
  total urinary output, 76(fig.)
  replacement therapy, 315,
    383(table), 386–7, 387(table)
Oestrogen–progestogen
  combinations, 220–4,
    223–4(table)
  contraindications in, 223
  hazards of, 221–2

  medical care in, 222–3
  neoplasia in, 222
Oestrone, 76
Older primigravida, 135–6
Oligohydramnios, 125, 132
Oligomenorrhoea, 291–2, 300
Oligospermia, 241–2, 248–9
Omnopon, 158
Oncogenesis, gonadal, 17
Oocytes, 50, 53, 244
Oogenesis, 50–1
Oophorectomy, 427
OP, *see* Occipitoposterior position
Oral contraception, *see* Hormonal
    contraception
Organogenesis, 85, 104
Orgasm, 354
Orgasmic dysfunction, 359
Orgasmic organs, 355(fig.)
Osteoporosis, 378–9
O'Sullivan's hydrostatic method,
    193
Ova, 50
Ovarian artery, 37
Ovarian cycle, follicular phase of,
    61(fig.)
Ovaries, 36
  cancer, 389–90, 425–7, 426(table)
  cysts, 420–5
  differentation of, 16(fig.)
  dysgenesis, 25
  endocrine cycle, 63–4
  failure, 277, 280
  follicular maturation, 52(fig.)
  function, 199
  hormones, 60–5
  ligaments, 32
  neoplasms, incidence of,
    422(table)
  polycystic, *see* Polycystic ovary
  steroid cycles, 63(fig.)
  tumours, 420–9
  ultrasound scan of, 284(fig.)
Oviducts, *see* Fallopian tubes
Ovulation, 243
  see also Endometrial cycles;
    Menstrual cycles
  control of, 54–7
  failure of, 249–51
  hormonal stimulants of, 250–1

pain, 342
  suppression of, *see* Hormonal
    contraception
Oxytocin (syntocinon), 62, 119, 131,
    162, 163, 164, 170, 172, 183,
    189, 196, 211

Pain relief
  in cancer, 396(table)
  in labour, 156–8
Palmar erythema (liver palms),
    82
Panhypopituitarism (Sheehan
    syndrome), 124, 282
Papanicolaou smear, 403
Paramesonephric ducts, 19, 20–1,
    23
  anomalies in, 25
Parametrium, 32
Partogram, 162
PCO, *see* Polycystic ovaries
PCT, *see* Postcoital test
Pediculosis pubis, 321
Pelvic congestion syndrome, 342
Pelvic diameters, 43(fig.)
Pelvic fascia, 32–3
Pelvic floor, 31–3
Pelvic infective damage, 251–2
Pelvic inflammatory disease (PID),
    328–31
  differential diagnosis of, 331
Pelvic organs, 33(fig.), 33–40
  see also individual organs
  orientation of, 40–2
Pelvic pain, chronic, 336–45
  classification of, 338
  factors influencing, 337(fig.)
  and retroversion of the uterus,
    343–4
Pelvic pain syndrome, 342
Pelvic peritonitis, *see* Pelvic
    inflammatory disease
Pelvic shape, abnormalities of, 44
Pelvic-sacral hold, 177
Pelvis, bony, 43–4, 47(fig.)
Penicillin, 104, 334
Penis, 21, 22
Perinatal mortality, 94, 136,
    212(fig.), 215–17
  see also Neonatal deaths

Perineal deficiency, 364
Perineal muscles, 31
Perineal oedema, 192
Perineum, 191–2, 197–8
Peritoneum, 24, 307
Peritonitis, 259
Persistent occipitoposterior (POP)
    delivery, 171
Pessaries, 235
Pethidine, 158
Phaeochromocytoma, 141
Phenothiazine, 105
Phenytoin, 118
PID, *see* Pelvic inflammatory
    disease
Pinard fetal stethoscope, 159
Pituitary
  failure, 278–9
  hormones, *see* Luteinizing
    hormone; Follicle-
    stimulating hormone
  necrosis, 124
  tumours, 279, 282
Placenta, 84
  accidental haemorrhage, 120–1
  abruption, 120–1, 120(fig.),
    123–4, 433
  blood flow, 91
  failure, 96
  in twin pregnancy, 112(fig.)
  insufficiency, 131–35, 216
  retained, 187, 189–90
  separation, site of, 207
Placenta accreta, 187
Placenta praevia, 120
  bleeding from, 120(fig.)
Placental lactogen, 258
Plasma osmolality, 81
Plasmapheresis, 139
  and rhesus disease, 140
PMS, *see* Premenstrual syndrome
Polycystic ovary (PCO), 249, 273,
    284–9
  pathogenesis of, 285
  pathophysiology of, 285
  treatment of, 287–8
  ultrasound scan of, 284(fig.)
Polyhydramnios, 100, 124–5
  with diabetes, 8–10(table)
Polymenorrhoea, 297

Polyps, benign, of the uterine body, 414
Pomeroy method, of sterilization, 232
Postcoital bleeding (PCB), 301
Postcoital contraception, 225–6
Postcoital test (PCT), 242
Postmenopausal bleeding (PMB), 301
  causes of, 303(fig.)
Postmenopause
  definition of, 375–7
  time scale of, 377(table)
Postnatal care
  see also Puerperium
  ascending genital tract infection in, 197
  blood, changes in, 200
  bonding, 202
  depression in, 209–10
  feeding, 202–4
  gastrointestinal tract in, 200–1
  genital tract infection in, 207–8
  home going, 204–5
  lochia, 197
  metabolism in, 201
  ovarian function in, 199
  perineum, 197–8
  psychology in, 201
  puerperal pyrexia in, 206–7
  sepsis in, 206
  thromboembolism in, 208–9
  urinary tract in, 200, 208
Postnatal exercises, 209
Postovulatory syndrome, 346
Postpartum haemorrhage (PPH), 187–91, 205–6
  anaesthesia and examination, 190
  causes of, 187–8, 188(fig.)
  clotting defects in, 190–1
  diagnosis of, 188
  management of, 189–90
  sequelae of, 191
Pouch of Douglas, 34, 41, 310
PPH, see Postpartum haemorrhage
Pre-eclampsia, 96, 116–19
  emergency treatment of, 118–19
  management of, 117–19

Precocious puberty, 68, 274–5
  see also Puberty
Pregnancy
  with active interauterine devices, 229
  acute fatty liver of, 144
  advice in, 101
  and AIDS, 335–6
  and amniotic fluid, 88
  anaemia in, 148–9
  antenatal complications of, 106–35
  biparietal diameter in, 86(fig.)
  and cardiovascular system, 80
  diabetes in, 77, 141–3
  diagnosis of, 82–3
  drugs in, 104–5
  early loss, 263
  ectopic, 229, 261–3
  endocrine changes in, 78–9
  financial benefits in, 103
  gastrointestinal system in, 81–2
  genital tract in, 88–92
  haematological changes in, 80
  heart disease in, 143–4
  and human chorionic gonadotrophin (hCG) levels, 70
  immunological changes in, 82
  incidental preparation for, 246
  after infertility treatment, 255–6
  investigations critical to, 10
  jaundice in, 144–5
  liver disease in, 144–5
  liver function in, 82
  medical abnormalites complicating, 140–9
  metabolic changes in, 78–9
  multiple, see Multiple pregnancy
  nausea and vomiting in, 107
  placenta in, 84
  with progestogen-only pills, 225
  psychological aspects of early loss, 263
  radiology in, 105–6
  renal function in, 81
  reproductive hormone changes, 74–8
  respiratory system in, 81
  thyroid disease in, 145–6

urinary tract disease in, 146–8
vaginal termination of, 437
water handling in, 81
Preinvasive carcinoma, cervical, 405–10
Premature delivery, 139
and rhesus disease, 139
Premature ejaculation, 358
Premature labour, 129–31, 431
causes of, 129
management of, 129–30
rupture of membranes, 130
Premenstrual syndrome, 346–52
aetiology of, 349
behavioural symptoms of, 348
diagnosis of, 350
historical and legal aspects, 346–7
management and treatment of, 350–2
prevalence of, 349
symptoms of, 347–8
Prepubertal maturation, 72
Presentations, fetal
see also Malpresentation
breech, see Breech presentation
brow, 45, 175(fig.)
cephalic, 89, 100
face, 173–5, 174(fig.)
shoulder, 178–9
vertex, 46
Primigravidae, 135–6, 152–3
Primolut N, 104
Primordial urogenital structures, 15(fig.)
Progesterone, 61, 68–9, 75(fig.), 198, 246, 258
Progestogen, 104, 220
see also Hormonal contraception
hazards of, 225
only pills, 224–5
Prolactin, 65, 67, 77, 199, 204
levels in suckling, 92
Prolactinoma, 283
Prolapse, 363–9
case presentation of, 11–13 (table)
cord, 176
operations, 438–9
urethra, 395

uterus, see Uterine prolapse
vaginal wall, 361
Prostaglandins, 75, 167, 168
pessary, 235
synthetase inhibitors, 311
Proteinuria, 116
Protozoal infections, 264
Pruritus vulvae, 318
types of, 317(table)
Pseudohermaphroditism, 265–6
Psoriasis, 396
Psychological aspects, 201
amenorrhoea, 280–2
early pregnancy loss, 263
premenstrual syndrome, 349
psychoprophylaxis, 156
Puberty, 266–9
delayed, 272–4
endocrine events in, 267–8
physical events of, 268–9
precocious, 274–5
problems of, 270–5
Pubic hair
development, 271(fig.)
shaving, 154
Pudendal block, 181
Puerperal complications, 205–10
Puerperal pyrexia, 206–7
Puerperal sepsis, 211
Puerperium
see also Postnatal care
care objectives in, 201–4
physiological changes in, 196–201
uterine rupture in, 194
Pulmonary embolism, 214, 221
Pulsatile GnRH secretion, 73
Pyelonephritis, 147
Pyometra, 414
Pyrexia, puerperal, 208
Pyridoxine, 222

Quinagolide, 283

Radical hysterectomy, 409
Radical surgery, 313–14
Radioiodine, 146
Radiology, in pregnancy, 105–6

Radiotherapy, 426
Rapid eye movement (REM) sleep, 72
RDS, *see* Respiratory distress syndrome
Rectocele, 361
Rectum, 40
Relate (*formerly* Marriage Guidance Council), 359
Relaxation techniques, 103
Relaxin, 62, 78
Renal agenesis, 125
Renal damage, 191
Renal disease, 223
Renal failure, 124, 259
Renal function, 81
Renal tuberculosis, 148
Respiratory distress syndrome (RDS), 88
Respiratory system, 81
Rest, during pregnancy, 102
Retention cysts, 401
Retroversion of uterus, 343–5, 345, 372–4
Retzius, cave of, 440
Rhesus disease, 137–40, 140
    prediction of, 139(fig.)
    prevention of, 137–40
Rhesus sensitization, 431
Rhesus-negative woman, risk of sensitization owing to CVS, 428
Rhythm method, of contraception, 231
Rickets disease, 127
Right occipitoposterior (ROP) position, 171
Ring pessary, 366
Ritodrine, 130
'Rose' salpingostomy, 441(fig.)
Rotational forceps, 182–3
Round ligaments, 32
Rugae, of vagina, 33, 378

Sacroiliac joints, 44
Safe period, 231
Salbutamol, 130
Salpingitis, 328, 329, 330
Salpingostomy, 440
    'rose', 441(fig.)

SANDS, *see* Stillbirth and Neonatal Death Society
Scar dehiscence, 194
Scar rupture, 193–4
Screening, routine, in pregnancy, 108
Scrotum, 21
Sedatives, in pregnancy, 105
Semen, 230
    see also Spermatozoa
    antisperm antibodies, 242, 248
    microscopy, 241
    plasma, 242
Semmelweis, Albert, 206, 211
Sepsis, 166, 206
Septic miscarriage, 259
Septicaemia, 259
Serosanguineous discharge, 197
Serous cysts, 421
Sertoli cells, 16, 17, 53
Sex in pregnancy, 102
Sex cord
    cells, 16
    tumours, 420, 422
Sex education, 270
Sex hormone-binding globulin (SHBG), 61
Sex steroid cycles, and gonadotrophin, 70–3
Sexual differentiation, abnormal, 264–6
Sexual dysfunction, 357–60
    female, 358
    male, 358
    treatment and referral, 359–60
Sexual function, 354–7
    in loving relationships, 353–6, 354(fig.)
    masturbation, 356
    health education, 360
Sexual response, 354–6, 355(fig.)
    clinical factors affecting, 356–7
    orgasm, 354
Sexual stimulation, physiological response to, 354
Sexually transmitted diseases, 331–2
    see also Venereal infection
SHBG, *see* Sex hormone-binding globulin

Sheath, 230
Sheehan's syndrome
    (panhypopituitarism), 124, 282
Shock, 193
    in obstetrics, 194–5
Shoulder
    dystocia, 432
    presentation, 178–9
'Silent abortion', 257
Sinovaginal bulbs, 20(fig.), 23
Skin
    collagen, 378
    diseases, in vulvitis, 321
Small-for-dates, 132
Smoking
    and fertility, 246
    in pregnancy, 101
    risk of thromboembolic disease
        and ischaemic heart disease,
        223
Spasmodic dysmenorrhoea, 339–40
Sperm, see Spermatozoa
Spermatids, 52
Spermatocytes, 52
Spermatogenesis, 51–3
    failure of, 248
Spermatogonia, 52
Spermatozoa, 50, 53, 57, 58
    see also Semen
    disorders, 247–9
    DNA, 410
    function, 242
    production of, 241
    transport, 57–8
Sphyngomyelin, 88
Spider naevi, 82
Spina bifida, 98, 108, 111, 216
Spiral arterioles, 69
Squamous carcinoma, 397
    cervical, 402(table), 408–9
Squamous epithelium, 33, 34
Squamous metaplasia, 400–1
Stamey procedure, 371
STD, see Sexually transmitted
    disease
Sterilization, 232–4
    counselling for, 233–4
    reversibility in, 233
Steroids, 60
Stilboestrol, 104

Stillbirths
    causes of, 216(table)
    management of, 217–18
Stillbirth and Neonatal Death
    Society (SANDS), 217
Streptomycin, 104
Stress incontinence, 372–3
Strokes, 221, 380
Stromal cells, 60
Subfertility
    see also Infertility
    advice to couples in, 245–6
    causes of, 238–9
    conception rates, 247(fig.)
    definition of, 237–8
    endometriosis in, 252–3
    history and examination in,
        240–1
    investigations of, 239–45
    ovulation failure in, 249–51
    ovulation in, 243
    sperm disorders in, 247–9
    treatments, 247
    tubal/pelvic infective damage
        in, 251–2
Suckling, 196
Suction evacuation, of uterus,173
    hydatidiform mole, 417
Sulphonamides, 104
Symphysis pubis, 41, 44, 48, 49
Syntocinon (oxytocin), 62, 119, 131,
        162, 163, 164, 170, 172, 183,
        189, 196, 211
Syntometrine, 164
Syphilis, 240, 331, 333–4, 395
Systolic murmurs, in pregnancy,
        80

Tachycardia, 130
Tay–Sachs disease, 109
TENS, see Transcutenous electrical
    nerve stimulation
Teratogenic substances, 85
Teratomas, 17, 422
Termination of pregnancy, 234–5
    see also Abortion
Testes, 70
    descent of, 24
    differentation of, 16(fig.)
    undescended, 265

Testicular feminization, 22, 266, 274
Testosterone, 17, 19, 70
Tetracyclines, 104
Thalassaemias, 148
Thalidomide, 104
Theca-lutein cysts, 421
Thecal cells, 60
Thecoma-fibromas, 17, 425
Thiazide diuretics, 105
Threadworms, 321
Thromboembolism, 208–9, 221
Thyroid, 78
    disease, in pregnancy, 145–6
    disorder, 289
    tumours, 174
Thyroid stimulating hormone
    (TSH), 65, 78
Thyrotoxicosis, 145–6
Thyroxine, 146
Thyroxine binding globulin, 78
TORCH (Toxoplasmasis, rubella,
    cytomegalovirus and herpes)
    335
Transcutenous electrical nerve
    stimulation (TENS), 158
Travel in pregnancy, 102
Trichomonas vaginalis, 316, 320,
    322–4, 323(fig.),402
Trimethoprim, 104
Trophoblast, 59
    disease, 260, 415–17
Tryptophan metabolism, 222
TSH, *see* Thyroid stimulating
    hormone
Tubal ectopic pregnancy, clinical
    features of, 261–3
Tubal infective damage, 251–2
Tubal lumen, 329
Tubal state, 243–4
Tubal surgery, 261, 442
Tuberculosis, 434
    renal, 148
Tumours
    Brenner, 422
    connective tissue, 423
    dermal, 394, 423
    endometrioid, 421
    fallopian tube, 418
    germ cell, 422–3
    granulosa cell, 17

    metastatic, 423
    ovarian, 418–27
    pituitary, 279, 282
    sex-cord, 422
    thyroid, 174
    trophoblastic, 415–17
    uterine body, 409–18
    vagina, 398
    vulval, 394–8
Turner syndrome, 15
Twins
    see also Multiple pregnancy
    diagnosis of, 179–80
    ultrasound, 134(fig.)
    undiagnosed, 181
    uniovular, 111

Ultrasound, in pregnancy, 106,
    133–4
    twins, 134(fig.)
Umbilicus, 49, 164
Unstable lie, 126
Upper genital tract infections,
    327–35
    AIDS, 334–5
    gonorrhoea, 332–3
    HIV infection, 334–5
    pelvic inflammatory disease,
        328–31
    and pregnancy, 334–5
    sexually transmitted disease,
        331–2
    syphilis, 333–4
    uterus, 328
Uraemia, 394
Ureter, 33
Urethra, 38–40
    cysts, 396, 398
    prolapse, 395
Urethral syndrome, 372
Urethrocele, 361
Urinary bladder, 38–40
Urinary incontinence, 39, 40, 200,
    370–1
    types of, 371(table)
Urinary nitrogen, 201
Urinary problems, 367–72
Urinary tract, 200
    disease in pregnancy, 146–8
    infection, 208

Urine, retention of, 345(fig.), 368
Urodynamic studies, role of, 370
Urogenital sinus, differentation of,
    18(fig.)
Urogenital structures, primordial,
    15(fig.)
Urogenital system
    development of, 18(fig.),
        19–20(table)
    ontogeny of, 22–3(table)
Uterine artery, 36
Uterine prolapse, 362
    clinical features of, 364–5
    degrees of, 363(fig.)
    treatment of, 365–7
Uterus, 34–6, 42–3, 328
    see also Endometrium
    abnormal activity, 170
    anomalies of, 26(fig.)
    atony, 187
    bicornuate, 260
    bleeding, 225, 298
    cancer of, 413–18
    contractions, 90, 153
    evacuation of, 435
    fibroids, 188, 421(fig.)
    fundus, height of, 41(fig.)
    hypertonic action, 170
    hypertrophy, 412
    inversion of, 193
    involution of, 198(fig.)
    positions of, 343(fig.)
    prolapse of, see Uterine
        prolapse
    retroversion of, 343–4, 345,
        372–4
    rupture, 190, 193, 194
    size, 99, 132
    tumours of, 409–18

Vagina, 20–21, 33–4, 192
    anomalies of, 26(fig.)
    atresia, 273
    cancer, 400–1
    discharge, 318, 341(table)
    haematoma, 190, 192
    intraepithelial neoplasia (VAIN),
        20(fig.), 399
    prolapse, 361, 362(fig.)
    soreness, 326

    squamous dysplasia, 401
    tumours, 398
    wall prolapse, see prolapse
Vaginal termination of pregnancy,
    437
Vaginitis, 322–7
    atrophic, 325–6
    bacterial vaginosis in, 324–5
    causes of, 323(table)
    chemical, 326
    excretions causing, 326–7
    by foreign body, 326
    fungal infections in, 324
    infections in, 322–5
    secretions in, 326
Vaginosis, bacterial, 324–5
VAIN, see Vaginal intraepithelial
    neoplasia
Variable lie, of fetus, 126, 178–9
Varicocele, 248
Vas deferens, 242
Vasa praevia, 121
Vasectomy, 233
Vasocongestion, 354
Vasomotor flushes, 376
Vault caps, vaginal, 231
Vault prolapse, vaginal, 362
Velamentous insertion of cord,
    122(fig.), 122(fig.)
Venereal Disease Research
    Laboratory (VDRL) test, 97
Venereal infection, 230
    see also Sexually transmitted
        diseases
Venereal warts, 320, 395, 400
Venogram, 209
Venous drainage, of vulva, 30
Venous embolization, 307
Venous engorgement, 80
Ventilation/perfusion scan, 209
Ventouse, 173, 184, 185(fig.)
Ventrosuspension, 345
Vertex presentation, 46
Vestibular bulbs, 29
Vimule caps, cervical, 231
VIN, see Vulval intraepithelial
    neoplasia
Viral hepatitis, 145
Vitamin E, 248
Vomiting, in pregnancy, 107

Vulva, 29(fig.), 29–30, 191, 394–8
    cancer, 397–8
    deep structures of, 30(fig.)
    dermatoses, 396–7
    intraepithelial neoplasia (VIN),
        396–7
    itching, 318
    tumours, 394–8
Vulvitis, 320–22
    Bartholin's cyst, 320–1
    skin diseases in, 322
Vulvovaginitis, 320

Warts, venereal, 400
Water handling, in pregnancy, 81
Weight loss, in amenorrhoea,
    280–2

Wertheim's hysterectomy, 372, 411,
    437–9
'Witch's milk', 264
Withdrawal, as contraceptive
    method, 231
Wolffian ducts system, 17
Working in pregnancy, 102
Wrigley's forceps, 181

X chromosome, 15
X-ray examination, 105
Xiphisternum, 42

Y chromosome, 15
Yeast infections, 264

Zygote, 59